Contemporary Health Informatics

Mark L. Braunstein, MD

Associate Director for Health Systems,
Institute for People and Technology
Professor of the Practice, School of Interactive Computing
College of Computing, Georgia Institute of Technology

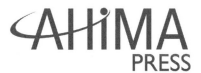
PRESS

ISBN: 978-1-58426-031-8
AHIMA Product No.: AB102913

AHIMA Staff:
Jessica Block, MA, Assistant Editor
Lesley Kadlec, MA, RHIA, Reviewer
Jason O. Malley, Vice President, Business Innovation
Ashley R. Sullivan, Production Development Editor
Diana Warner, MS, RHIA, CHPS, FAHIMA, Reviewer
Pamela Woolf, Director, Publications

For more information, including updates, about AHIMA Press publications, visit http://www.ahima.org/education/press.

American Health Information Management Association
233 North Michigan Avenue, 21st Floor
Chicago, Illinois 60601-5809
ahima.org

I have had the privilege of teaching health informatics since coming to Georgia Institute of Technology a number of years ago. It has been gratifying to see our computer science and other graduate students grow excited about a field they had not been previously exposed to. I wrote this text in the hope that it will assist others to teach and enter this dynamic and rapidly changing field. I joined it myself a long time ago and in a very different time with the help of two teachers who supported me at the onset of my career and to whom I dedicate this book:

Drs. Hiram B. Curry, Chairman of Family Medicine and
JFA (Joseph Forde Anthony) McManus
Dean of the College of Medicine
Medical University of South Carolina

Contents

Detailed Contents

Chapter 5

PART III   Real World Applications

Chapter 6

Chapter 10

Mark Braunstein is a professor of the practice in the School of Interactive Computing at Georgia Institute of Technology (Georgia Tech). Before joining Georgia Tech, Dr. Braunstein started and ran several HIT companies. His goal in this text is to give you a pragmatic and contemporary survey of the exciting field of health informatics based as much on practice as on theory.

Dr. Braunstein was a medical student in the early 1970s and was one of the early researchers to get interested in developing an ambulatory electronic medical record. At the Department of Family Medicine of the Medical University of South Carolina, his early EMR supported 32 simultaneous terminals scattered around a state-of-the-art clinic that in many ways resembled today's patient-centered medical home model (all serviced by a single PDP-15 computer using MUMPS). He was able to give them something similar to contemporary results. Figure 0.1 shows an electronic patient summary, called a Continuity Care Document (CCD). It is actually a machine-readable XML document being rendered here for viewing by people. The CCD and its underlying technologies will be discussed in detail in chapter 5. Figure 0.2 is part of a very similar patient summary from one of the ancient EMR systems of the 1970s. Perhaps more surprisingly, the clinic where the author was working had the concept of population health, something that is "cutting edge" today and that will be discussed in detail in chapter 8.

Dr. Braunstein shows that the technology to do many of the things that are needed to improve healthcare has been around for quite some time and, in fact, the opportunity to use that technology to increase the efficiency of healthcare; to monitor and evaluate the quality of services; and to supply data for research was understood a long time ago. A 1977 report to Congress by the Office of Technology Assessment clearly illustrates this when it says:

> Medical information systems can be used to educate and assist medical professionals during clinical care, reducing the need to rely on memory. Potentially, they can increase efficiency and reduce or contain institutional costs. They can provide a way to monitor and evaluate the quality of medical services. They can eliminate duplication of data collection and can provide accurate, accessible data for evaluating and planning medical care services. Finally, they can be used to supply data that have previously been unavailable to researchers and policy makers. (OTA 1977)

Despite the early recognition of its potential role, 30 years later in 2008 (DesRoches et al. 2008) and then in 2009 (Jha et al. 2009), two landmark studies published in the *New England Journal of Medicine*, arguably the leading journal in healthcare and medicine, showed that a very tiny percentage of physicians' offices and an even smaller percentage of non-federal US hospitals (federal hospitals like those run by the military and the VA had been automated for quite some time) had an electronic medical records system capable of improving care quality.

Why this dichotomy between the recognition and the realization of the potential role of health informatics? This will be discussed in detail in chapter 1.

Figure 0.1   A visualization for use by providers of a contemporary patient summary, the Continuity of Care Document (CCD).

Continuity of Care Document

Created On: September 30, 2010

Patient:	Jeffery Surrett 347 Grove Street Williamsport, PA, 17701 tel: +1-(570)837-9933	MRN: 00004201
Birthdate:	September 24, 1960	Sex: Male

Allergies and Adverse Reactions

Substance	Adverse Event Type	Reaction	Status	Note
CODEINE PHOSPHATE POWDER	Drug allergy	allergic drug reaction	Active	Hives
AMPICILLIN TR 250 MG CAPSULE	propensity to adverse reactions		Active	Diarrhea, nausea, vomiting

Medications

Medication	Instructions	Start Date	Status
Atorvastatin (LIPITOR 10 MG TABLET)	1 tablet(s), oral, QD	2002/05/05	Active
Potassium Chloride (KLOR-CON 10 MEQ TABLET)	1 tablet(s), oral, BID	2002/05/05	Active
Furosemide (LASIX 20 MG TABLET)	1 tablet(s), oral, BID	2002/05/05	Active
Glyburide (DIABETA 2.5 MG TABLET)	1 tablet(s), oral, QD, AM	2009/09/16	Active

Problems

Problem Name	Type	ICD-9-CM	Status
DIABETES UNCOMP TYPE II UNCONT	Diagnosis	250.02	Active
401.9 - HYPERTENSION ESSENTIAL	Symptom	401.9	Active
CAD	Finding	414.01	Chronic
272.4 - HYPERLIPIDEMIA OTH/UNSPEC	Condition	272.4	Active

Results

Test	LOINC	Sep 16, 2009
HDL Cholesterol (40 - 999mg/dl)	14646-4	43mg/dl
Total Cholesterol (0 - 200mg/dl)	14647-2	162mg/dl
Creatinine (0.5 - 1.4mg/dl)	14682-9	1.0mg/dl
Fasting Blood Glucose (70 - 100mg/dl)	14771-0	178mg/dl*
Triglycerides (0 - 150mg/dl)	14927-8	177mg/dl*
BUN (7 - 30mg/dl)	14937-7	18mg/dl
LDL cholesterol (0 - 100mg/dl)	2089-1	84mg/dl
Chest X-ray, PA	24648-8	No disease is seen in the lung fields or pleura

Reproduced with the permission of ABEL Medical Software.

Figure 0.2   A similar patient summary using the technologies of the 1970s.

```
STATUS REPORT                UN:1036X
DEMO,ABRAHAM LINCOLN (M) 66 YRS    (2/12/12)
PENNSLYVANIA AVE, WASHINGTON, D.C.   00011
                                 INS:UNKNOWN

NO PRIMARY PROVIDERS

BHAE1      COMPLETE HISTORY AND PHYSICAL EXAM      DOE,JUDY,MD 3/2/78
             LOOKS REASONABLY WELL CONSIDERING HIS MANY PROBLEMS. IS
             WORRIED ABOUT DOMESTIC STRIFE.

                      --MAJOR PROBLEMS--

YJSN1      DEPRESSION                          DOE,JUDY,MD 4/15/78
             INTERMITTENTLY BECOMES VERY WITHDRAWN AND UNHAPPY

                      --MINOR PROBLEMS--

MHAB1      HYPERTENSION              DOE,JUDY,MD 3/2/78-2-4/15/78
             BP CONTINUES ELEVATED.  SUGGEST EXERCISE PROGRAM
CGDC2      WEIGHT LOSS                          DOE,JUDY,MD 4/15/78
             20 LBS IN PAST YEAR WITH NO CLEAR CAUSE EXCEPT
             ANXIETY ABOUT COMING ELECTION
QGAA7      HEARTBURN                            DOE,JUDY,MD 3/2/78
             PARTICULARLY AGGRAVATING AFTER CABINET MEETINGS

                      --PHYSICAL EXAM--

CAEF1      BLOOD PRESSURE       * 4/15/78      165/100 RIGHT ARM
CAKH1      WEIGHT                 4/15/78      162

                      --THERAPIES--

TTAX1      CHLOROTHIAZIDE                              3/2/78
             100MG PO QD TAKE WITH ORANGE JUICE
             QTY:100 REFILL:2
CWMF1      EXERCISE                                   4/15/78
             RUN 2 MILES EACH DAY
CWBB1      SYMPTOMATIC THERAPY                        3/2/78
             TRY GLASS OF MILK FOR HEARTBURN
QWDN1      SALT RESTRICTION                           3/2/78

                      --PROCEDURES--

BTTK5-N    SMALLPOX VACCINE INJECTION                 3/2/78

                      --TESTS--

CHEMISTRY
  CNCJ1      BLOOD UREA NITROGEN        3/2/78            23
  FNCW5      FREE THYROXINE [ORDERED]   4/15/78
  KQBA1      STOOL OCCULT BLOOD         3/2/78          NEG
HEMATOLOGY
  MNBN3 *  HEMATOCRIT                   3/2/78        * 35
MISCELLANEOUS
  WPAN1      ELECTROCARDIOGRAM          4/15/78
             NSR  LOW T WAVES OVER PRECORDIUM
```

In the spring term of 2013 (and again in the fall term that year), I taught one of Georgia Tech's first Mass Open Online Courses (MOOC), and the first I believe, in health informatics. Twelve thousand students registered in the first MOOC, and I was fascinated by the interesting mix of backgrounds they represented. A third of the students who responded to a post-course survey were healthcare professionals. Of these, 17 percent were physicians, and nearly 7 percent were nurses. The rest were about equally divided between information technology professionals and students with a wide range of other professions and backgrounds.

This was of particular interest to me because I had anticipated it as best I could in the design of the course. Specifically, I tried to present the material so that it would be relevant and comprehensible to exactly such a diverse group of learners with highly variable technology skills. The very positive feedback we got from the students suggests that this approach worked, and many of the survey respondents said that would be interested in a text that mirrored the approach of the MOOC. The feedback encouraged me to create this book. It mirrors the organization of the MOOC but often provides more detail but with fewer graphic images given the inevitable space limitations of print.

This book is divided into four sections:

Problems and Policies (chapters 1 and 2): We begin by discussing the unique, complex, and often perplexing US healthcare delivery system (readers from other countries should note that many of these same problems exist to one degree or another in most of the industrialized nations). It is so complex and perplexing that many people object to even using the term "system" to describe it. I will introduce you to an alternative term, complex adaptive system, which seems to fit it quite well. This complexity, as is so often the case, creates many difficult and intractable problems, and we will look at some of them with a particular emphasis on those for which health informatics can be a key part of the solution. We will then discuss recent new programs and incentives the federal government has created in an attempt to get the healthcare system to adopt health IT and to use it in ways that it is believed will help solve many of the problems that we will have previously discussed.

Key Technologies (chapters 3–5): Here we will discuss some of the key technologies and tools that drive modern health informatics. This is the most technically complex part of the book, but I have made an effort to focus on key concepts rather than getting into a great deal of detail that most readers will not need. Of course, those readers seeking careers in HIT software development or technical support will require that detail and I would advise them to seek it in other books, from the many resources available on the Internet and from courses aimed at those professions.

Real World Applications (chapters 6–8): In this section we will examine the real world applications of health information technology. This will include provider facing tools such as electronic health records and population health management systems. It will also include personal health records for use by patients as well as technologies aimed at helping people stay healthy or management disease should they have it. This is currently a particularly intense area for innovation and entrepreneurial activity. It will also include the management of health and disease at the population level rather than the traditional one-patient-at-a-time approach to care.

Health Data and Analytics (chapters 9–10): In this final section, we will then look at how the data derived from the use of health informatics in practice can be used to increase medical knowledge, improve the diagnosis and treatment of disease, and even help design an improved healthcare delivery system. This is an area of intense research and innovation as we enter a period of exploration of the vast quantities of digital health data now available because of increased adoption of the tools we will have covered earlier in this section.

In the final two sections I will illustrate the real world use of health informatics by profiling a number of organizations that either develop or utilize the technologies as well as some interesting future-facing research projects. My choice of what to profile is based on my own experience and specific contacts and knowledge of the industry. While in all cases I believe the profiles represent outstanding examples of their genre, there may be better examples I am unaware of. In no case should my choice be construed by readers in clinical practice as specific advice or recommendations with respect to their best choice of commercial systems or products. Finally, I have no financial interest in or business relationship with any of the companies I have profiled with the sole exception that some of them are partners in our efforts here at Georgia Tech to promote HIT research and adoption. I was personally involved in the research project at the joint Emory-Georgia Tech Predictive Health Institute.

Throughout the book I will provide references to relevant article or publications. They are virtually all freely available on the Internet, and I have provided URLs when available in the chapter references and encourage you to read any that interest you. I also offer suggested and supplemental readings and resources at the end of each chapter. At the end of this foreword I point you to some of the best health IT blogs. I require students in my health IT graduate seminar here at Georgia Tech to subscribe to *iHealthBeat*, a free daily e-newsletter published by the California Health Foundation. I feel that it provides a good, impartial summary of current events in health informatics, so I urge you to subscribe to it as well.

Finally, this book will mainly focus on healthcare and health IT in the ambulatory environment, healthcare delivery outside of institutions such as hospitals and nursing homes but including the care of patients living in their homes. There are two reasons for this. My career has been mostly spent in this environment and, since most healthcare is delivered outside of institutions, I feel it represents many of the greatest and potentially most impactful challenges and opportunities in health IT.

Mark L. Braunstein, MD

Acknowledgments

A text that seeks to cover an entire discipline is a substantial undertaking that few people could accomplish without help. I am certainly not one of those exceptional people, so I am indebted to my Georgia Tech colleagues Rahul Basole, Myung Choi, Vikas Kumar, Phil Lamson, and Steve Rushing for reviewing all or parts of the book and for their many helpful suggestions. Dr. Frank Clark, Chief Information Officer and Vice President for Information Technology at the Medical University of South Carolina, reviewed the book and provided many important suggestions, particularly with respect to health information exchange. Dr. David Kibbe of DirectTrust and Greg Meyer of Cerner were invaluable in helping to expertly guide me through the rapidly changing Direct landscape. Each of the researchers whose work is profiled in chapter 10 reviewed my drafts and invariably provided useful suggestions.

I am, of course, solely responsible for any remaining errors. While I attempted to assure that the text was up-to-date as of the time I submitted it to the publisher (not an easy task given the rate on change in this field), I am sure that I did not do a perfect job and apologize for any statements or sections that are already out-of-date.

Healthcare and Health Informatics Are Different

Healthcare is an unusually complex industry so, to appreciate and more fully understand health informatics[1], you will need to understand its connections to that industry and its many problems. Health (actually "medical" was the term used at the time) informatics was defined by two of its pioneers as "the science that deals with the structure, acquisition, and use of patient data to orchestrate an ever changing evidence base toward the goal of efficiently improving health outcomes" (Greenes and Shortliffe 1990).

Health informatics, like any technology, is also a tool intended to solve certain problems. Ideally these solutions should be designed and implemented in a manner that will facilitate innovation. The development of app marketplaces by some suppliers of personal and medical record systems is a good example of this. The potential impact on outcomes and cost of healthcare through innovative health information technology (HIT) is the subject of an interesting and insightful Tom Friedman article in the *New York Times* (Friedman 2013). In it Mr. Friedman discusses specific start-up HIT companies whose creation is based, at least in part, on some of the new federal laws and regulations discussed in Chapter 2.

The trend toward open software platforms is a another example of health informatics approaches that spur innovation but, today, the majority of health information systems—particularly the large enterprise systems designed to provide integrated support for an entire health system consisting of hospitals, clinics and other specialized facilities—are based on closed, proprietary technologies that may even be uniquely used in healthcare.

A prime example of this is the Massachusetts General Hospital Utility Multi-Programming System (MUMPS), a unique programming language and file system (once with its own operating system) designed specifically to support HIT development in the late 1960s. For decades this unique-to-healthcare technology has been the basis for some of the most widely deployed enterprise health information systems (commercial systems from EPIC and MEDITECH and the Veteran's Administration's VistA electronic health record system).

This provides a clue that the healthcare industry and the specific informatics systems and tools that support it are different from most industries you may be familiar with and encounter from day-to-day. However, this is definitely starting to change. As the Friedman article discusses, the federal government is aggressively promoting the adoption of health informatics tools and systems by care providers and their patients through new incentives and approaches to care delivery (Friedman 2013). Over the past few years health informatics has begun to seriously embrace technologies developed elsewhere and used, in particular, on the Internet. The long-time and related challenges of interoperability and health information exchange may finally be yielding to these new approaches and incentives.

This rapidly changing environment was the inspiration for writing a textbook based on the contemporary landscape in healthcare and health informatics.

AHIMA provides supplementary materials for educators who use this book in their classes. Visit http://www.ahimapress.org/Braunstein0318 and click the link to download the files. If you have any questions regarding the instructor materials, contact AHIMA Customer Relations at (800) 335–5535 or submit a customer support request at https://secure.ahima.org/contact/contact.aspx.

[1] In this text, HIT, health IT, health information technology, and health informatics are used interchangeably.

REFERENCES

DesRoches, C.M., E.G. Campbell, S.R. Rao, K. Donelan, T.G. Ferris, A. Jha, R. Kaushal, D.E. Levy, S. Rosenbaum, A.E. Shields, and D. Blumenthal. 2008. Electronic Health Records in Ambulatory Care—A National Survey of Physicians. *N Engl J Med.* 359:50–60. http://www.nejm.org/doi/full/10.1056/NEJMsa0802005

Friedman, T. 2013 (May 26). Obamacare's other surprise. *The New York Times.* http://www.nytimes.com/2013/05/26/opinion/sunday/friedman-obamacares-other-surprise.html

Greenes, R.A., and E.H. Shortliffe. 1990. Medical Informatics: An Emerging Academic Discipline and Institutional Priority. *JAMA.* 263(8):1114–1120.

Jha A.K., C.M. DesRoches, E.G. Campbell, K. Donelan, S.R. Rao, T.G. Ferris, A. Shields, S. Rosenbaum, and D. Blumenthal, 2009. Use of Electronic Health Records in U.S. Hospitals. *N Engl J Med.* 360:1628–38. http://www.nejm.org/doi/pdf/10.1056/NEJMsa0900592

Office of Technology Assessment. 1977. *Policy Implications of Medical Information Systems.* http://ota-cdn.fas.org/reports/7708.pdf

Suggested Health Informatics Blogs

http://geekdoctor.blogspot.com/

John D. Halamka, MD, MS, is Chief Information Officer of the Beth Israel Deaconess Medical Center, Chief Information Officer and Dean for Technology at Harvard Medical School, Chairman of the New England Health Electronic Data Interchange Network (NEHEN), CEO of MA-SHARE (the Regional Health Information Organization), Chair of the US Healthcare Information Technology Standards Panel (HITSP), and a practicing Emergency Physician.

http://blogs.gartner.com/wes_rishel/

Wes Rishel is a vice president and distinguished analyst in Gartner's healthcare provider research practice. He covers electronic medical records, interoperability, health information exchanges and the underlying technologies of healthcare IT, including application integration and standards.

http://www.emrandhipaa.com/

John Lynn has written over 1,500 articles on the topics of EMR, EHR, HIPAA, and healthcare IT. He was the EMR Manager for the University of Nevada Las Vegas' Health and Counseling Center. In this capacity he led the conversion from paper charts to a full electronic medical record. He has also worked on a variety of EMR consulting opportunities.

http://histalk2.com/

Anonymous, the author says he works for a non-profit hospital that has vendor relationships with some of the companies he writes about. He says that his objectivity (and potentially his job security) could be compromised if vendors or anybody else worked that connection to muzzle him.

http://hitsphere.com/

This is an attempt to create a one-stop shop where people can get blogs, news, tools, and other items of interest to the healthcare IT community. It was founded and is operated by Shahid N Shah, an enterprise software analyst who specializes in healthcare IT. Over the past 15 years he has been CTO for CardinalHealth's CTS unit (now CareFusion), CTO of two Electronic Medical Records (EMR) companies, a Chief Systems Architect at American Red Cross, Architecture Consultant at NIH, and SVP of Healthcare Technology at COMSYS.

Some of these blogs may accept advertising from the HIT industry.

Suggested Health Informatics Newsletters

http://www.ihealthbeat.org/

iHealthBeat is a daily e-newsletter published as a service by the California HealthCare Foundation and an almost indispensable source of up-to-date information on health informatics.

http://www.fiercehealthit.com/

Another very useful and informative daily e-newsletter published by FierceHealthcare. It does accept advertising.

Part

I

Problems and Policies

Chapter 1

The US Healthcare System

To put health informatics in the proper perspective, this text explores the connections between problems, policy, incentives, technology, and innovation. This chapter focuses on problems.

The Problems

When many people think about healthcare, particularly in the United States, they think of it in terms of dramatic, high-technology care for people who are acutely ill and may die without that care. Brent James, MD, MStat, executive director of the Institute for Health Care Delivery Research, Intermountain Healthcare, points out that the United States excels at this kind of care, which he terms "rescue care" (Kline 2008). Figure 1.1 shows

Figure 1.1 The US healthcare system produces lower mortality rates for acute life-threatening problems requiring high technology "rescue care."

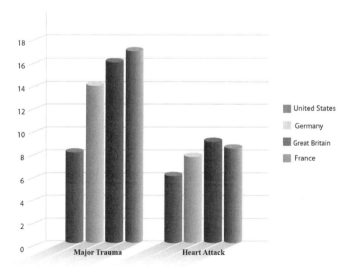

Source: James 2008

mortality rates; low numbers are better. The United States, when compared to other advanced industrial nations, gets much better results treating conditions like heart attack and major trauma (Kline 2008). Yet, paradoxically, the same high-technology system that produces such dramatic rescue care results falls short on fundamental issues, such as quality, outcomes, cost, and equity, according to the Institute of Medicine (IOM), the healthcare part of the National Academy of Science, which is the advisory body to the US Congress for scientific matters (IOM 2001).

Over the last decade or more, IOM has stimulated a revolution in thinking about US healthcare, its problems, and their solutions. This arguably began with the publication of *Crossing the Quality Chasm: A New Health System for the 21st Century*, a book that is freely available online and is a recommended reading for students of healthcare (IOM 2001).

What are the problems faced by our healthcare system? The United States spends a lot more than other countries on healthcare. The United States is one of the world's largest countries and has the largest gross domestic product of any country (World Bank 2013), but data from the Organisation for Economic Co-operation and Development (OECD) shows that, even on a proportionate basis, correcting for population or gross domestic product, the United States spends significantly more money for health than any other country (OECD 2011). Figure 1.2 is from the OECD and shows per capita spending on healthcare; the United States is a significant outlier, well above all other advanced industrialized countries. The OECD data would look much the same based on gross domestic product. So, no matter how one corrects for US income levels, the size of the US economy, or its population, it is an outlier with respect to healthcare costs. Moreover, US costs are rising faster than in other countries. Figure 1.3 compares healthcare cost growth in the United States to other advanced industrialized countries, and shows that the slope of the US cost curve is steeper, indicating more rapid growth. However, according to the Congressional Budget Office

Figure 1.2   The US healthcare system costs far more per capita (y-axis is dollars spent annually per capita) than the healthcare systems of other advanced industrialized countries.

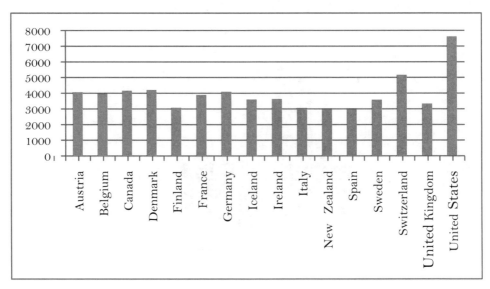

Source: OECD 2011

Figure 1.3   US healthcare system costs have historically grown faster than costs in other nations.

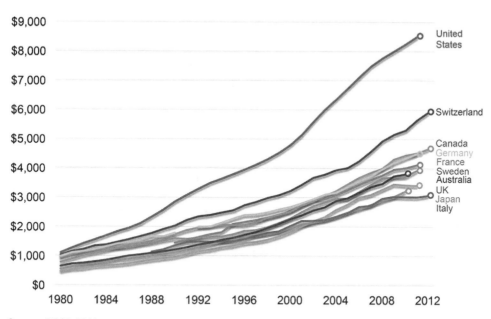

Source: OECD 2011

(CBO), "spending for health care in the United States has grown more slowly in recent years than it had previously" but the CBO forecasts increased spending as a percentage of GDP in the future (CBO 2013). There is no consensus yet as to the reasons for this recent slower growth but some experts suggest it may be due to the changes in medical practice which will be discussed in chapter 2 (Lowry 2013).

Of course there are reasons for growing healthcare costs. People are living longer. The life expectancy for both males and females has increased over the past few decades. But, despite the high level of spending, Americans die younger than the citizens of most other advanced industrialized countries (OECD 2011). So, in business terms, the United States obtains a poor return on investment for healthcare spending.

To summarize, the United States spends a greater proportion of its national wealth on healthcare; however, despite this fact, in most of the advanced industrial countries people live longer. Those countries where people do not live longer have much lower incomes and smaller economies than the United States.

The United States also has significant health disparities within the country, as shown in figure 1.4. Although there are numerous statistics like this, infant mortality is a good illustration. Figure 1.4 shows infant mortality rates in the United States are much greater for African Americans. Mortality rates are much lower for college graduates, suggesting that income and education have an enormous impact on the quality and availability of healthcare. Where you live also matters, as people in many poor and rural parts of the country have limited access to even basic healthcare.

Many Americans also lack health insurance, and the country's health insurance system is uniquely complex, two problems that can contribute to long term health costs because uninsured or underinsured patients may avoid treatment, due to economic considerations, until their problems become too severe to ignore. This was a key finding of a 2013

Figure 1.4   The US healthcare system has significant health disparities based on socio-demographic factors such as race, ethnicity, and educational level.

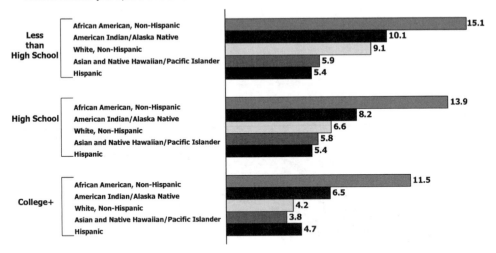

Infant deaths per 1,000 live births:

Source: NCHS 2009

Commonwealth Fund survey (Schoen et al. 2013), which was summarized by the Commonwealth Fund as having found that "more than one-third (37%) of US adults went without recommended care, did not see a doctor when they were sick, or failed to fill prescriptions because of costs, compared with as few as 4 percent to 6 percent in the United Kingdom and Sweden" (Commonwealth Fund 2013).

Finally, the United States faces huge future spending increases. It is important to explain Medicaid and Medicare to understand these increases. Medicaid is the federally sponsored program for the care of the poor and some disabled people. Currently, 16 percent of Americans are Medicaid recipients. The cost of Medicaid is shared by each state with the federal government, depending on that state's economic situation (Kaiser Family Foundation 2011). Each state manages its own Medicaid program, under a certain degree of federal guidance. Medicare provides health insurance to people after they are presumed to be no longer working, typically when they are age 65 and older; currently, 16 percent of Americans fall into that group (Kaiser Family Foundation 2011). Medicare is fully funded and managed by the federal government.

In 2011 healthcare spending was 16.4 percent of the total gross domestic product (GDP) (CBO 2011). However, over the next 60 years, projections show an enormous increase in Medicare spending along with a not-nearly-so-dramatic increase in Medicaid spending (see figure 1.5). All other healthcare spending also increases, but not at the same rate.

If the economics are not bad enough, care is often not optimal. Assessing Care of Vulnerable Elders (ACOVE) was a study done by RAND Health researchers, with support from Pfizer Pharmaceuticals, that looked at care of the most vulnerable, elderly populations. One of the key questions explored was what percentage of the time these patients get the best known care for their problem. Receiving any other care does not imply that the treatment will damage patients but that it is not the best and most effective currently available therapy. A key conclusion was that "Vulnerable elders receive about half of the recommended care, and the quality of care varies widely from one condition and type of care to another" (Rand Health 2004, 1).

Figure 1.5 Projected US federal healthcare spending is driven predominantly by the anticipated growth in Medicare spending.

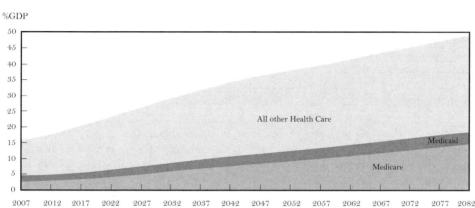

%GDP

Source: CBO 2007

The ACOVE report goes on to say that our health system is far more attuned to the management of acute rather than chronic conditions.

> What's more, providers administered proper care to patients with conditions that demanded immediate treatment (acute conditions) far more frequently than to those with chronic health problems. Indicators for treatment of acute general medical conditions had an adherence rate of 83 percent, compared with only 51 percent for chronic conditions. Treatment of acute and chronic geriatric conditions showed a similar disparity: 41 percent for acute conditions compared with 29 percent for chronic conditions. (Rand Health 2004, 3)

A 2003 patient survey found somewhat different results and suggested that patients received only slightly more than 50 percent of the recommended treatments for their conditions. However, the results were virtually the same for either preventative care or for the treatment of acute or chronic diseases (McGlynn et al. 2003).

If this were not bad enough, the IOM said American medicine is not always safe, killing between 44,000 and 98,000 patients annually for preventable problems in US hospitals. Several causes are cited for medical errors, both inside and outside of hospitals, and they mirror the discussions here. The following quote emphasizes care coordination as a root cause and suggests the potential role of health informatics in facilitating solutions: "When patients see multiple providers in different settings, none of whom has access to complete information, it becomes easier for things to go wrong" (IOM 1999).

So how is this possible? How can one of the world's richest countries, which spends such an extraordinary amount of money on healthcare, still have these profound problems? One of the root causes is that the US healthcare system was not engineered as an effective, efficient system. Rather it is what system scientists call a complex adaptive system. In such a system, there are multiple independent agents—each acting in their perceived self-interest (Rouse 2008). Moreover, those self-interests are often in conflict. Also, the agents adapt their behavior, if there is an external attempt to influence it, to continue to maximize their perceived interests. An often cited example is the tension between pharmaceutical companies, which want physicians to prescribe their latest, patented and most highly profitable medications; the payers (employers and government), who want more use of less expensive generic medications (medications that are no longer patented and can be produced by other companies, typically lowering their price); and patients, whose preference may be influenced by what is called direct-to-the-consumer advertising (allowed only in the United States and New Zealand) particularly, if they only pay a small part of the cost of their prescriptions (World Health Organization 2009).

Finally, no person or entity is ultimately in charge. Many observers feel this is an appropriate framework from which to consider the US healthcare system and its many problems. For example, the IOM says "One oft-cited problem arises from the decentralized and fragmented nature of the health care delivery system—or 'non-system,' to some observers" (IOM 1999).

There is also the problem of perverse financial incentives. Robert Doherty, the American College of Physicians' (ACP) senior vice president for governmental affairs and public policy has said, "We need to move away from the piecemeal approach: how many visits you can generate, how many tests you can order" (Carroll 2007). ACP is the leading organization of internal medicine physicians, so it is striking that they are calling for change in the incentives their own members have historically worked within.

Taken together, these problems and others lead to a high level of waste, inefficiency, and excessive cost in the US healthcare system. Figure 1.6 is the IOM's attempt to summarize this, and it shows 30 percent of the $2.5 trillion the United States spends each year on healthcare represents unnecessary, wasteful, fraudulent, or overpriced services.

Figure 1.6   Waste, excessive administrative costs, inefficiency, and other factors are estimated to account for around approximately a third of US healthcare spending.

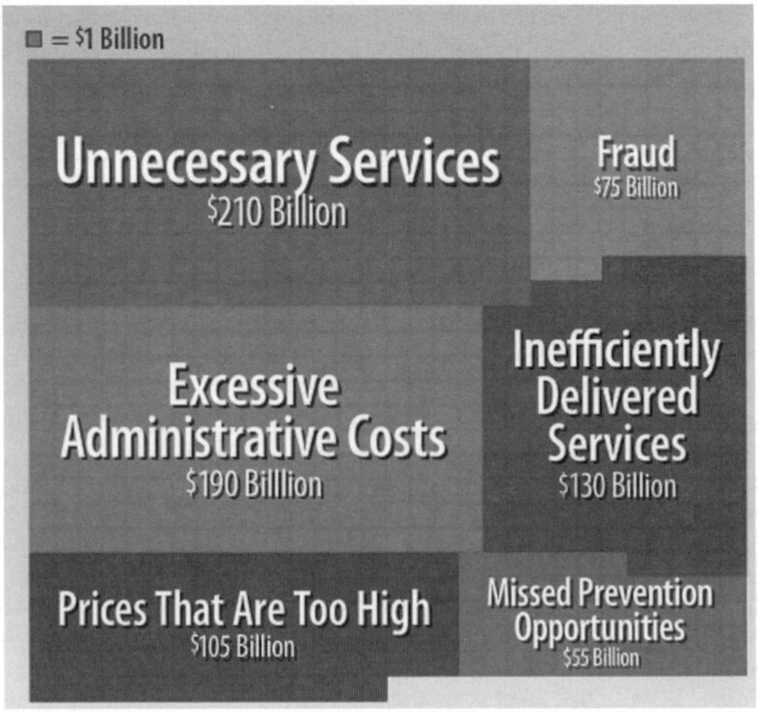

```
■ = $1 Billion

Unnecessary Services        Fraud
$210 Billion                $75 Billion

Excessive                   Inefficiently
Administrative Costs        Delivered
$190 Billlion               Services
                            $130 Billion

Prices That Are Too High    Missed Prevention
$105 Billion                Opportunities
                            $55 Billion
```

Reprinted with permission from the National Academy of Sciences. Courtesy of the National Academies Press, Washington, D.C.

The Challenge of Chronic Disease

Figure 1.5 shows that Medicare is the main driver of projected enormous future increases in healthcare costs. To understand why this is the case, medicine will be divided, in a simplistic way, into two kinds of problems: acute and chronic medical problems. Acute medical problems include common conditions—like a viral upper respiratory infection (cold)—and also less common problems, such as appendicitis, that may require surgery but where patients typically have a short and full recovery. Acute medical problems, by definition, are curable or self-limited. For example, viral infections usually go away on their own in a few days even without treatment.

The second kind, chronic medical problems, are almost by definition incurable, so the goal of the healthcare system is control and optimal management to avoid complications that can lead to serious issues, including death. Examples of chronic diseases include diabetes, hypertension (high blood pressure), chronic lung disease, and congestive heart failure. These problems are quite different from acute medical problems. The first difference, previously discussed, is that they typically last for the balance of a patient's lifetime. The second difference is they can cause each other. For example, if hypertension is not properly controlled, the patient is at risk for stroke, heart disease, and other problems. If diabetes is not properly controlled, the patient is at risk for kidney disease and many other problems. The third difference is that behavior is often causal for chronic diseases. A few people may swallow a seed and cause appendicitis by blocking the outlet of the gland, but that is rare. In virtually all cases, it is hard to say that the patient's behavior caused the appendicitis. By contrast "a number of studies have shown that most chronic conditions are preventable through behavior change" (Anderson and Horvath 2004). Moreover, once the patient has a chronic disease, changing their behavior is crucial to successfully managing it.

A key connection to make is that optimal treatment of chronic medical problems ultimately requires a different healthcare system than the United States has today. Such a system would focus not just on patients when they come to the provider's office and not just on the diagnosis and treatment of diseases once they occur. The system needed would provide what is often called "continuity of care" and place significant emphasis on wellness and prevention of chronic disease. The current system does not do this because, at present, the financial incentives most often point elsewhere and do not reward practicing medicine this way. If the United States is going to contain the massive escalation of costs that is projected for the next few decades, it will need a new healthcare system. That recognition reinforces the ACP's position that we need a new approach.

The largest behavior causing chronic disease is obesity. Figure 1.7 presents data from the Centers for Disease Control and Prevention (CDC). The acronym for this agency reflects its original name: Communicable Disease Center. The subsequent name changes, first to Centers for Disease Control and then to the current name, presumably reflect the shift in morbidity from infection to chronic diseases since CDC's founding in 1946 and in the agency's increasing recognition that prevention is a key goal for controlling chronic diseases. Figure 1.7 illustrates that 20 years ago no state in the United States had an obesity rate as high as 15 percent. Of its latest data, from 2011, the CDC says:

> By state, obesity prevalence ranged from 20.7% in Colorado to 34.9% in Mississippi in 2011. No state had a prevalence of obesity less than 20%. 39 states had a prevalence of 25% or more; 12 of these states had a prevalence of 30% or more: Alabama, Arkansas, Indiana, Kentucky, Louisiana, Michigan, Mississippi, Missouri, Oklahoma, South Carolina, Texas, and West Virginia.
>
> The South had the highest prevalence of obesity (29.5%), followed by the Midwest (29.0%), the Northeast (25.3%) and the West (24.3%). (CDC 2013)

Figure 1.7   The United States has experienced an obesity epidemic over the 20 years illustrated by these state maps. Obesity rates are particularly high in the southeastern United States.

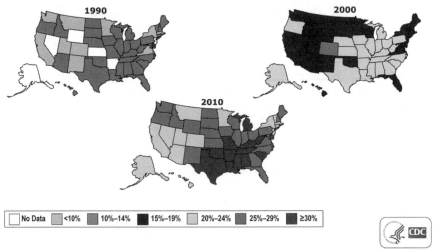

Obesity Trends* Among U.S. Adults
BRFSS, 1990, 2000, 2010
(*BMI ≥30, or about 30 lbs. overweight for 5'4" person)

No Data   <10%   10%–14%   15%–19%   20%–24%   25%–29%   ≥30%

Source: CDC 2013

This may sound ominous, but it pales in comparison to projections for the future according to *F as in Fat: How Obesity Threatens America's Future*:

> If obesity rates continue on their current trajectories, by 2030, 13 states could have adult obesity rates above 60 percent, 39 states could have rates above 50 percent, and all 50 states could have rates above 44 percent.
>
> By 2030, Mississippi could have the highest obesity rate at 66.7 percent, and Colorado could have the lowest rate for any state at 44.8 percent. (Levi et al. 2012)

Obesity is now understood to be causal for a whole range of problems, including many types of cancer. As behavior has led more people to be more obese, and as they also become more sedentary, they are at increased risk of developing chronic disease. The *F as in Fat* report provides these estimates of state-specific potential disease prevalence reductions if the average weight of Americans could be reduced by 5 units in terms of a measure of obesity called the body mass index (BMI), a number calculated from a person's weight and height:

- **Type 2 diabetes:** 14,389 in Alaska to 796,430 in California;
- **Coronary heart disease and stroke:** 11,889 in Alaska to 656,970 in California;
- **Hypertension:** 10,826 in Alaska to 698,431 in California;
- **Arthritis:** 6,858 in Wyoming to 387,850 in California; and
- **Obesity-related cancer:** 809 in Alaska to 52,769 in California. (Levi et al. 2012)

The United States is a world leader in obesity and long had the highest obesity rate among the developed nations. (OECD 2011) As a result, the United States has more chronic disease. Figure 1.8 compares the diabetes[1] rates in the United States with those in India and China, correcting for the populations. The United States has almost twice the rate of India and nearly four times the rate of China. Both countries have much lower obesity rates than the United States; hence their much lower rates of diabetes.

Figure 1.9 is a comparison of the annual cost of caring for people based on whether they are underweight (BMI less than 18.5), normal weight (BMI 18.5–24.9), overweight (BMI 25.0–29.9), obese (BMI 30.0–39.9), or morbidly obese (BMI of 40 or more). The costs are substantially greater for the morbidly obese group than for the group with normal weight. It is also shown that the percentage of the population that is morbidly obese has tripled in less than 15 years.

Figure 1.8   The rate of diabetes in the United States is substantially higher than in India or China.

	Population	Diabetes Rate
India	1.155 billion	0.0274
China	1.331 billion	0.0156
USA	307 million	0.0576

Source: IDF 2013

Figure 1.9   Obesity, particularly morbid obesity (a BMI in excess of 35 with symptoms or 40 without them), drives increased healthcare costs.

Weight Category	1987		2001	
	% of Population	Per Capita Spending	% of Population	Per Capita Spending
All persons	100	$2,400	100	$3,200
Underweight	4	$2,700	2	$3,100
Normal	52	$2,300	39	$2,800
Overweight	31	$2,300	36	$3,100
Obese	12	$2,700	21	$3,700
Morbidly Obese	1	$2,700	3	$4,700

Source: CBO 2008a

[1]Type 1 diabetes is not usually associated with obesity and is an inherited autoimmune process that destroys the specialized beta islet cells in the pancreas that produce insulin, the critical hormone for glucose metabolism. In this text, diabetes refers to Type 2, which is a relative insulin deficiency for which excessive body mass is an accepted risk factor.

Figure 1.10   United States obesity rates in girls aged 12 to 19 have grown dramatically, particularly in minorities. Rates for males are even higher.

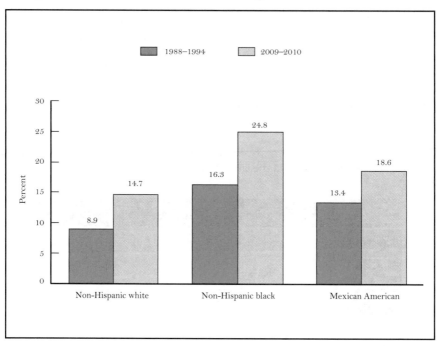

Source: Fryer et al. 2012

"The greatest single cause of rising healthcare spending in the United States is the growing prevalence of chronic disease" (Kumar and Nigmatullin 2010). Because of behavior change—escalating rates of obesity due to poor diet and lack of exercise—it is not just that the United States has *more* chronic disease, the *rate* of chronic disease is growing and "chronic conditions in the U.S. are projected to grow at alarmingly large rates" (Kumar and Nigmatullin 2010).

Finally, people are getting obese at a younger age, suggesting there may be additional decades of caring for chronic diseases that will develop in them at an earlier age than before. There will also be more complications of those diseases given the longer time frame for them to develop. Figure 1.10 from the CDC shows the growth in obesity among children in the United States. In the 6- to 11-year-old group, the United States now has obesity rates approaching 20 percent, around twice the rates of 15 to 20 years ago.

A Brief Review of the Current US Healthcare System

The greatest cause of rising healthcare spending in the United States is the growing prevalence of chronic disease. "The current healthcare delivery system is designed for treating acute illnesses." (Kumar and Nigmatullin 2010) So the root cause of the problems that have been discussed at least in part, is that the current US healthcare delivery system is designed to treat acute illnesses but 84 percent of all US healthcare spending is for chronic disease. The US system excels at treating life-threatening high technology acute problems. Chronic disease is a different kind of problem, is the principle cost driver, and treating it requires a different kind of healthcare system, a system that the United States does not have.

Another key insight is that the US system was not engineered. It was not designed to a purpose. It evolved as the complex adaptive system described earlier. What does the current system look like? A simple working description is that providers—this term encompasses physicians, hospitals, and various other health professionals—are typically paid for providing services. In other words, when the patient is in their presence, they are paid for a physical service, such as the office visit and any tests or procedures. In many contexts, even though the technology exists to do visits remotely via telemedicine, providers are not paid if it is done that way. Depending on what the test is, providers may make more money doing it in their office. If they are a provider that does surgery or interventional procedures, they are paid each time they do them. In most cases, these payments are not sensitive to outcomes. If they do a good job and get a great outcome, providers do not make more money than if they do a bad job and have a poor outcome. If they get a good outcome very expensively, by doing way more tests and procedures than are really necessary, they do not get paid less than a provider who gets the same outcome much less expensively by doing only the procedures and tests that are actually required. In fact, under the traditional fee-for-service payment model, the latter provider might actually make less, even though they are providing more cost effective care.

Moreover, there is no incentive for care coordination. The critical topic of care coordination is discussed at length later but, for now, it is important to recognize that under traditional reimbursement models, providers lack financial incentives to cooperate with each other. As a result, if it is not easy to get the results of a lab test done elsewhere, they may just repeat it driving up costs.

There is also typically no incentive to focus on wellness and prevention. The US healthcare system is configured to treat a disease once it happens. It usually provides no incentives to prevent that disease from occurring.

Other Models

There are other, more innovative models for healthcare in the United States. Health maintenance organizations (HMOs) are the most common. HMOs have different goals than exist in the traditional fee-for-service US healthcare system. One example is to substitute less expensive forms of care for more expensive forms by using providers in the clinic more and hospitals less. An HMO is a complicated topic that this text covers very simply. It is a form of what is more generically called managed care. Typically there is a primary care physician (PCP): a family physician, a general internist, a pediatrician, or an obstetrician gynecologist (or, in some cases, a nurse practitioner or physician's assistant). These are generalists—the providers who are prepared to take on and manage all of each patient's problems. In an HMO, the PCP is typically also the gatekeeper who decides when more expensive tests, procedures, and specialist referrals are needed. This need to access specialists only through a PCP is a concern sometimes cited by patients as a reason for preferring traditional care.

HMOs typically audit their providers' performance. This requirement, and their early recognition of the need for care coordination, led HMOs to become early adopters of health information technology (HIT). One example of the early adoption of HIT by HMOs was when Kaiser, by far the largest US HMO, installed clinical pharmacy systems long before that technology was the norm. The most recent CDC data on electronic health record (EHR) adoption (see figure 2.13) shows that physicians working within an HMO are the only identified subset with 100 percent adoption (Jamoom et al. 2013).

In an HMO, a provider who gets good results but at very high cost, might show up on a report and may even be asked the reason for this performance because the HMO is typically reimbursed at a fixed per member, per month rate. The HMO is getting the same amount of money whether the care costs more or less, so it is critical that PCPs deliver quality results at the lowest reasonable cost.

There are a number of variations of the HMO model. In a staff model HMO—these exist in a very few places in the United States—the providers work for the HMO, and the hospitals and other facilities are owned by the HMO. A network-model HMO contracts with independent providers for many of those same services. There is also a point-of-service model HMO, which provides greater choice of providers for the covered members.

Incentives are different in any HMO for both the patient and their providers. In most HMO models, the patient must seek care from physicians who are employed by the HMO (staff model) or are in the contracted HMO network. If patients go elsewhere, they may need to pay for the care themselves. If PCPs keep costs below what they would have been expected by the HMO, they typically receive or share in a bonus. These incentives do seem to reduce costs; a major study of HMOs showed that incenting PCPs to reduce costs appears to reduce them about 5 percent (Gaynor et al. 2001). A comprehensive study of HMOs suggests that increasing HMO enrollment growth has led to substantial reductions in hospital and other healthcare costs (Markovich 2003). These reductions are within an overall healthcare system where costs are growing every year, so the result is actually more significant than might appear be the case.

At the same time, "physician groups that were best at keeping costs below 'target' levels were also best at hitting their quality targets" (Gaynor et al. 2001). This is sometimes surprising, but experts in quality improvement will not be surprised to learn that the physicians who are best at keeping their costs low also produce the best quality. Quality does not need to cost more and it may even cost less because of the avoidance of wasteful practices. There are, however, some limitations to quality of care studies that derive from HMO data. The quality measures used by HMOs are standard and tend to focus on preventive care practices (Gaynor et al. 2001). In fact, as discussed in chapter 2, measuring healthcare quality is far from a precise science.

There are many similarities between the HMO model and the new Accountable Care Organization (ACO) model that is part of the Obama Administration's effort at healthcare reform and the Affordable Care Act (ACA). If HMOs have been successful at reducing costs and increasing quality (at least in so far as it can be measured), why introduce new models? The answers, in part, deal with practical aspects of implementing a full staff model HMO. Many people want a wide choice of providers or may already have a provider they wish to keep seeing. Also, it can be difficult to implement the staff model in rural areas where there is a far more geographically dispersed population. This can even be an issue in some sprawling urban areas. These new efforts, while they have many of the characteristics of an HMO, are to be implemented by self-aggregating groups of existing providers in the community, making them more acceptable and, the hope is, attracting enough providers to create needed coverage even in rural areas.

How Did US Healthcare Evolve?

An understanding of how the United States developed such a mismatch between its healthcare system and what is needed requires consideration of the evolution of the current system from a number of perspectives. The first is morbidity, the reasons people die.

Antibiotic medications became widely available after World War II. For eons before, most people died of infectious diseases. As a result of antibiotics (along with vaccinations and improved sanitation, changes that began around the beginning of the last century) and lifestyle changes over the ensuing three or four decades, more and more people died of chronic disease. Overall, people are living longer, so the death rates per 100,000 people in a given year has come down. Figure 1.11 presents data from the CDC, which shows that in 1900 a majority of people died of an infectious disease. Today, of the most common causes of morbidity in the United States, only one—pneumonia—is an infectious disease, and it is a small component of overall morbidity.

In short, why people die has changed dramatically over a period of a century. The United States has also changed substantially as to how the healthcare system cares for disease. For the period before about 1975, medicine was relatively low technology. Most of the technology people take for granted today—CAT and MRI scanners, advanced robotic surgery, sophisticated ICU monitoring equipment—did not exist before 1975. Over the 25-year period after 1975, the United States evolved from a low-tech to an extremely high-tech healthcare system. Now, yet another revolution has started toward what is called personalized medicine in which treatments are individualized based on sophisticated analysis of genomic and other digital data that is specific to each patient. This is discussed in chapter 10.

Figure 1.11   Mortality in the United States in 1900 versus 2010 reflects a dramatic shift from infectious causes to chronic disease.

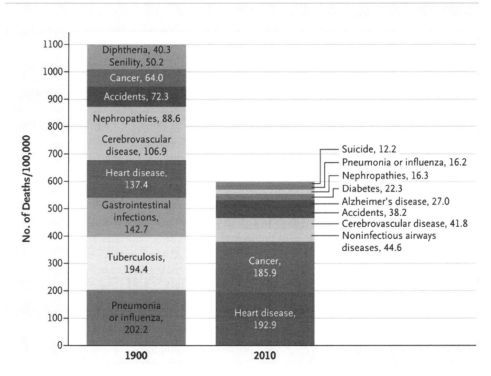

From *The New England Journal of Medicine*, D.S. Jones, S.H. Podolsky, and J.A. Greene, The Burden of Disease and the Changing Task of Medicine, Volume No. 336. Copyright © 2012 Massachusetts Medical Society. Reprinted with permission from Massachusetts Medical Society.

In most industries, technology reduces cost. For example, people have been replaced by robots in manufacturing, lowering the cost of the goods that are produced. People do their own banking using ATMs, often check themselves out in the grocery store using self-checkout scanners, and make their own airline reservations and print their boarding pass using the Internet.

Yet, a compilation of studies by the CBO shows that the advent of technology-based medicine has been a leading driver of increased healthcare costs (CBO 2008b). An often cited reason is the overuse of expensive tests and procedures when simpler, less expensive options would be an acceptable substitute. In support of this view, data from the OECD shows that the United States has more MRI machines per million people than any country except Japan. The United States performs more MRI exams per thousand people than any country except Greece (OECD 2011). What will happen as the United States evolves toward personalized health, where disease will be treated and health will be maintained based on the individual genomic makeup of each patient, remains to be seen. Many people argue this change will have a dramatic impact by improving the quality and reducing the cost of care, but that is not clear yet. Similar claims have been made in the past for earlier new medical technologies.

Another large change since World War II is in who pays for healthcare. Prior to then most healthcare was paid for by the patient. That may sound onerous, but remember, it was low tech. There was much less chronic disease, so it was mostly acute, self-limited care. As a result it was inexpensive compared to today, so paying for it was not as difficult for many people as it would be today. During World War II, wage and price controls were placed on American employers. To compete for workers, companies began to offer health benefits, giving rise to the employer-based system in place today. After the war the US economy was growing at a rapid rate. Because it was the only major economy not largely destroyed in the war, the United States was supplying the whole world with products. Employers were desperate to hire people, so more of them developed new incentives, one of which was healthcare benefits. In thinking about this, it is important to keep in mind that employers back then were not looking at today's health system. They were looking at a low-tech healthcare system that was relatively inexpensive, and chronic disease was not yet a major problem, so these benefits did not seem like an expensive thing to offer, even to retirees. Also in 1965, Congress passed the Medicare and Medicaid programs, the two federally sponsored programs mentioned earlier.

As a result of those programs, some 72 percent of healthcare costs in the United States are paid for by either private health insurance provided by employers or by federal/state programs (Wilson 2013). As compared to other advanced industrialized nations, a great deal more of healthcare costs are born in the United States by private companies. In fact, the United States is virtually the only industrialized country that does not have a single payer system under which the government manages a single nationwide health benefit (the exact approach to this varies widely). One of the results is that the relatively high cost of healthcare has become a competitiveness issue for many US companies (Johnson 2012). This is only one aspect of the significant economic consequences of our overly complex healthcare system.

The current trend is for a smaller share of healthcare costs to be paid by employer sponsored health insurance, shifting more of the cost to employees. Some companies have stopped offering health insurance. An increased percentage of healthcare costs are being born over time by Medicare and Medicaid because of demographic and economic trends. These are not yet dramatic shifts, but they are shifts that have clearly been considered in developing the policies discussed in chapter 2.

REFERENCES

Anderson, G. and J. Horvath. 2004. The growing burden of chronic disease in America. *Public Health Reports* 119:263–270.

Carroll, J. 2007. How doctors are paid now, and why it has to change. *Managed Care*. http://www.managedcaremag.com/archives/0712/0712.docpay.html

Centers for Disease Control and Prevention. 2013. Adult Obesity. Facts. http://www.cdc.gov/obesity/data/adult.html

Commonwealth Fund. 2013. http://www.commonwealthfund.org/Publications/In-the-Literature/2013/Nov/Access-Affordability-and-Insurance.aspx

Congressional Budget Office. 2013. Federal Spending on the Government's Major Health Care Programs Is Projected to Rise Substantially Relative to GDP. http://www.cbo.gov/publication/44582

Congressional Budget Office. 2008a. Growth in Health Care Costs. http://www.cbo.gov/sites/default/files/cbofiles/ftpdocs/89xx/doc8948/01-31-healthcareslides.pdf

Congressional Budget Office. 2008b. Technological Change and the Growth of Health Care Spending. http://www.cbo.gov/sites/default/files/cbofiles/ftpdocs/89xx/doc8947/01-31-techhealth.pdf

Congressional Budget Office. 2007. The Long-Term Outlook for Health Care Spending. http://www.cbo.gov/sites/default/files/cbofiles/ftpdocs/87xx/doc8758/11-13-lt-health.pdf

Fryar, C.D., M.D. Carroll, and C.L. Ogden. 2012. Prevalence of Obesity Among Children and Adolescents: United States, Trends 1963–1965 Through 2009–2010. Centers for Disease Control and Prevention. Division of Health and Nutrition Examination Surveys. http://www.cdc.gov/nchs/data/hestat/obesity_child_09_10/obesity_child_09_10.htm

Gaynor, M., J.B. Rebitzer, and L.J. Taylor. 2001. Incentives in HMOs. *National Bureau of Economic Research Working Paper No. 8522*. http://www.nber.org/papers/w8522

Institute of Medicine. 2013. US Healthcare Costs—Where is the money going? http://resources.iom.edu/widgets/vsrt/healthcare-waste.html

Institute of Medicine. 2001. Crossing the Quality Chasm: A New Health System for the 21st Century. http://www.iom.edu/Reports/2001/Crossing-the-Quality-Chasm-A-New-Health-System-for-the-21st-Century.aspx

Institute of Medicine. 1999. *To Err Is Human: Building a Safer Health System*. National Academy Press. http://www.nap.edu/openbook.php?isbn=0309068371

International Diabetes Federation. 2013. IDF Diabetes Atlas, 6th edn. Brussels, Belgium: International Diabetes Federation. http://www.idf.org/diabetesatlas

James, B.C. 2008. Building Quality Health Care for the 21st Century" (presentation, Institute of Medicine Roundtable on Evidence-Based Medicine Engineering a Learning Healthcare System: A Look at the Future The Keck Center of the National Academies, Washington, DC Tuesday, 29 April 2008)

Jamoom, E., P. Beatty, A. Bercovitz, D. Woodwell, K. Palso, and E. Rechtsteiner. 2013. Physician adoption of electronic health record systems: United States, 2011. *NCHS Data Brief* (98). http://www.cdc.gov/nchs/data/databriefs/db98.pdf

Johnson, T. 2012. Healthcare Costs and U.S. Competitiveness. http://www.cfr.org/competitiveness/healthcare-costs-us-competitiveness/p13325

Jones, D.S., S.H. Podolsky, and J.A. Greene 2012. The burden of disease and the changing task of medicine. *N Engl J Med* 366:2333–2338.

Kaiser Family Foundation. 2011. Federal and State Share of Medicaid Spending. http://kff.org/medicaid/state-indicator/federalstate-share-of-spending/

Kline, M.A. 2008. In Sickness and In Health. Accuracy in Media. http://www.aim.org/aim-column/in-sickness-and-in-health/

Kumar, S. and A. Nigmatullin. 2010. Exploring the impact of management of chronic illnesses through prevention on the U.S. healthcare delivery system: A closed loop system's modeling study. *Information Knowledge Systems Management* 9:127–152.

Levi J., L. Segal, R. St. Laurent, A. Lang, and J. Rayburn. 2012. *F as in Fat: How Obesity Threatens America's Future*. Trust for America's Health/Robert Wood Johnson Foundation. http://www.rwjf.org/en/research-publications/find-rwjf-research/2012/09/f-as-in-fat--how-obesity-threatens-america-s-future-2012.html

Lowrey, A. 2013 (February 12). Slower growth of health costs eases budget deficit. *The New York Times*. http://www.nytimes.com/2013/02/12/us/politics/sharp-slowdown-in-us-health-care-costs.html

Markovich, M. 2003. The Rise of HMOs. RAND Corporation Document RGSD-172. http://www.rand.org/pubs/rgs_dissertations/RGSD172.html

McGlynn, E.A., S.M. Asch, J. Adams, J. Keesey, J. Hicks, A. DeCristofaro, and E.A. Kerr. 2003. The quality of health care delivered to adults in the United States. *N Engl J Med* 348:2635–2645. http://www.nejm.org/doi/full/10.1056/NEJMsa022615

National Center for Health Statistics. 2009. Health, United States, 2008 With Chartbook. Hyattsville, MD. http://www.cdc.gov/nchs/data/hus/hus08.pdf

OECD. 2011. Health at a Glance 2011: OECD Indicators. http://www.oecd.org/els/health-systems/49105858.pdf

Rand Health. 2004. The Quality of Health Care Received by Older Adults. http://www.rand.org/content/dam/rand/pubs/research_briefs/RB9051/RB9051.pdf

Rouse, W.B. 2008. Health Care as a Complex Adaptive System: Implications for Design and Management. The Bridge, NAE. http://www.nae.edu/File.aspx?id=7417

Schoen C., R. Osborn, D. Squires, and M.M. Doty. 2013. Access, affordability, and insurance complexity are often worse in The United States compared to 10 other countries. *Health Affairs* 32:12. http://content.healthaffairs.org/content/early/2013/11/12/hlthaff.2013.0879.full.pdf+html?ijkey=7LvT

Wilson K.B. 2013. Health Care Costs 101: Slow Growth: A New Trend? California HealthCare Foundation. http://www.chcf.org/publications/2013/09/health-care-costs-101

The World Bank. 2013. GDP by Country (current US$). http://data.worldbank.org/indicator/NY.GDP.MKTP.CD

World Health Organization. 2009. Direct-to-Consumer Advertising under Fire. http://www.who.int/bulletin/volumes/87/8/09-040809/en/

RECOMMENDED READING AND RESOURCES

For more information on obesity:

Visit the CDC site at http://www.cdc.gov/obesity/.

Read the full *F Is for Fat* report at http://healthyamericans.org/report/100/.

This video produced by the CDC with HBO shows the obesity problem in the United States http://theweightofthenation.hbo.com.

The OECD health data can be accessed at http://stats.oecd.org/index.aspx?DataSetCode=HEALTH_STAT.

State specific healthcare facts can be found here: http://kff.org/statedata/.

Additional resources:

Centers for Disease Control and Prevention. 2013. Children and Diabetes—More Information. http://www.cdc.gov/diabetes/projects/cda2.htm

Young, P.L. and L. Olsen. 2010. The Healthcare Imperative: Lowering Costs and Improving Outcomes: Workshop Series Summary. National Academies Press. http://www.ncbi.nlm.nih.gov/books/NBK53920/pdf/TOC.pdf

Chapter 2

Current US Federal Policies and Initiatives

Electronic medical records and other health informatics offer the potential to help with the problems cited in chapter 1. However, to do that, they must be adopted by healthcare providers who have historically lacked real financial incentives to make the investment in these systems and tools. This chapter begins by looking at the incentives in healthcare, the models of care, and the adoption of health information technology (HIT). The connections among these have not yet been made explicit but the current hope is that some combination of these three elements will provide a solution to the problems described in chapter 1.

In the supply chain world, there is a concept of rating organizations by their skill at managing a global logistics network. A mark of 4P is the highest rating for an organization's ability to design, build, and run a comprehensive supply chain that cost effectively brings together products and services in a carefully orchestrated and often global manner. Wal-Mart is an oft cited example that uses IT extensively, making sure they have an adequate winter supply of snow shovels in Minnesota but not too many beach balls in Florida at that time when they are not in great demand (Johnson 2006). They do it so seamlessly that a shopper in their stores would hardly notice what is going on, but there is an enormously complex IT-driven logistics organization behind every purchase. Similar approaches are also very commonplace today in manufacturing, where the next part going into a car being manufactured in Michigan may have come from China. It is not just that the part came from China, but it arrives at just the point in time when it is needed (a characteristic of just-in-time manufacturing). In fact, it may have been customized for that car; so it is not just any car part, it is the specifically tailored part for the car into which it will be installed (a concept often called mass customization).

Both of these examples require an enormously complex IT-based logistics supply chain. So what about healthcare? What sort of job does healthcare do in managing logistics? First, why do we need a health data logistics solution in the first place?

Medicare beneficiaries with five or more chronic conditions are an interesting and often studied group of patients. One of the key characteristics of chronic diseases is that they can cause each other. Partially as a result, roughly 20 percent of the 40 million Medicare patients have five or more chronic diseases, and they account for half of all Medicare costs. In an average year, each of those patients sees almost 14 different providers (Andersen and Horvath 2004). One might ask if those providers are part of a seamlessly integrated supply and logistics chain. According to the Institute of Medicine (IOM), the answer is a clear no. In fact, the IOM says "they operate as silos often providing care without the benefit of complete information about the patient's condition, their medical history and what others are doing to care for that patient" (IOM 2001).

One might think that the patient can convey the needed information and it is not uncommon for patients suffering from major diseases, such as cancer, to perform that role. However, studies show that patients are often unable to list their medications, diagnoses, treatment plan (names and purposes of medications), and common side effects of prescribed medications when they are discharged from the hospital (Rosenow 2005). This problem is further illustrated in figure 2.1, based on a few studies that, taken together, show what the care logistics network (in this case, it conveys data, not goods) looks like for the average primary care physician (PCP). PCPs are often the gatekeepers; the key coordination point in the management of chronic disease. Typically a PCP will care for older Medicare patients, many of whom have multichronic diseases. Each of these patients is seen, on average, by 14 providers, including their PCP. Taken together, all of the multi-chronic disease patients for our hypothetical PCP will be seen in total by 86 providers. On average, this typical PCP's entire referral network consists of 229 providers (Pham et al. 2009; Andersen and Horvath 2004). This is clearly quite a complex care network. It is very difficult to understand how it can be managed very effectively or efficiently without using some of the same information sharing techniques and technologies that are used in retailing and manufacturing. To make matters worse, the United States has a smaller percentage of primary care physicians (12.3 percent) and a greater percentage of specialists (65 percent) than most other advanced industrialized nations voluntarily represented in The Organisation for Economic Co-operation and Development (OECD) databank, as shown by figure 2.2. As a result, the United States has a highly specialized healthcare system, so referrals to physicians who

Figure 2.1   The care logistics network of the typical PCP involves nearly 100 other physicians for the care of multichronic disease patients and over 200 other physicians in total.

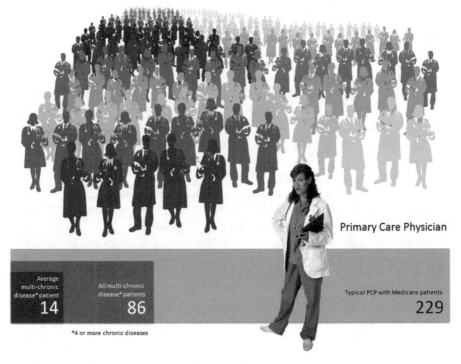

Primary Care Physician

| Average multi-chronic disease* patient | All multi-chronic disease* patients | | Typical PCP with Medicare patients |
| 14 | 86 | | 229 |

*4 or more chronic diseases

Source: Pham et al. 2009 and Andersen and Horvath 2004

focus on only one aspect of the patient's care are quite common, which is a factor in creating such complex data logistics issues.

As a result of the lack of coordination among US physicians, 54 percent of the time, test results and records were not available during an appointment; doctors ordered test(s) that had already been done; providers failed to share important information with each other; specialists did not have information about medical history; or the regular doctor was not informed about specialist care. The percentage dropped to 33 percent for patients receiving care under a medical home model (Schoen et al. 2011). This model will be discussed later in the chapter, but it is a an increase in organized and systematic approach to managing chronic disease. Another result is an increase in medical errors as patients are cared for by more physicians in a system with inadequate care coordination, as shown in figure 2.3.

Figure 2.2   The United States has a greater percentage of specialists and a smaller percentage of primary care physicians than most other advanced countries.

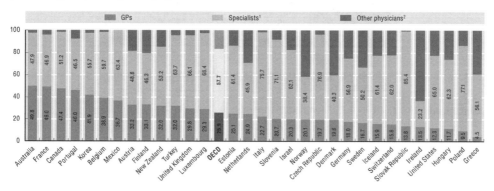

Source: OECD 2011

Figure 2.3   This data from this survey of sicker patients shows a positive correlation between the number of physicians caring for a patient and the number of patient-reported medical errors.

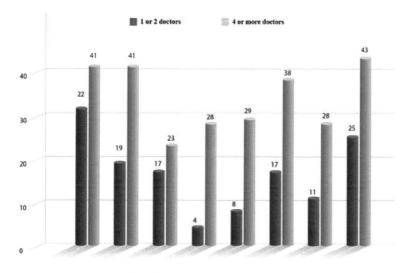

Used with permission from OECD (2011), *Health at a Glance 2011: OECD Indicators*, OECD Publishing, http://dx.doi.org/10.1787/health_glance-2011-en

Figure 2.4   Despite progress, a substantial percentage of sicker patients report that no provider has reviewed their medications with them in the past year.

	% of Patients With No Medication Review in the Past Year	
	2011	2008
France	58	68
Netherlands	41	62
Australia	34	41
New Zealand	31	48
Germany	29	49
United States	28	41
Canada	28	40
UK	16	48

Source: Commonwealth Fund 2011 and 2008

Figure 2.4 shows the United States, in 2011, compared favorably to most other industrialized countries in physician review of medications with their patients, as compared to the same data in 2008. This progress may be at least in part as a result of programs that will be discussed later in this chapter. Keep in mind, however, that the patients in this survey were all "sicker adults" defined as those in fair or poor health; had surgery or been hospitalized in past two years; or had received care for serious or chronic illness, injury, or disability in past year. Presumably the healthcare system would make a special effort with such patients, but with 28 percent of complex chronic disease patients reporting no review of their medications in the prior year, healthcare in the United States is still a long way from the kind of quality that other industries have achieved (Schoen et al. 2011).

A Case Study: Informatics for Improved Use of Medications

Prescriptions are a relatively simple use case[1] to illustrate the potential applications of IT to coordinate care among many providers. As compared to most other clinical documents, a prescription is quite simple. There are only a few data elements: the date; the physician's name (the term "physician" is used even though patients are increasingly cared for and prescriptions are written by other care providers, such as nurse practitioners); their drug enforcement administration (DEA) number, if required (for controlled substances like narcotics); the patient's name; the name of the drug; the quantity; how it should be taken; and how many times it can be refilled.

---

[1]A use case is a specific, realistic patient care scenario that is used to inform the design and development of health IT tools and solutions to support that scenario.

Prescriptions may be relatively simple, but not managing them correctly can lead to serious problems. For example, as an unintended negative result of their medication therapy, many patients experience adverse drug events that can be caused by allergies to drug components, interactions between drugs, an incorrect dosage, or side effects of their medications. Patients who have an adverse drug event can be hospitalized 8 to 12 days longer than patients who do not, and this can cost $16,000 to $24,000 more per patient (AHRQ 2001). Adverse drug events result in over 700,000 injuries and deaths each year and cost as much as $5,600,000 per hospital, depending on its size (AHRQ 2001). Admission to the hospital is a known risk factor for increasing the number of adverse medication events and errors in the patient's medication regime (Murray and Kroenke 2001). This is largely due to problems caused by not performing medical reconciliation, a process for assuring the continuity of each patient's medication regimen as they move from one care venue to another (a special case of care coordination).

All of these problems occur despite very extensive use of technology to manage medications in hospitals. Virtually every hospital in the country with more than 100 beds has a specialized information system that is used by their pharmacy (Davis 2009). Most have automated dispensing systems and some even have specialized systems to manage compliance with the physicians' orders as medications are administered to the patient. These typically involve bar codes on each dose of the medication (medications are usually administered in unit dose packages in most hospitals) and another bar code, usually on a wristband, that identifies the patient. A third bar code or badge (via an RFID signal) may identify the person administering the medications. This helps make sure that each patient actually gets the appropriate medication at the appropriate time. It also provides an audit log and accountability record for medication administration.

Medication reconciliation involves comparing the medications the patient was taking at home with those ordered when they are admitted to the hospital and repeating that process at discharge. The goal is for patients to stay on the maintenance medications that they should be on when they go into the hospital and that they are still on those medications when they leave. A key study of hospitalized patients shows how important this process is. It found that

> 60% of patients had at least one unintended variance and 18% at least one clinically important unintended variance. None of the variances had been detected by usual clinical practice before reconciliation was conducted. Of the 20 clinically important variances, 75% were intercepted by medication reconciliation before patients were harmed. (Vira et al. 2006)

There are also many potential sources for medication errors in ambulatory care outside of the hospital. For example, the doctor can prescribe the wrong medication. The pharmacist may misread a prescription if it is handwritten, or they may dispense the wrong medication even if they read the prescription correctly. The patient can administer the medication in the wrong dose or at the wrong interval. The patient may not even fill the prescription for economic reasons or because they do not understand its importance. How likely is this to happen? Those patients with five or more chronic conditions on average fill 50 prescriptions in a year that can be written by 14 different providers (Andersen and Horvath 2004). Most of these are elderly patients, with multiple medical problems, who are trying to manage a very complicated medication regimen. There is plenty of room for mistakes. It is widely accepted that adverse drug reactions are more likely in patients taking many medications (Koper et al. 2013).

The result is that medications are often not managed well. There are over 700,000 emergency department visits and over 120,000 hospitalizations in the United States each year due primarily to medication errors (CDC 2010). There is also a growing trend for children to be taking prescription medications, suggesting that these numbers may only increase in the future.

Improved electronic coordination of medications is now widely available in the United States. Surescripts, a private entity that is owned by a number of stakeholders in the healthcare system operates what it describes as "the nation's largest health information network." Using Surescripts, any provider who can legally prescribe in the United States can do it electronically and that prescription will appear electronically in the pharmacy that the patient chose to fill it. In 2012 some 788 million prescriptions were routed from the prescribing provider to the patient's pharmacy (Surescripts 2012). The network also provides information on refill intervals, a marker for compliance since patients cannot be consuming medications as prescribed if they do not refill them on time. Finally, providers can access Surescripts to get a relatively complete medication record for their patients, a use of the service that has grown from a small number in 2008 to some 586 million histories accessed in 2012 (Surescripts 2012). These histories can also indicate potential problems such as drug interactions and potential adverse drug reactions (Surescripts 2012). As a result of these services, this network is widely used. Today, according to Surescripts, around 58 percent of all office-based physicians and virtually all pharmacies in the United States are connected. Utilization grew 75 percent from 2010 to 2011 (Surescripts 2012). A lot of this growth is driven by federal policies and incentives that will be discussed later.

The federal government wants prescriptions to be prescribed electronically for several reasons. It is more convenient for patients, so they are more likely to actually get the prescription. Only about 70 percent of patients who have a prescription written actually pick it up at their pharmacy. The number goes up by about 10 percent with electronic prescribing, presumably because of increased patient convenience (Surescripts 2012). Since everyone is connected to a network, many of the problems related to coordination of medications, such as prescribing duplicate medications when patients complain about the same problem to more than one physician, can be avoided. Academic studies also show that e-prescribing reduces errors dramatically, as compared to manual prescribing (Kaushal et al. 2010). Medication errors before and one year after e-prescribing was initiated are shown in figure 2.5. These are dramatic results that clearly support the case for e-prescribing in the community as a means of reducing medication errors and the resultant impact on patient morbidity, care quality, and cost.

Figure 2.5   Medication errors declined rapidly within a year of introducing e-prescribing.

	Outset	One Year
e-Prescribing	42.5/100	6.6/100
Manual Prescribing	37.3/100	38.4/100

Source: Kaushal et al. 2010

Why Coordinated Care?

It should be clear by now that managing chronic disease, particularly in patients with multiple chronic diseases is a complex data logistics problem. This problem can be solved by mimicking other industries and using information systems that allow clinicians to communicate with each other on a timely basis.

This section will explain the specific programs and policies the federal government has adopted to promote the adoption of HIT systems. The link between their design and what is needed for improved health data logistics should be clear. The management of chronic disease is a very significant challenge for Medicare, the program that provides care to the older patients most likely to have these problems. *Making the Case for Ongoing Care* is a report by Partnership for Solutions, which provides a wealth of information on chronic disease and its impact (Anderson 2010). It states that in 2009 "145 million people—almost half of all Americans—live with a chronic condition. This represents an increase of 10 million people over the estimate that was made in 2002 for the year 2009" (Anderson 2010). Figure 2.6 shows the growth in chronic disease as people age (and that the overall rate has increased over time), and since Medicare pays for the care of older patients, this helps explain why virtually all Medicare spending is for chronic care management.

Fixing the management of chronic disease is the central priority for improving the efficiency and effectiveness of US healthcare. The key tactic must be coordinating care among the many providers involved in the care of these patients, particularly those with multiple chronic diseases. Doing this requires the use of clinical information systems.

This is not a new insight. The preface mentioned early work on the development of electronic medical records in the 1970s. These early systems were studied in *Policy Implication of Medical Information Systems*, a 1977 report to Congress that is quoted in the preface. As this report demonstrates, electronic medical records existed decades ago, however as recently as a few years ago only "four percent of physicians reported having an extensive, fully functional electronic-records system, and 13% reported having a basic system" (DesRoches et al. 2008; Jha et al. 2009).

Figure 2.6   Chronic disease rates increase with age and have increased over time.

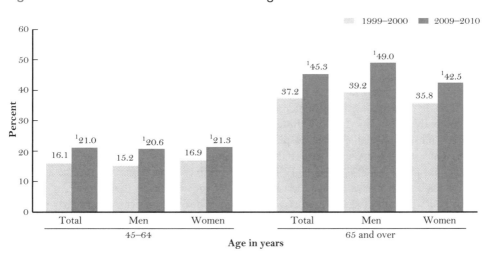

Source: Freid et al. 2012

The Growing Burden of Chronic Disease in America says that "we need to align financial incentives to promote coordination within the medical care system" (Andersen and Horvath 2004). For the most part (HMOs are an exception and there are others) there are no financial incentives to coordinate care in the healthcare system.

To review, chronic disease, and multiple chronic diseases in particular, drive most healthcare costs particularly among elderly populations. Success in managing them requires coordination among and between the many providers who care for these patients. The connection between this need and HIT was made over 40 years ago. However, physicians and hospitals have had no meaningful financial incentive to coordinate care (and can even benefit financially from the duplicative and unnecessary services that they often provide because they are unaware of the overall care of their patients). Remember, as well, the nature of a complex adaptive system—no one is in charge. "The United States is the only western industrialized nation that fails to provide universal coverage and the only nation where health care for the majority of the population is financed by for-profit, minimally regulated private insurance companies" (Quadango 2004). In the United States control of healthcare is spread widely among millions of employers and many federal and state sponsored programs. This has, in part, led to the uncoordinated and largely paper-based system of care that has been described. In such a fragmented payment system, no one entity has usually had sufficient market share to afford or to be able to provide significant enough financial incentives to spur adoption. Almost certainly only the federal government, the single largest payer, could have created the needed incentives. Starting in 2004 under President George W. Bush, adoption of HIT became a national priority. President Obama created actual financial incentives. This will be discussed in detail later in this chapter.

New Care Models Require Health Informatics to Succeed

The current healthcare delivery system is designed to treat acute illnesses and most of healthcare is managing chronic diseases. Several new and innovative care models are designed to align healthcare with the needs of chronic disease patients. Perhaps the best known is the Patient Centered Medical Home (PCMH). The PCMH is a specific example of the new care models primarily for the management of chronic disease that all emphasize a more team-oriented approach to care, more continuous involvement with the patient between physical visits, and the widespread use of HIT, which is essential to operating successfully in these new care models.

There are numerous industry studies that suggest that these new care models work to improve outcomes and lower costs. One study shows increases in quality and even greater decreases in cost and in the utilization of hospitals, in favor of providing care in less expensive outpatient settings (Horizon Blue Cross 2012). Another study looks specifically at a PCMH and shows a reduction in hospital readmissions and improvement in quality against specific measures (MetCare 2012). It also shows improved satisfaction both among patients and among the providers (remember the PCMH involves a team approach, so these are not just physicians), who had a much greater sense of satisfaction in their work. An effect of these positive results is growth in the conversion of health practices, particularly primary care practices, to new practice models, such as the PCMH. Data from the National Committee for Quality Assurance (NCQA), a major supporter of this change, shows a significant increase in the number of novel practice sites (NCQA 2011). However, these data are still relatively small numbers and are only through 2010.

HIT is crucial to operating a fully functional PCMH, although there are still issues with using it. For example, an article in the *Annals of Family Medicine* describes a current hodge-podge of IT that includes systems that are often not well-integrated, in large part because they were not designed to be "interoperable" (Nutting et al. 2009). The concept of interoperability is a key idea in HIT and has been its long time goal. It implies that diverse systems from different sources can seamlessly share data almost as if they were all parts of a single system. The technologies to support interoperability will be a major focus of chapters 3 through 5. It is also often difficult, using electronic medical record (EMR) systems alone, to do population health management, which is why new systems have been developed that can sit over a diverse set of EMRs and provide management tools largely through solving the data integration and specialized visualization issues. These technologies will be the focus of chapter 8.

Accountable Care

In chapter 1, Robert Doherty of the American College of Physicians was quoted as saying that the United States needs to move away from reimbursing physicians based on how many patient visits they do, how many tests they order, or how many procedures they do. A common term for the alternate approach is "pay-for-performance." There have been numerous pay-for-performance studies and trials performed involving both physicians and hospitals. A paper in the *Annals of Internal Medicine* said that five of six studies of physician-level financial incentives and seven of nine studies of group-level financial incentives found partial or positive effects on measures of quality (Petersen et al. 2006). This suggests a positive relationship between the way physicians are paid and quality of care. A similar study from the *New England Journal of Medicine* looked at heart failure, acute myocardial infarction, community-acquired pneumonia, coronary artery bypass, and hip and knee replacement using a composite of 18 quality measures in hospital care (Lindenauer et al. 2007). In all cases, the quality of care being delivered improved under pay-for-performance. Evidence like this led to the Physician Group Practice (PGP) demonstration conducted by Medicare at 10 sites (CMS 2011). The goal was to look at the potential to improve care quality and save money through a reimbursement model that involved sharing savings created by the physicians "by proactively coordinating their patients' total health care needs, especially for beneficiaries with chronic illness, multiple co-morbidities, and transitioning care settings" (CMS 2011).

PGP was a two-year project and at the end of the second performance year, all 10 of the participating physician groups achieved benchmark or target performance on at least 25 out of 27 quality metrics. Five of the groups achieved benchmark quality performance on all 27 quality measures (CMS 2011). Unsurprisingly, the metrics related to the management of diabetes, congestive heart failure, coronary artery disease, and preventive care. The measures are similar to those that were later adopted for Meaningful Use.

Notable improvements included:

- 11.0 percent in diabetes
- 12.4 percent in heart failure
- 6.0 percent in coronary artery disease
- 9.2 percent in cancer screening
- 3.8 percent in hypertension (CMS 2011)

Four sites did well enough to earn bonus payments because of quality improved *and* reduced costs. One site, the Marshfield Clinic, earned half of the total rewards paid, and in explaining how they did it on their website, the first reason they list is a well-developed electronic health record (E.H.R.) [through which] All Clinic physicians have access to patient records from all Clinic centers through the E.H.R., which helps to eliminate duplication of services, like lab tests and imaging. The E.H.R. helps plan visits; addresses care at the time of the visit; and assures appropriate monitoring of chronic conditions is performed. (Marshfield Clinic 2013)

This pilot program led to the accountable care concept for Medicare. At present, it is voluntary, and any group of providers can create an Accountable Care Organization (ACO). Currently "about four million Medicare beneficiaries are now in an ACO, and, combined with the private sector, more than 428 hospitals have already signed up. An estimated 14 percent of the U.S. population is now being served by an ACO" (Gold 2013).

The basic requirements include enrolling 5,000 or more Medicare beneficiaries. Providers are still paid under fee for service, but they can earn a performance bonus based on a combination of quality improvement and cost savings. In fact, they can earn 50 to 60 percent of the savings after the first 2 percent; although the bonus is capped at 10 to 15 percent of their targeted spending level, which is the estimated amount of money they would have spent under the a traditional Medicare model (Commonwealth Fund 2011).

An interesting characteristic of ACOs is that the configuration of providers is generally up to the ACO. It must include primary care. It may include a hospital, but that is not required. This freedom to configure an ACO has already led to some interesting innovations. Providers will be seeking help in managing their patients in a more continuous and coordinated way. Beyond the obvious incentives to employ advanced HIT, underutilized community resources, like pharmacies and home care agencies, may play an important part in these novel care delivery networks. Interestingly, both of these industries were relatively early adopters of HIT, so they should be generally well prepared for a new role in community-wide care managed through and coordinated by IT.

There are also 32 Pioneer ACO programs created by the Centers for Medicare and Medicaid Services (CMS) to investigate the next stage beyond the current ACO program. These are said to be already high performing sites that must have 15,000 beneficiaries enrolled (5,000 if they are rural) (CMS *Pioneer ACO Model* 2013). They have a more aggressive reward system, with the concept of shared losses as well as shared savings. In year three they can move to a population-based payment model that may be a flat payment per beneficiary per year, similar to the way HMOs are paid. The application for an ACO must be made by the actual providers or suppliers of the services, not by an insurance company or some other organization that would sit between them and Medicare. Finally, and of particular interest, there is a requirement that 50 percent of the primary care providers in the Pioneer ACO must have achieved Meaningful Use (CMS *Pioneer ACO Model* 2013). Medicare very specifically states that, in selecting Pioneer ACO sites, it will give preference to those organizations with advance HIT capabilities including:

- Population-based management tools
- Electronic exchange of healthcare data
- Ability to share performance feedback with participating providers
- A portal providing patients with access to their data
- A demonstrated ability to coordinate care (CMS *Pioneer ACO Model* 2013)

These are the essential tools that it is believed will help facilitate organizing care according to the right models IT to more successfully manage chronic disease.

Policy Overview

The first government to try to organize its own healthcare system was Germany in 1883, when Chancellor Bismarck introduced a nationwide healthcare program. He was concerned about workers and their ability to get care. The program was not terribly generous by today's standards—employers contributed a third, and the workers contributed two-thirds—but it was a big step forward. Three decades later, in 1912, President Theodore Roosevelt, became the first US President to say that the United States had reason to be concerned about sickness, irregular employment, and old age and should adopt a system of special health insurance. Despite his interest, nothing happened. After World War II, President Harry Truman said many of the same things, but once again, nothing happened. In 1971 President Nixon put forward a very ambitious agenda for improving healthcare in this country. He was concerned about equal access to care, something we mentioned briefly earlier. He felt that the system needed to grow to meet the demand, as people were living longer, and he wanted to do this in part by HMOs, the form of healthcare delivery we discussed earlier. This was very advanced thinking for the day, but once again, nothing happened. In 1994 President Clinton reintroduced the notion of healthcare reform. A very contentious debate ensued, and nothing happened.

Then in 2004, although President George W. Bush did not propose healthcare reform, he did propose that the country adopt a 10-year goal of universal computerization of health records and specifically linked achieving that goal to reducing medical errors, reducing healthcare costs, and improving care quality. Moreover, he did this in the State of the Union Address, a highly visible presidential address. To accomplish the goal he created the Office of the National Coordinator for Health IT (ONC).

By 2008, when President Obama took office, the adoption of HIT by both hospitals and physicians in the United States was low, and only 4 percent of physicians and 1.5 percent of hospitals had electronic medical systems capable of helping to improve the quality of care (DesRoches et al. 2008; Jha et al. 2009). Many more had a "basic" system that was essentially the digital equivalent of paper records, a passive system for recording care. In 2009, President Obama and Congress passed the Health Information Technology for Economic and Clinical Health (HITECH) Act as part of the American Recovery and Reinvestment Act (ARRA) economic stimulus program. HITECH's purpose was to provide funding to spur adoption by paying a substantial amount (that could even exceed the cost of purchasing an EMR) to those providers who met certain criteria. Significant adoption has occurred under these programs, particularly in hospitals. The Department of Health and Human Services (HHS), the agency of the federal government that manages Medicare and the federal components of Medicaid said in May 2013 that

> more than half of all doctors and other eligible professionals have received Medicare or Medicaid incentive payments for adopting or meaningfully using electronic health records (EHRs). HHS has met and exceeded its goal for 50 percent of doctor offices and 80 percent of eligible hospitals to have EHRs by the end of 2013. (CMS 2013a)

In 2010, as part of the Patient Protection and Affordable Care Act, there was a significant attempt to change the financial incentives in healthcare.

The overall goals of these two measures were universal adoption of HIT by 2014, which was the same goal put forward by President Bush four years earlier, and moving healthcare to new outcome-based incentives (as called for from the American College of Physicians) such as the Medicare ACOs we discussed earlier. These two programs ultimately depend on each other. HIT is virtually mandatory to operate in an outcome-based reimbursement environment, but adoption must first be "jump started" by offsetting the cost of HIT under the current system, in which there is little financial incentive for physicians and hospitals to make the needed investment.

Reimbursement depends on meeting certain criteria that will be discussed in more detail later. However, the federal program to spur HIT adoption is implemented in three parts:

- **EHR certification** defines the minimal acceptable requirements for an EHR that, if used according to the requirements of Meaningful Use, would qualify the provider for incentive payments.

- **Meaningful Use** defines what the provider has to do with their certified EHR in order to be eligible to receive incentive payments.

- **Incentive payments** allows providers to apply to either Medicare or Medicaid to receive payments under a schedule as compensation for implementing a certified EHR and achieving Meaningful Use.

ONC also funded some interesting research and demonstration projects to showcase and promote innovative use and further development of HIT. It also specifically promoted the adoption of HIT in small primary care practices (mostly rural) through regional extension centers. These are the practices that are the most resistant to automation, in part because they feel they lack the technical support to successfully select and deploy systems (DesRoches et al. 2008). ONC is also advancing data and interoperability standards by facilitating work groups around a number of key remaining challenges, such as aggregating data across EMRs and health information exchanges. Some of this work will be discussed in detail in chapters 3 through 5.

Another major ONC effort has been the technical development and promotion of a national health information exchange (HIE). The proposed national HIE has had several names. The latest is eHealth Exchange, which is now operated by a public-private partnership called Healtheway. Using ARRA money, ONC provided 50 awards, totaling over $500 million to states, to get HIEs up and running (ONC 2010).

The demonstration and research projects funded by ONC fall into three groups:

- **Beacon Communities** are places where groups of healthcare providers propose to show advanced use of HIT to support patient centered care.

- **SHARP** was awarded to several university consortiums that proposed to work on very specific problems that ONC felt impeded the adoption of HIT.

- **HIE Challenge Grants** were awarded to promote innovative use of HIEs.

EHR Certification

The ONC HIT website has comprehensive information to provide an overview of the certification criteria and process for verifying them in an individual EHR (healthit.gov 2013). There are a number of domains in which the certification program specifies what electronic medical records should do:

- They should record demographic and clinical health information.
- They should provide many of the tools we discussed earlier to improve care.
- They should do this in a way that protects confidentiality, integrity, and availability of the data they record.

For example, certification criteria, in the privacy, security, and trust domain, are further subdivided into:

- Access control
- Emergency access
- Automatic log-off
- Audit log
- Integrity
- Authentication
- General encryption
- Encryption when exchanging electronic health information
- Accounting of disclosures (optional)

Each of these, and a matching testing procedure, is defined in detail. For example, integrity is defined as meaning that the EHR must be able to create a message digest, must be able to verify that information is unaltered in transit, and must be able to detect the alteration of audit logs. In short, the system must have a comprehensive set of tools to manage the transfer of information. Certification testing is designed to verify that a system can do these things.

Another key functional area is supporting clinical practice. This is defined by a set of very specific things that a certified EHR must do and that are directly aligned with the Meaningful Use criteria for eligible providers:

- Record and chart vital signs
- Record smoking status
- Maintain a current problem list
- Maintain an active medication list
- Maintain an active medication allergy list
- Record laboratory test results
- Perform drug formulary checks
- Generate patient lists

Quality improvement is another key area, and there are a number of very specific functions that must be done there as well:

- Electronic prescribing
- Drug-drug and drug-allergy interaction checks
- Medication reconciliation
- Computerized provider order entry
- Patient reminders
- Patient-specific education resources
- Automated measure calculation
- Ability to calculate and submit clinical quality measures

"Calculate and submit clinical quality measures" is particularly critical for the next phase, Meaningful Use, which is largely about submitting these measures.

A key element of EHR certification (and Meaningful Use) is care coordination, so the system must be able to make an electronic copy of health information (particularly electronic clinical summaries). It must be able to provide timely access to that information. Finally, it must be able to exchange clinical information. The technologies to support doing these things are a major focus of chapters 3 through 5.

The characteristics that an EHR must have to be certified are closely aligned with the information capture, exchange, management, and reporting capabilities that are necessary for success in achieving a coordinated, non-episodic care system that can manage chronic disease successfully. Finally, a certified EHR must be able to submit data to public health for immunization registries, for surveillance of infectious diseases and disease outbreaks, and to help detect potential bioterrorism attacks as early as possible.

The National Institute of Standards and Technology (NIST) has been designated to develop the procedures for verifying certification. Requirements and detail analysis fed a process that developed the necessary testing materials, a small sample of which is shown here.

> **Test Data: ICD-9 Problems:**
> Cerebrovascular Accident, ICD-9 Code: V12.54
> Recurrent Urinary Tract Infection, ICD-9 Code: V13.02
> Chronic Obstructive Pulmonary Disease, ICD-9 Code: 496.0
> Essential Hypertension, ICD-9 Code: 401.9
>
> **Status:** Vendor-supplied (for example, Active)
> **Date Diagnosed:** Vendor-supplied (for example, May 22, 2010)

In this example, the vendor is supplied (by NIST) with four ICD-9 codes. ICD codes will be discussed in chapter 5 but these codes are the accepted international standard for coding diagnoses (problems) for healthcare claims and for other purposes throughout the healthcare industry. As shown, in addition to the code, the vendor must provide a mechanism for assigning a status to each problem: Is it active? Has it been resolved? There must also be a date when the problem was initially diagnosed.

Alternatively, as shown here, NIST allows the vendor to use Systemized Nomenclature of Medicine (SNOMED CT), an even more comprehensive system for categorizing healthcare data, which will also be discussed in chapter 5.

> **Test Data:** SNOMED Problems:
> Cerebrovascular Accident, SNOMED CT Code: 230690007
> Recurrent Urinary Tract Infection, SNOMED CT Code: 197927001
> Chronic Obstructive Lung Disease, SNOMED CT Code: 13645005
> Essential Hypertension, SNOMED CT Code: 59621000
>
> **Status:** Vendor-supplied (for example, Active)
> **Date Diagnosed:** Vendor-supplied (for example, May 22, 2010)

The testing procedure involves demonstrating that the system can display the correct problems, the history of those problems, and, using a NIST-supplied Inspection Test Guide, verify that they are displayed correctly without omission. The next step in a typical testing procedure involves modifying data. An example of this is changing the urinary tract infection problem from active status to the vendor supplied code for a resolved status and then verifying that this change is appropriately illustrated in the various displays of the patient's problems, such as the problem list and the problem histories, along with a date when that change was made.

Quality reporting is a particularly interesting example of EHR certification testing. To facilitate testing for this, ONC has developed an open source system called Cypress that creates synthetic quality data that can be provided to an EHR vendor. Cypress indicates what the quality reports should say, and this is compared to what the EHR reports. This example is a good point from which to discuss the problem of creating realistic synthetic clinical test data. Real patient data (called Protected Health Information [PHI]) is protected by a strict law call the Health Insurance Portability and Accountability Act of 1996 (HIPAA). HIPAA violations can bring severe penalties, including imprisonment. To avoid the complex and expensive procedures needed to protect PHI, researchers and others often use "deidentified" patient data, from which all fields that could be used to link back to the individual patient have been removed. Alternately, but less commonly, they use synthetic data that requires no safeguards at all. While much easier to work with administratively, since no HIPAA safeguards are required, "clinically realistic" synthetic data can be very hard to produce. In this instance, it is less important that the quality metric be realistic than it is to show that, given a known test data set, the EHR will produce the mathematically correct result. Given the issues with creating realistic synthetic clinical data, synthetic data is often used for prototyping, in order to show that a system works, but not to show that the results are actually valid in an absolute sense.

There is a surprisingly large number of certified EHRs, divided into two groups. Complete EHRs should, on their own, be sufficient for a provider to achieve Meaningful Use. Modular EHRs might be something like an e-prescribing system and need to be combined with other modular EHRs to achieve Meaningful Use. As of publication there were a total of over 3,300 certified EHRs equally divided into complete and modular. Selecting the best EHR for any particular provider practice can be a daunting undertaking given this huge number of product offerings. Chapter 6 will discuss often overlooked but key usability issues for those providers contemplating an EHR purchase.

Quality Measurement in Healthcare

Certification is an EHR technical specification developed by ONC. To earn incentive payments the provider must purchase a certified EHR, but they must also use it in a manner that achieves Meaningful Use. The criteria for this were developed by CMS and are largely based on quality reporting, so before we can discuss the Meaningful Use program, it is important to understand what quality means in healthcare, and how it can be measured.

This is not a simple topic and people do not necessarily even agree on how to define healthcare quality. The IOM provides a working definition that says that healthcare quality measures should indicate "the degree to which health services for individuals and populations increase the likelihood of desired health outcomes and are consistent with current professional knowledge" (IOM 2001). Under this definition, improved outcomes are achieved by delivering care based on research-derived medical evidence.

To further explore this, we will use the common chronic disease diabetes. Diabetic patients have an abnormal blood glucose (sugar) regulatory mechanism. In type 2 diabetes, the most common form, this is often caused, at least in part, by excessive body mass. The major goal of diabetes care is to keep blood glucose as close to normal levels as possible. Extended abnormally high blood glucose levels can cause serious medical problems, including heart and kidney disease. Measuring blood glucose is simple and can even be done by patients at home. However, an isolated glucose reading is of little value, since glucose levels will vary significantly, depending on when and what the patient has eaten, when they took their medications, the amount of exercise they have had, and other factors. Moreover, the goal is to keep the glucose level within normal bounds over an extended period of time, so ideally, a test that measured control over time would be highly desirable. It turns out that there is a blood test—hemoglobin a1c (HbA1c)—that is essentially a surrogate for the average blood glucose level over the prior two to three months. HbA1c is formed when glucose enters the red blood cells and binds with the oxygen carrying protein hemoglobin, forming its a1c variant. The higher the glucose level, the more binding with hemoglobin, and the percentage of HbA1c goes up.

As a result, HbA1c provides a measure of the average blood glucose over time, as illustrated in figure 2.7. Although the *current* blood glucose level varies a great deal, the HbA1c level remains constant, so long as the *average* blood glucose level over the recent past remains the same. Not only is HbA1c a useful measure in clinical practice, it can be used to illustrate the two major types of quality measures (metrics): process and outcome. Today, there are many more process measures than outcome measures, but both exist. A *process* quality metric involving HbA1c might be the percentage of a provider's diabetics that have had this test done in some specified time period, typically the last year. Using paper records, the percentage is typically around 50 percent. In other words, only half of the diabetic patients in the average practice using paper records have this important and useful test done annually, as recommended. Therefore, the HbA1c process measure is, was the test done?

The *outcome* measure is whether the provider's diabetic patients are adequately controlled. This might be stated as the percentage of diabetics above or below some specified HbA1c threshold level that represents adequate control of their diabetes. (The Mayo Clinic uses 7 percent as the goal, representing an average glucose level of 154 milligrams per deciliter [8.5 millimoles per liter], but many others use 9 percent.) As part of Meaningful Use, one of the required quality measures is the percentage of 18 to 75 year old diabetics in the practice whose HbA1c level is above 9 percent, indicating that they are not under adequate control.

Figure 2.7   The HbA1c level reflects the average blood glucose level of the past two or three months and, in this illustration, remains constant even though individual blood glucose levels vary significantly.

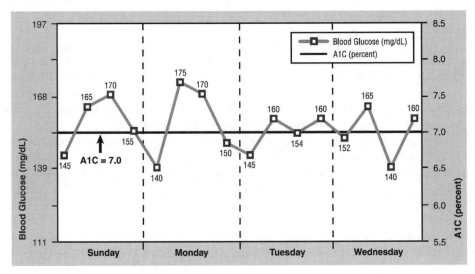

Source: HHS 2011, 4

Electronic Health Records

It is important to have a basic understanding of electronic records and new care models before we go into the federal initiatives and policies designed to promote adoption of those electronic records and these new care models. This section will begin with an EMR overview and then go through three federal HIT programs:

- EHR certification
- Meaningful Use
- Incentive Payments

To appreciate electronic records, it is important to discuss what physicians actually do. (The term physician is used, but there are a number of other licensed health professionals involved in patient care and these federal programs.)

Physicians are in the data business; they collect data, make decisions and act on that data, follow what happens, and then adjust accordingly. For example, a patient who is first seen for a problem, such as hypertension, will be evaluated to try to determine a cause that requires a particular approach to treatment. An appropriate treatment will then be prescribed that might consist of exercise and dietary changes, but it will almost certainly include medications. The patient will return at intervals, his or her hypertension will be assessed, and any needed changes will be made to the prescribed treatments. Historically physicians have done this on paper, which can and has caused numerous problems. To illustrate this, we will again turn to medications. Figure 2.8 is an example of a paper prescription. This happens to be a particularly important prescription. Look carefully at the name of the drug and decide whether it is Isordil or Plendil. The pharmacist thought it was Plendil, and dispensed that drug. The physician who wrote the prescription intended it to be Isordil. This patient died, and there was a successful law suit, the first in the United States, for illegible handwriting in a medical record.

As discussed earlier, healthcare providers often operate in silos. There can be insufficient communication and cooperation among them, particularly with respect to the sharing of detailed electronic clinical data. Healthcare is also often episodic and is organized around physical visits of patients to their physician, with very little interaction in between those visits. HIT has the clear potential to bridge both of these data gaps.

Figure 2.9 is a representation of the key elements of contemporary HIT, with EMRs at the bottom to indicate their foundational role in supporting all that is above them. EMRs, along with personal health records for patients and HIEs allowing the secure and private sharing of protected health data, provide the technology and sources of data to comprise

Figure 2.8   For which medication was this prescription written—Isordil or Plendil?

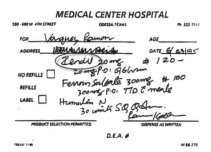

Reprinted with permission from Buckingham Barrera, PLLC.

Figure 2.9   The spectrum of contemporary HIT begins with the individual provider electronic medical record (EMR) and the patient's personal health record (PHR) as the source of most patient data. Data are aggregated across providers and from the patient, via HIEs, to create an EHR. It can then also be aggregated for population health management and for secondary use, such as clinical research or public health surveillance.

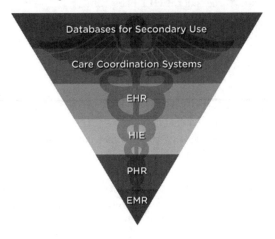

an EHR. Increasingly, specialized cloud-based population management systems sit above EMRs. Their role is to aggregate data usually from many providers that have contracted with one or more payers that provide incentives for them to deliver superior clinical outcomes. Sometimes these incentives reward efficiency and incent providers to routinely perform certain well defined process measures that are believed to lead to improved clinical results and/or reduced costs. These systems will be the focus of chapter 8.

From this whole spectrum of records, there is the increasing capability to aggregate data for secondary uses, such as studying how to most cost-effectively diagnose a problem, which treatments work best, or which are the most cost effective. This will be discussed more specifically in chapters 9 through 10.

If EMRs are thought of as the places where clinical data are stored as a part of patient care, they can be divided into four broad categories, although there are not always sharp delineations between them. These include enterprise EMRs used within hospitals and health systems, EMRs for office-based providers, personal health records for use by patients, and population health management systems for managing quality and other care issues across a large cohort of patients.

Hospitals are complex entities consisting of various departments, such as pharmacy, radiology, or clinical laboratory. Each of those have their own departmental systems, and the goal of an enterprise EMR is to bring together data from all of those entities, maybe even across multiple hospitals and associated provider practices, to give an integrated view of each patient's medical record no matter where in the health system they have received care. The 10 most commonly installed hospital enterprise EMRs account for 94 percent of all installations, according to Modern Healthcare using data from HIMSS Analytics (Modern Healthcare 2012).

The physician's office is a much simpler environment but one where adoption has historically been a significant challenge. There are hundreds of EMRs for physician practices, and according to a 2012 Medscape survey, the top 10 vendors have 69 percent of all installed systems (Medscape 2012). Increasingly physicians are being employed by hospitals, and those hospitals are often now looking for EMR solutions that scale across an entire enterprise, including physicians in office practice.

The third type is the personal health record (PHR). The target user is not a provider but the patient. PHRs are a new component of the EHR. Like population health management systems, another new component, the leading PHRs are cloud-based, although for the most part, hospital and physician systems are based on the traditional client-server architecture, with the computer systems, including the servers, installed either in the hospital or at a hosting facility under contract to the hospital.

EMRs for physicians often mimic the sections of a paper chart, such as demographic data, laboratory tests, imaging studies, or medications. The functionality of a physician practice oriented EMR is almost always designed to support the predominant practice model—the care of patients one at a time. As a result EMRs are typically used to track individual patients over time but not manage patients as groups, which is therefore more typically done by population health management systems. They can often trend key measures, such as blood pressure or lab results. They can identify patients due for visits or procedures. They can provide remote access to care providers if, for example, they are "on call" (interacting after normal office hours with patients of the practice). In this situation the physician may have to deal with patients they have not previously seen, a use case that showcases the advantages of electronic records. More advanced EMRs monitor the quality of care across patients and providers within a practice.

The distinction that is made between EMRs and EHRs is important. The EMR is essentially the digital version of the traditional paper chart, the electronic record of a particular physician's office. The EHR ideally represents the total health of the patient across *all* providers. Patients with multiple chronic diseases may be seeing many providers, so the EHR would ideally bring data together from all of them to create a single, unified view of each patient's care. Ideally it would also include data from the patient's PHR and from other sources, such as physiologic measurement devices in the home that provide up-to-date information on key measures, such as blood pressure, weight, or blood glucose.

A distinction is often made between basic and more advanced EMR functionality. Advanced functionality includes the capability of reminders for such things as routine screening or performing tests important to long-term patient management; for direct support of clinical decisions through practice guidelines; or, in the most advanced EMRs, for automated clinical decision support. The basic distinction is that the advanced EMR, unlike the paper chart and its basic EMR equivalent, is no longer a passive component of care delivery. These advanced functions all involve the electronic chart effectively reaching out to the provider in order to help improve the quality and efficiency of care. EHRs and population health management systems introduce the opportunity to provide advanced functionality across many EMRs, to facilitate care coordination, to manage care quality across and among practices, and increasingly, to allow patients to retrieve and record their own health data.

There is some early data to show that physicians that use EHRs provide better care. A review of the literature on computerized reminders for routine diabetes care (Boren et al. 2009) concluded that "Twelve of the 15 studies (80%) measured a significant process or outcome" and that "Thirty-five of 50 process measures (70%) were significantly improved." The hope is that improved process measures will lead to improved clinical outcomes but, to date, this has not been demonstrated nearly as convincingly as the impact of EHRs on improved process measures. Some would argue that improved outcome measures depend on more widespread use of clinical decision support where, it is presumed, physicians will make better, more evidence-based care decisions.

PHRs began as a way for patients to record their own data, but they have grown tremendously in functionality. Patients can now upload data from EMRs into their PHR (discussed in further detail later in this chapter), and they effectively provide a platform for patients to manage their own healthcare through associated applications that are beginning to become available as PHRs become "app platforms." These apps can obtain access to each patient's clinical data and use it to personalize that patient's app experience. This will be discussed in more detail in chapter 7.

HIE is yet another key element of HIT. It is the secure transport of critical and protected health data among and between providers and is the topic of chapter 3.

Meaningful Use

There are three key objectives in Meaningful Use. The first is that the certified EHR is being used in a meaningful manner, a somewhat circular definition. The second is that health information is being exchanged. And the third is that clinical quality measures are being collected and submitted. Based on this, Meaningful Use takes place in three stages, as shown in figure 2.10.

Stages 1 and 2 have been defined and stage 3 discussions are being facilitated by the HIT Policy Committee of ONC including the solicitation of comments from the public. Stage 1 focuses on capturing and sharing data, essentially the use of electronic records as the means for documentation in clinical practice and care coordination. Stage 2 focuses on using that data to improve clinical processes. Reminders and clinical decision support may help accomplish this. Stage 3 begins focusing on the ultimate objective, which is improving outcomes. The next section will discuss the incentive payments that providers can earn. They are tied to achieving the three stages of Meaningful Use creating a direct connection between Meaningful Use and the Incentive Payments program.

Figure 2.10   Meaningful Use is defined and implemented in three stages reflecting an increase in the clinical impact of electronic records over time as providers become accustomed to using them and health information exchange becomes more widespread.

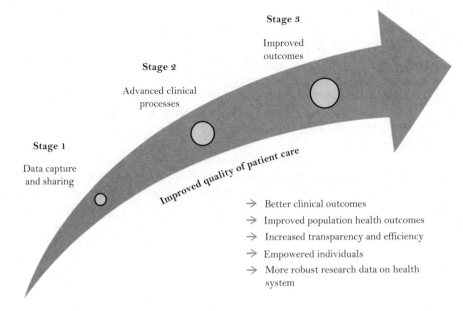

Source: ONC 2013c

Stage 1

The first stage consists of measures divided into three categories:

- Core measures
- Menu set measures
- Clinical quality measures

There are 15 mandatory core measures. Providers in stage 1 must also submit 5 of the 10 "menu set" measures, as well as six clinical quality measures. Three of these are mandatory, and providers can choose three more from a list of 41.

The core measures are divided into four groups:

- **Improve quality, safety, and efficiency, and reduce health disparities**
  - *Example*: Transmit at least 40 percent of prescriptions electronically to patients' pharmacies.
- **Engage patients and families**
  - *Example*: Provide patients with clinical summaries within three business days for more than 50 percent of all office visits.
- **Improve care coordination**
  - *Example*: Perform at least one test to demonstrate the ability to exchange key clinical information with other providers.
- **Privacy and security**
  - *Example*: Conduct or review a security risk analysis and implement security updates as necessary.

Note that, under care coordination, the provider has to perform one test to demonstrate their ability to share key clinical information. Presumably the assumption here is that all providers won't yet be in an area where the HIE infrastructure exists to actually share the data.

Menu set measures are divided into similar groups:

- **Improve quality, safety, and efficiency, and reduce health disparities**
  - *Example*: Generate at least one report listing patients with a specific condition.
- **Engage patients and families**
  - *Example*: Send reminders, if desired, for preventive/follow-up care for specified minimum percentages of adult and pediatric patients.
- **Improve care coordination**
  - *Example*: Perform medication reconciliation for more than 50 percent of patient transitions in the care of the physician.
- **Improve population and public health**
  - *Example*: Perform at least one test of the EHR's capability to provide electronic syndromic surveillance data to public health agencies, and perform a follow-up submission if the test is successful.

Under quality, safety, and efficiency, a provider might produce a report listing patients with a specific condition, such as all the diabetic patients in a practice. This would be a useful tool to help assure that all these patients had a hemoglobin a1c test done in the past year if the provider's EHR did not check for that automatically. Under public health, it might be the ability to provide surveillance data, such as patients with the flu, to a public health agency.

The three mandatory clinical quality measures that are core measures are screening for weight; screening for, and diagnosing patients with hypertension; and preventive care and screening for smoking. Providers must submit 3 of the 41 other quality measures. These include clinical issues such as cancer screening or prescribing antiplatelet therapy for patients with coronary artery disease, something that is known to reduce the chance of heart attacks.

Stage 2

The second stage raises the goals for quality measures similar to those in stage 1. The menu set in stage 2 is all new and it is more clinically sophisticated. The stage 2 quality measures are unchanged, but the number of measures required of the provider is increased.

Three new stage 2 measures that focus on patient access to their data are particularly important and worth emphasizing. Doing this requires some technical terms that will not be fully explained until later, but a simple understanding of them will suffice for now. The first is that at least 50 percent of patients seen by a provider within a reporting period must have been provided electronic access to their data within four days of when the data become available to the provider. There is a similar requirement for emergency department visits and inpatient hospital stays. The second is that at least five percent of the patients seen by a provider within the reporting period (or their designated representative) must have digitally accessed their health information. This metric now has the acronym VDT (view, download, or transmit), and any one of these—viewing, downloading, or transmitting the data—counts *toward* the requirement. There is a similar requirement post hospital discharge. It is insufficient under stage 2 to simply provide patients with a means of accessing their digital health data, some of them must do it. This essentially mandates that providers educate and encourage patients to become involved in their own care by at least looking at their data. For many patients, downloading it into a PHR or into other patient-facing tools may be preferable. PHRs will be discussed in detail in chapter 7, but once the data is in the patient's PHR, they can also use it to personalize many apps that are provided using the PHR as a platform. The transmit option means patients can send their data to a third party. This could even be a family member helping care for them, and with patient authorization, that person could actually do the viewing or downloading of the data (Morris et al. 2013).

Providing the ability for patients to view the data is relatively straightforward. Many EHRs include a "patient portal" specifically to support this via the web. This is not a new idea, although the specific data requirements are newly defined by Meaningful Use stage 2.

More interesting issues are the formats in which the information could be downloaded or transmitted and the means for that transmission. The format can be either human readable, for example a PDF, or it can be machine readable. The machine readable documents must be in the XML-based Consolidated Clinical Document Architecture (CCDA) format, discussed extensively in chapter 5. For now it is sufficient to know that the clinical data in such a document can be identified and properly classified by a computer. The degree typically depends on whether it is coded or not. The means of transmission from the patient to a third party might be the Direct SMTP standard (or Blue Button +, which uses Direct for this purpose). The details of Direct are discussed in chapter 3, but for now it is sufficient to know that it is a simple but secure way of sending protected health information using appropriate Internet standards, including secure e-mail.

Stage 2 of Meaningful Use also specifies that providers involved in "transitions of care" scenarios (such as a referral to another provider) transmit a document containing information appropriate to the specific scenario in a CCDA defined format (ONC 2013b). These and the VDT scenarios are summarized in figure 2.11. The technical details of this will be discussed in far more detail in chapter 5.

Figure 2.11   Meaningful Use Stage 2 defines what CCDA clinical summaries should be transmitted in various care scenarios.

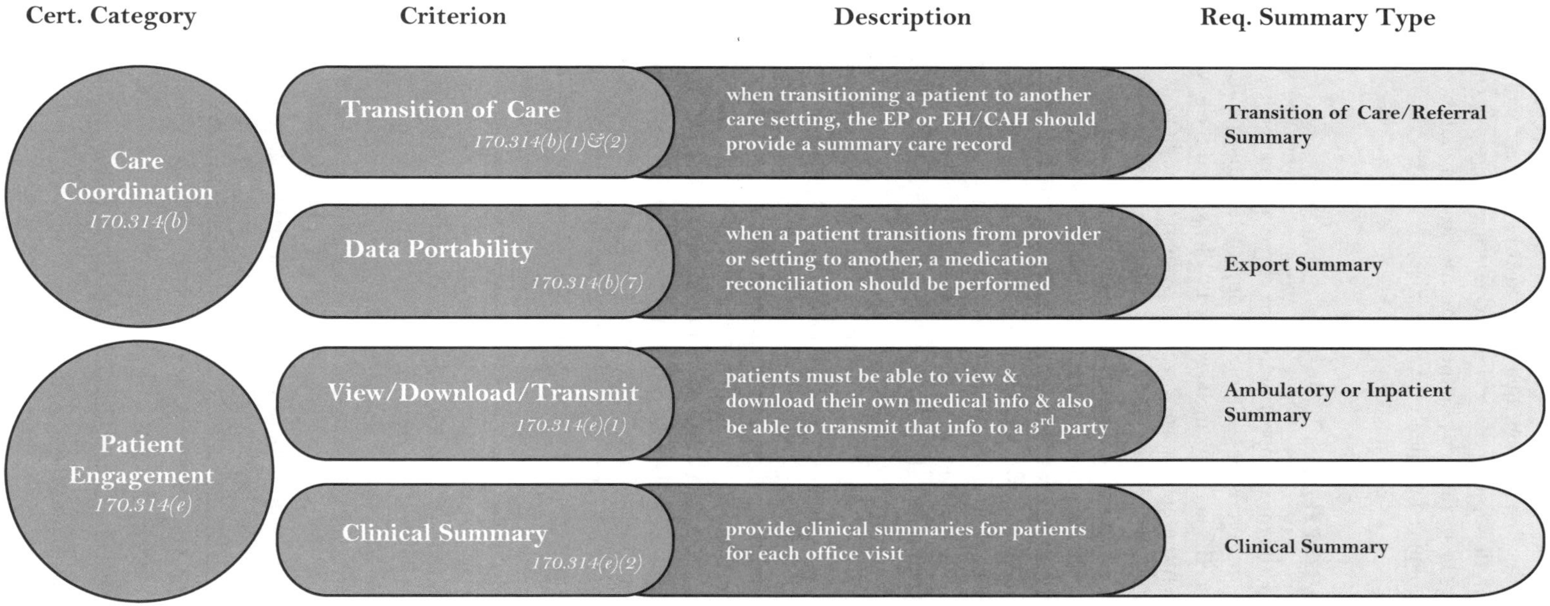

Cert. Category	Criterion	Description	Req. Summary Type
Care Coordination 170.314(b)	Transition of Care 170.314(b)(1)&(2)	when transitioning a patient to another care setting, the EP or EH/CAH should provide a summary care record	Transition of Care/Referral Summary
	Data Portability 170.314(b)(7)	when a patient transitions from provider or setting to another, a medication reconciliation should be performed	Export Summary
Patient Engagement 170.314(e)	View/Download/Transmit 170.314(e)(1)	patients must be able to view & download their own medical info & also be able to transmit that info to a 3rd party	Ambulatory or Inpatient Summary
	Clinical Summary 170.314(e)(2)	provide clinical summaries for patients for each office visit	Clinical Summary

Stage 3 of Meaningful Use has yet to be defined, but the stated overall goal is improved clinical outcomes, so developing new quality measures and reporting requirements for them is a clear focus in developing stage 3 (ONC 2013a). Stage 3 is currently planned for 2016 but this date may be pushed out further into the future to allow providers more time to implement what is required in the first two stages.

Incentive Payments

The last, and arguably the most important, of the three programs designed to incent providers (which may be hospitals or a defined group of "eligible professionals" out in the community) to adopt EHRs is the financial reward. Why should the government reimburse providers for implementing an electronic record system? The hope is that improved care quality and coordination will lead to improved quality at lower cost. It was mentioned in chapter 1 that the growth in US healthcare costs has slowed in recent years, but the relationship, if any, to HIT adoption of new care models is not yet clear. In any case, as healthcare is currently structured, if savings materialize they accrue to the entities that pay for care (for the most part the federal and state governments and private employers) and not to the providers who installed and have traditionally had to pay for their EHR systems. It is not difficult to understand why most providers have been unwilling to make this investment and to go through the very real pain and expense of implementing a new system if they have no prospect of seeing a financial gain from it. The incentive payments largely overcome the cost of implementing the system. In fact, a provider who contracts for a relatively inexpensive cloud-based EHR might make a profit, at least over the first few years.

There are two incentive programs that pay for the adoption and Meaningful Use of EHRs. One is through Medicare, the other through Medicaid. These payment programs are not operated by the ONC. As discussed, ONC defined EHR certification criteria and CMS defined Meaningful Use. The incentive payments come to providers through either the Medicare (CMS) or Medicaid (state) payments to that provider. Each provider can only be eligible for one program. Under the Medicare program, the amount of money that can be earned is based on the quantity of Medicare patients in the provider's practice. Under Medicaid this must be at least 30 percent of their patients or 20 percent if they are pediatricians. The term Eligible Professional (EP) designates those providers that qualify for either the Medicare or Medicaid incentive payment program (CMS 2013b).

Figure 2.12 shows that the payments that can be earned under the Medicare program decrease the later a provider starts the program. The similar numbers are larger for Medicaid. The payments are also tied to achieving the stages of Meaningful Use. If a provider has not achieved Meaningful Use by 2015, their Medicare payments are reduced by small percentage amounts, which the Secretary of Health and Human Services could increase if he or she chooses. There are no penalties or reimbursement reductions under the Medicaid program since these providers are already taking care of the most disadvantaged patients, often in difficult situations and usually for very low reimbursement rates.

The December 2013 CMS incentive monthly program report shows that program-to-date active registrations were 440,988 including:

- 63 percent of Medicare- and Medicaid-eligible professionals
- 90 percent of eligible hospitals (CMS 2013b)

Figure 2.12   Incentive payments are based on when an individual eligible provider enrolls and achieves the three stages of Meaningful Use.

Maximum Payment	Medicare Incentive Payment by Meaningful Use Stage					
by Start Year	2011	2012	2013	2014	2015	2016
2011	1	1	1	2	2	3
$44,000	$18,000	$12,000	$8,000	$4,000	$2,000	
2012		1	1	2	2	3
$44,000		$18,000	$12,000	$8,000	$4,000	$2,000
2013			1	1	2	2
$39,000			$15,000	$12,000	$8,000	$4,000
2014				1	1	2
$24,000				$12,000	$8,000	$4,000

Source: CMS 2014

Moreover, 60 percent of Medicare-eligible professionals and 20 percent of Medicaid-eligible professionals were Meaningful Users of EHRs and 88 percent of eligible hospitals and 78 percent of Medicaid-eligible professionals had received an EHR incentive payment. CMS also says that the 2013 National Electronic Health Records Survey found that 19 percent of physicians who plan to participate in the Meaningful Use program had adopted 14 of 17 Meaningful Use Stage 2 objectives. (CMS 2013b)

In total some $19.2 billion in meaningful-use incentive payments have been distributed to eligible hospitals and healthcare professionals (CMS 2013b).

A December 2012 CDC survey asked providers whether they intended to enroll for Meaningful Use, and on average, 65 percent said yes (Hsiao and Hing 2012). According to this more recent CMS report, 60 percent of Medicare-eligible professionals and 20 percent of Medicaid-eligible professionals were Meaningful Users of EHRs and 88 percent of eligible hospitals and 78 percent of Medicaid-eligible professionals had received an EHR incentive payment. CMS also says that the 2013 National Electronic Health Records Survey found that 19 percent of physicians who plan to participate in the Meaningful Use program had adopted 14 of 17 Meaningful Use Stage 2 objectives. (CMS 2013b) Medicaid providers can earn an adopt, implement, or upgrade (AIU) payment for adopting, implementing, or upgrading an EHR ahead of achieving Meaningful Use (CMS 2013b).

There are state-by-state variations posted on the ONC HIT Dashboard. The CMS reports provide up-to-date data on the ability of eligible providers to use their installed EHRs to actually meet meaningful-use criteria (CMS 2013c). The percentages vary from over 97 percent for basic functions, such as patient problem, medication, or allergy lists, to 82 percent for e-prescribing, or 63 percent for patient reminders. The corresponding data was reported for eligible hospitals (CMS 2013c).

The CDC study also looked at the demographics of physician adopters (figure 2.13). Unsurprisingly younger physicians have a higher percentage of adoption. but physicians age 50 and over are approaching 50 percent (Hsiao and Hing 2012). It was mentioned earlier that the single biggest factor affecting adoption by physicians in independent practices may be the size of their practice. The bigger the practice, the more likely they are to have implemented an EHR, with practices of 11 or more physicians at 86 percent (Hsiao and

Figure 2.13 Provider demographics, practice size and ownership, and provider specialty have an influence on EMR adoption rates.

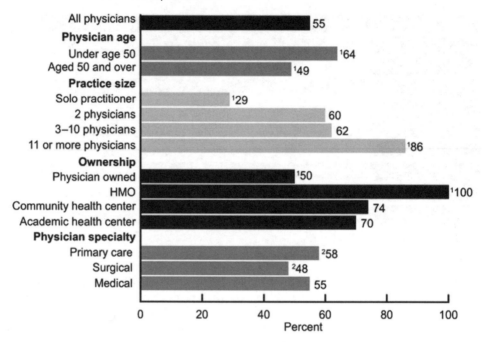

Source: Jamoom et al. 2013

Figure 2.14 Physicians that have achieved Meaningful Use Stage 1 report various benefits of using their EHRs.

% Strongly Agree or Agree	Total	PCP	Surgical Specialist	Non-surgical Specialist	Other
Administrative/Financial Benefits:					
Faster and more accurate billing for services	74	80	67	77	72
Time savings through e-prescribing	67	78	64	64	71
Savings from not managing/storing paper	59	66	51	58	66
Practice/worksite efficiency increase	53	61	50	51	60
Clinical Benefits:					
Improved communication and care coordination	67	56	64	70	76
Immediate data availability	59	63	53	56	77
Guideline prompts and timely lab results	56	64	49	55	63
Patient submission of information	41	43	42	38	51

Hing 2012). Small practices have much lower implementation rates (30 percent) (Hsiao and Hing 2012), which is why ONC funded the Regional Extension Centers (this program is now largely over) to help small practices, particularly primary care practices in rural areas, implement EHR systems. Ownership of the practice also affects adoption. As was mentioned earlier, HMO adoption is 100 percent (Hsiao and Hing 2012). These physicians, like an increasing number of physicians in other settings (who may now work for a hospital), are employees of the HMO. In physician owned practices, adoption is about 50 percent. Academic medical centers and community health centers are roughly in the middle. Physician specialty was not a significant factor (Hsiao and Hing 2012).

How are physicians actually using these EHRs? Does this use align with the problems and solutions that have been discussed? The Deloitte Center for Health Solutions' 2013 Survey of US Physicians provides recent data from 613 randomly selected physicians (margin of error +/− 3.89 percent at the 95 percent confidence level) (Deloitte 2013). For the purposes of this text, it is particularly interesting to look at data from physicians whose practices have an EHR that meets Meaningful Use stage 1 requirements, where the data are based on experience to date with their EHR (figure 2.14). The greatest percentage (two-thirds) of these physicians cited improved communication and care coordination as a clinical benefit (Deloitte 2013). However, it is important to remember that these are physicians who have achieved stage 1 of Meaningful Use and not physicians as a whole. In the executive summary of this study, Deloitte comments that:

> U.S. physicians who use HIT are optimistic about its prospects for better care and lower administrative costs once fully integrated. Physician non-adopters accept HIT as an inevitable requirement for practicing medicine in the future. However, they may be skeptical about clinical value and concerned about implementation costs. As a result, care coordination via cross-practice clinical data sharing is not widespread. And the clinical impact of HIT on population health outcomes is not readily apparent in many communities. In our view, this skepticism is likely to change. Powerful market forces exerted by health plans and consumers are accelerating HIT adoption. HIT adoption is expected to promptly move from Wave One—use for outcome improvement—to Wave Two—use for coordination of care in risk-sharing relationships with payers. (Deloitte 2013)

The Healthcare Information and Management Systems Society (HIMSS) has developed a 7-stage model for EHR adoption with stage 7 representing the most broad and deep EHR adoption. Since Meaningful Use began, there has been a dramatic increase in the hospitals that are in stages 5, 6, and 7, and a substantial decrease in the hospitals that are in the lower stages, indicating a clear trend for hospitals to move towards more advanced EHR implementation. This rate of change is illustrated by a 2009 survey of hospital adoption found only 1.5 percent of hospitals had EHRs capable of some of this advanced functionality (Jha et al. 2009).

REFERENCES

AHRQ. 2001. Reducing and Preventing Adverse Drug Events to Decrease Hospital Costs. Agency for Health Policy and Research Fact Sheet # 01-0020. http://www.ahrq.gov/research/findings/factsheets/errors-safety/aderia/index.html

Anderson, G. 2010. Making the Case for Ongoing Care. Robert Wood Johnson Foundation. www.rwjf.org/pr/product.jsp?id=50968

Andersen, G. and J. Horvath. 2004. The growing burden of chronic disease in America. *Public Health Reports* 119. http://www.ncbi.nlm.nih.gov/pmc/articles/PMC1497638/pdf/15158105.pdf

Boren, S.A., A.M. Puchbauer, and F. Williams. 2009. Computerized prompting and feedback of diabetes care: A review of the literature. *J Diabetes Sci Technol* 3(4):944–950. http://www.ncbi.nlm.nih.gov/pmc/articles/PMC2769983/#!po=30.0000

The Buckingham Law Firm. 1999. Illegible Prescription. http://www.medmal-law.com/illegibl. htm

Centers for Disease Control and Prevention. 2010. Medication Safety Basics. http://www.cdc.gov/ medicationsafety/basics.html

CMS. 2014. An Introduction to the Medicare EHR Incentive Program for Eligible Professionals. http://www.cms.gov/Regulations-and-Guidance/Legislation/EHRIncentivePrograms/ Downloads/Beginners_Guide.pdf

CMS. 2013a. Doctors and Hospitals' Use of Health IT More Than Doubles since 2012. http:// www.hhs.gov/news/press/2013pres/05/20130522a.html

CMS. 2013b. Monthly EHR Incentive Payments Report. http://www.cms.gov/Regulations-and- Guidance/Legislation/EHRIncentivePrograms/Downloads/December2013_SummaryReport.pdf

CMS. 2013c. Medicare & Medicaid EHR Incentive Programs. http://www.cms.gov/Regulations-and- Guidance/Legislation/EHRIncentivePrograms/Downloads/HITPC_Nov2013_Full_Deck.pdf

CMS. 2013c. EHR Incentive Programs. http://www.cms.gov/Regulations-and-Guidance/ Legislation/EHRIncentivePrograms/index.html?redirect=/EHRIncentivePrograms/

CMS. 2013d. Pioneer ACO Model. http://innovation.cms.gov/initiatives/Pioneer-ACO-Model/

CMS. 2011. Medicare Physician Group Practice Demonstration: Physicians Groups Continue to Improve Quality and Generate Savings under Medicare Physician Pay-for- Performance Demonstration. http://www.cms.gov/Medicare/Demonstration-Projects/ DemoProjectsEvalRpts/downloads/PGP_Fact_Sheet.pdf

Commonwealth Fund. 2011. The Final Rule for the Medicare Shared Savings Plan. http://www.commonwealthfund.org/~/media/Files/Publications/Other/2011/ ZezzasummaryfinalruleMedicaresharedsavingsv2%202.pdf

Commonwealth Fund. 2008. http://www.commonwealthfund.org/Surveys/2008/2008- Commonwealth-Fund-International-Health-Policy-Survey-of-Sicker-Adults.aspx

Davis, M.W. 2009. The State of U.S. Hospitals Relative to Achieving Meaningful Use Measurements. HIMSS Analytics 2009. http://www.himssanalytics.org/docs/HA_ARRA_100509.pdf

Deloitte Center for Health Solutions. 2013. Physician Adoption of Health Information Technology: Implications for Medical Practice Leaders and Business Partners. http://www.deloitte.com/ view/en_US/us/Industries/health-care-providers/46fb8ec4d1a8e310VgnVCM2000003356f7 0aRCRD.htm

Department of Health and Human Services. National Institutes of Health. 2011. The A1C Test and Diabetes. NIH Publication No. 11–7816. http://www.diabetes.niddk.nih.gov/dm/pubs/ A1CTest/A1C_Test_DM-508.pdf

DesRoches, C.M., E.G. Campbell, S.R. Rao, K. Donelan, T.G. Ferris, A. Jha, R. Kaushal, D.E. Levy, S. Rosenbaum, A.E. Shields, and D. Blumenthal. 2008. Electronic health records in ambulatory care: A national survey of physicians. *N Engl J Med* 359:50–60. http://www.nejm.org/doi/full/ 10.1056/NEJMsa0802005

Freid V.M., Bernstein A.B., and Bush M.A. 2012. Multiple chronic conditions among adults aged 45 and over: Trends over the past 10 years. NCHS data brief, no 100. Hyattsville, MD: National Center for Health Statistics.

Gold, J. 2013. ACO Is the Hottest Three-Letter Word in Health Care. Kaiser Health News. http://www.kaiserhealthnews.org/stories/2011/january/13/aco-accountable-care-organization-faq.aspx

Goldberg D.G. and A.J. Kuzel. 2009 (Jul–Aug). Elements of the patient-centered medical home in family practices in Virginia. *Ann Fam Med* 7(4):301–308.

Horizon Blue Cross. 2012. http://www.horizon-bcbsnj.com/eprise/main/SiteGen/horizon_bcbsnj/Content/old_news_room/news_releases/article.html?id=33878

Hsiao, C.J. and E. Hing. 2012. Use and characteristics of electronic health record systems among office-based physician practices: United States, 2001–2012. http://www.ncbi.nlm.nih.gov/pubmed/23384787

Institute of Medicine. 2001. Crossing the Quality Chasm: A New Health System for the 21st Century. http://www.iom.edu/Reports/2001/Crossing-the-Quality-Chasm-A-New-Health-System-for-the-21st-Century.aspx

Jamoom, E., P. Beatty, A. Bercovitz, D. Woodwell, K. Palso, and E. Rechtsteiner. 2013. Physician Adoption of Electronic Health Record Systems: United States, 2011. *NCHS Data Brief* No. 98. http://www.cdc.gov/nchs/data/databriefs/db98.pdf

Jha, A.K., C.M. DesRoches, E.G. Campbell, K. Donelan, S.R. Rao, T.G. Ferris, A. Shields, S. Rosenbaum, and D. Blumenthal. 2009. Use of electronic health records in U.S. hospitals. *N Engl J Med* 360:1628–1638. http://www.nejm.org/doi/pdf/10.1056/NEJMsa0900592

Johnson, P.F. 2006. Strategic Marketing. https://www.inkling.com/read/strategic-marketing-cravens-piercy-10th/comprehensive-cases/case-6-9-wal-mart

Kaushal, R., et al. 2010 (June). Electronic prescribing improves medication safety in community-based office practices. *J Gen Intern Med* 25(6): 530–536. http://www.ncbi.nlm.nih.gov/pmc/articles/PMC2869410/?tool=pubmed

Koper, D., et al. 2013 (June). Frequency of medication errors in primary care patients with polypharmacy. *Fam Pract* 30(3):313–319. http://fampra.oxfordjournals.org/content/30/3/313.long

Lindenauer, P.K., D. Remus, S. Roman, M.B. Rothberg, E.M. Benjamin, A. Ma, and D.W. Bratzler. 2007. Public reporting and pay for performance in hospital quality improvement. *N Engl J Med* 356:486–496. http://www.nejm.org/doi/full/10.1056/NEJMsa064964#t=article

Marshfield Clinic. 2013. Clinic Demonstrates Improved Quality of Care Resulting in Cost Savings for Medicare. https://www.marshfieldclinic.org/about-us/quality/medicare-savings

Medscape. 2012. EHR Report. http://www.medscape.com/features/slideshow/EHR2012

MetCare. 2012. http://www.metcare.com/care-model/results-pcmh-patient-centered-medical-home.php

Modern Healthcare. 2012. Top Vendors of Enterprise EMR Systems. http://ecom.datajoe.com/ecom/download/?sTNYlA58

Morris, G., S. Afzal, and D. Finney. 2013. Key Considerations for Health Information Organizations Supporting Meaningful Use Stage 2 Patient Electronic Access Measures. http://www.healthit.gov/sites/default/files/key_considerations_for_health_information_organizations_vdt.pdf

Murray, M. and K. Kroenke. 2001. Polypharmacy and medication adherence: Small steps on a long road. *J Gen Intern Med* 16(2): 137–139. http://www.ncbi.nlm.nih.gov/pmc/articles/PMC1495172/

NCQA. 2011. NCQA's Patient-Centered Medical Home 2011. http://www.ipfcc.org/advance/topics/PCMH_2011_Overview_White_Paper.pdf

Nutting, P.A., W.L. Miller, B.F. Crabtree, C.R. Jaen, E.E. Stewart, and K.C. Stange . 2009 (May). Initial lessons from the first national demonstration project on practice transformation to a patient-centered medical home. *Ann Fam Med* 7(3): 254–260 http://www.annfammed.org/content/7/3/254.full

OECD. 2011. "Medical doctors", in OECD, *Health at a Glance 2011: OECD Indicators*, OECD Publishing. doi: 10.1787/health_glance-2011-21-en

ONC. 2010. State Health Information Exchange Cooperative Agreement Program. http://www.healthit.gov/policy-researchers-implementers/state-health-information-exchange

ONC. 2013a. Meaningful Use Workgroup: Stage 3 Update. http://www.healthit.gov/facas/sites/faca/files/MUWG_Stage3_13_Sep_4_FINAL_0.pdf

ONC. 2013b. Implementing Consolidated-Clinical Document Architecture (C-CDA) for Meaningful Use Stage 2. http://www.healthit.gov/sites/default/files/c-cda_and_meaningfulusecertification.pdf

ONC. 2013c. Meaningful Use Definition and Objectives. http://www.healthit.gov/providers-professionals/meaningful-use-definition-objectives

ONC. 2013d. Meaningful Use Regulations. http://www.healthit.gov/policy-researchers-implementers/meaningful-use-stage-2

Petersen, L.A., T. Urech, K. Simpson, K. Pietz, S.J Hysong, J. Profit, D. Conrad, R.A. Dudley, M.Z Lutschg, R. Petzel, and L.D Woodard1. 2006 (August). Design, rationale, and baseline characteristics of a cluster randomized controlled trial of pay for performance for hypertension treatment: Study protocol. *Ann Intern Med* 145(4):265–272. http://www.ncbi.nlm.nih.gov/pmc/articles/PMC3197549/

Pham, H.H., A.S. O'Malley, P.B. Bach, C. Saiontz-Martinez, and D. Schrag. 2009. Primary care physicians' links to other physicians through Medicare patients: The scope of care coordination. *Ann Intern Med* 150(4):236–242.

Quadango, J. 2004. Why the United States has no national health insurance: Stakeholder mobilization against the welfare state, 1945–1996. *Journal of Health and Social Behavior* vol. 45 (Extra Issue): 25–44. http://www.asanet.org/images/members/docs/pdf/featured/JHSB04ExtraQuadagno.pdf

Rosenow, E. 2005. Patients' understanding of and compliance with medications: The sixth vital sign? *Mayo Clinic Proceedings* 80(8):983–987. http://www.mayoclinicproceedings.org/article/S0025-6196(11)61577-2/abstract

S&I Framework. 2014. "2014 Ed. CEHRT Criteria Requiring C-CDA." Companion Guide to HL7 Consolidated CDA for Meaningful Use Stage 2". http://wiki.siframework.org/Companion+Guide+to+ Consolidated+CDA+for+MU2

Schoen, C., R. Osborn, D. Squires, M.M. Doty, R. Pierson, and S. Applebaum, 2011. New 2011 Survey of Patients with Complex Care Needs in 11 Countries Finds That Care Is Often Poorly Coordinated, *Health Affairs* Web First, Nov. 9, 2011. http://www.commonwealthfund.org/Publications/In-the-Literature/2011/Nov/2011-International-Survey-Of-Patients.aspx

Surescripts. 2012. The National Progress Report on E-Prescribing Year 2012. http://www.surescripts.com/about-e-prescribing/progress-reports/national-progress-reports

Vira, T., M. Colquhoun, and E. Etchells. 2006 (April). Reconcilable differences: correcting medication errors at hospital admission and discharge. *Qual Saf Health Care* 15(2):122–126. http://www.ncbi.nlm.nih.gov/pmc/articles/PMC2464829/

RECOMMENDED READING AND RESOURCES

The Growing Burden of Chronic Disease in America (Andersen and Horvath 2004) is a discussion of the impact of chronic disease on US healthcare.

Elements of the Patient-Centered Medical Home in Family Practices in Virginia (Goldberg and Kuzel 2009) provides details about how HIT is key to operating successfully under the PCMH model of care.

For more details on ACO requirements, read Commonwealth Fund 2011's *The Final Rule for the Medicare Shared Savings Plan*. http://www.commonwealthfund.org/~/media/Files/Publications/Other/2011/ZezzasummaryfinalruleMedicaresharedsavingsv2%202.pdf.

Read *Reference Grids for Standards and Certification Criteria*, an online document on ONC's healthIT .gov site, for the details of certification for ambulatory EHR systems. There is a separate certification process for the enterprise EHR systems used by hospitals. http://www.healthit.gov/policy-researchers-implementers/reference-grids-standards-and-certification-criteria.

ONC Reference Grids for Standards and Certification Criteria. http://www.healthit.gov/policy-researchers-implementers/reference-grids-standards-and-certification-criteria.

ONC Certified Health IT Product List. http://oncchpl.force.com/ehrcert/ehrproductsearch.

ONC HealthIT Dashboard. http://dashboard.healthit.gov/

Current information on provider adoption should be available from the ONC's HIT Dashboard at http://dashboard.healthit.gov/ or from the CMS EHR Incentive Payment Program Data and Program Reports page at http://www.cms.gov/Regulations-and-Guidance/Legislation/EHRIncentivePrograms/DataAndReports.html.

Part II

Key Technologies

Chapter 3

Health Information Exchange

Health information exchange (HIE) is the key component of health informatics through which information from various electronic record systems is shared and is potentially transformative for the healthcare system. For example, with chronic disease, there is a need for coordinated care between the often large number of specialized providers caring for the same chronic disease patient. These providers need a way of synchronizing and coordinating their care by sharing information. This chapter will discuss the concept of HIE and the enabling technologies that facilitate this sharing while protecting the privacy and security of protected health information (PHI). If you drill down sufficiently, it is essentially digital plumbing that can get quite complex. The United States has struggled over the years with how to balance that complexity with the need for economic sustainability. This will be discussed further, but first we examine why HIE is important.

Overview

HIE is essential for coordinating healthcare, but it has other important and growing applications. As the United States moves toward Accountable Care Organizations (ACOs) and other outcome-based reimbursement systems, HIE is the way that patients can be managed at the population level and providers can be managed as a group against outcome measures that are going to determine how much each organization gets paid. It also provides a means for engaging patients through their typically cloud-based personal health records (PHRs) by facilitating two-directional communication between them and their providers' electronic medical records (EMRs). HIE can be used to aggregate clinical data for public health surveillance and, increasingly, for research purposes, as the amount of available digital clinical data grows exponentially.

HIE has other potential advantages. The way health information systems have historically communicated with each other is through point-to-point interfaces; this special software allows system A to exchange data with system B, typically using a technology called HL7 messaging that will be discussed in detail in chapter 5. Developing and maintaining these point-to-point interfaces was historically problematic and expensive. For example, the systems at either end kept changing, and the point-to-point interfaces had to change to adapt. If they did not, there were problems with interfaces that had once worked suddenly not working with new releases of the systems at either end. The people developing the systems often failed to consider the impact of changes on these interfaces, which were, at best, a peripheral consideration to them. Moreover, this was something talented programmers did not like to do, so it was difficult to interest them in working on it. The hope is that getting rid of these point-to-point interfaces and creating a utility will lower the cost of exchanging data, while still assuring privacy, security, and trust.

For many years the federal government has sought to promote national HIE and has recently created Healtheway, a public-private organization, to accomplish this. The proposed national HIE itself is now named eHealth Exchange. Previous attempts at regional and national HIE had a number of names, each with their own acronyms including: Regional Health Information Organization (RHIO), Regional Health Information Exchange (RHIE), National Health Information Network (NHIN), and Nationwide Health Information Network (NwHIN).

One early example, to illustrate just how old the concept is, was an effort to create a HIE in rural Hampton County, South Carolina, in 1974 (Schuman et al. 1976). A basic shared electronic patient summary record was to be shared by all the local primary care physicians, the hospital, and the pharmacies, so that, whenever and wherever a patient was seen, there was a complete up-to-date basic picture of what was going on with their care. Patients were not directly involved, since there was no practical way to do it in an era when they did not have computers, smartphones, other devices, or the Internet. Technically the HIE got up and working, but there was little utilization of it. This shows the importance of incentives. No one used the HIE because they had no financial incentive to change their behavior.

Figure 3.1 *The 2011 Commonwealth Fund Survey of Sicker Adults* shows the percentage of patients in several countries who reported care coordination problems, such as test results unavailable at the time of an appointment, the ordering of tests

Figure 3.1   Significant percentages of patients in most of the countries surveyed by the Commonwealth Fund reported care-coordination problems.

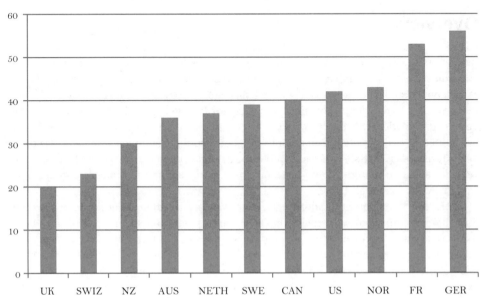

Source: Schoen and Osborne 2011

that had already been done, providers who failed to share important information with each other, specialists not having information about the patient's medical history, and patient's regular doctor not being informed about specialist care. (Schoen and Osborne 2011) While the United States has one of the higher reported problem rates, this actually represented an improvement from a prior survey in 2008 when the United States performed the worst among the surveyed countries. The United States needs more HIE to further improve.

Care coordination has been discussed as an essential concept for managing chronic disease. In practice, it can be challenging to do in the US environment in which every provider has their own EMR, and that EMR can come from any one of the hundreds of companies certified for Meaningful Use. A key issue is that there are currently no robust standards for how those EMRs represent clinical data. As a result, HIEs—at least the more robust HIEs—attempt to solve this "interoperability" problem using sophisticated approaches to normalizing and standardizing diverse data sets from different systems.

However, before data can be correctly normalized or standardized, the patient must be correctly identified. This can be a difficult issue, particularly if there are many people with the same or similar names in a community. How do you know for sure that this John Smith in one clinic is the same as that John Smith in another? They may have different medical record numbers in each practice, so this cannot be used as the key to link them. There is no national ID number in the United States that is permitted to be used (for example, the Social Security number). As a result, special technologies, often called master patient indexes (MPIs), have been developed. These look at a variety of factors about people (such as birth date, gender, race, ethnicity, and address) to try to make sure they are accurately matched with the same person in another care location. However, this is a complex issue, and a perfect technical approach does not exist. The problem would be simplified but not completely solved if the United States adopts a national ID number, at least for healthcare, as other countries, such as France, have done.

Interoperability is such a widespread issue that many health systems—typically consisting of multiple hospitals, provider practices and other care facilities, such as rehabilitation centers, nursing homes, and home healthcare—have their own enterprise master patient index (EMPI) to bring together patient data from the systems installed within their own enterprise. The term cross-enterprise master patient index (XMPI) designates even more sophisticated MPIs that are designed to deal with multiple healthcare enterprises, each consisting of a group of hospitals and clinics that are all under common ownership or management.

Integrating the Healthcare Enterprise (IHE) was founded in 1996 as a global effort specifically focused on these and other clinical integration issues across health enterprises. IHE USA was founded in 2010. IHE Profiles are the principle tool and provide a standards-based framework for sharing information by defining and specifying interoperability issues related to information access for both providers and patients. Each addresses workflow, security, administration, and information infrastructure issues by defining the actors, transactions, and information content required to address a specific clinical use case referencing appropriate standards.

Another issue is locating desired clinical data. For example, finding where a patient with chronic lung disease previously had x-rays taken is a requirement for the physician who is now seeing that patient and is interested in whether the finding in a current chest x-ray represents a change from before. One solution is to bring all the data to a central warehouse (centralized HIE). That approach is difficult politically, since competing health systems may not want to share their data this way and may worry about losing control of their data and how it will be used. It is also typically expensive. An alternative approach is a document locator or registry service. Under this approach, as each new document is created, the clinic or hospital that creates it sends a message in a specified format to a central database that is effectively an index of where all clinical data in the area it covers is located (a form of hybrid HIE).

Once the correct data has been assembled, using the tools just discussed, there is still the problem of cross-provider integration of clinical data. Providers who need to coordinate often have different EMRs, the way they describe data is often different and the way they configure and use even the same EMR can be different. Ultimately, the terms and even the way (for example, free text versus structured codes or terminology) providers describe the same clinical concept is often different. The historic approach is to standardize—or normalize—the data to facilitate presenting an accurate, integrated picture of the patient across the multiple providers caring for them. This facilitates care coordination and it can create a virtual community-wide EHR such as the one at the Indiana Health Information Exchange that will be discussed later in this chapter. Although the technologies exist to support this model, it is typically costly and there is not always some entity willing to pay for it to be done.

It may turn out that complex and expensive data normalization is not required. For example, Memorial Sloan Kettering Cancer Center (MSKCC) is using IBM's Watson system to help clinicians prescribe the most effective, personalized treatment for their patients. The approach is based in large part on Watson's powerful natural language processing (NLP) capabilities that allow it to relate those parts of each patient's clinical data that are unstructured text to its knowledge base from the medical literature. Interestingly and importantly, it is well known that the unstructured text in clinical notes may sometimes be important because busy clinicians do not have the time (or will not take the time) to accurately record their clinical findings in a structured manner. Moreover, there are often clinical nuances in the unstructured record that structured recording systems do not accommodate well. Despite this reliance on unstructured clinical data, Dr. Craig Thompson, president and CEO of MSKCC has said that "Watson's capability to analyze huge volumes of data and reduce it down to critical decision points is absolutely essential to improve on our ability to deliver effective therapies" (IBM 2013). This suggests that recent advances in both NLP and machine learning (ML) may be able to overcome the issues of non-standardization of clinical data that have plagued health informatics for decades. The application of Watson to cancer care at MSKCC is discussed further in chapter 10.

The amount of data to be exchanged will only grow over time. The rapid development of inexpensive sensors that are now even being built into smartphones or deployed in other ways suggests that monitoring millions of patients from home is becoming a reality. For example, the M7 coprocessor in the Apple 5s phone introduced in late 2013 specifically measures motion data from the accelerometer, gyroscope, and compass, even when the phone is not being used, thus enabling apps to know how much time the phone's user spent walking, running, or can be assumed to be sedentary. This has potential value for physicians to monitor patients with conditions, such as congestive heart failure, where activity can indicate a patient's cardiac status. It also has potential implications for wellness and prevention since "Physical inactivity is recognized as an important risk factor for multiple causes of death and chronic morbidity and disability" and "there were insufficient data available worldwide [to quantify physical inactivity]" (Bull et al. 2004). Wider use of these technologies will result in a significant expansion of the volume of data that could be shared, and many more issues of privacy, security, and trust will have to be addressed. There will also be the challenging issue of how to process this data usefully so that busy providers aren't overwhelmed with information they do not need.

HIE remains a matter of tradeoffs, as has been the case for many years. Ideally HIE would be capable of solving all the issues identified, and this can be done, given sufficient resources. Increasingly, a better approach seems to be identifying the critical subset of all possible capabilities that can be provided by efficient and affordable technology approaches.

Classifying Health Information Exchanges

HIEs are classified in different ways. Each of them will be discussed to include their scope (What is the geographic area [or healthcare service area] they cover?); their status (Where is each HIE in the process from an idea to full functionality?); their HIE architecture (How are the systems that support the exchange organized?); and their functionality (Of all the things that are possible, what does each HIE do?).

Three organizations are actively involved in HIE classification. eHealth Initiative (eHI) keeps track of the status of HIEs in the United States. The Health Information Management Systems Society (HIMSS), the largest organization of health informatics professionals, has developed a classification for the architecture of HIEs, and the Office of the National Coordinator for Health Information Technology (ONC) has developed a functional classification. There is no formal classification based on scope, but it is a very important attribute of HIEs that affects many aspects of their operation and financial sustainability, so it will be discussed first.

Scope of HIEs

A set of terms describe the scope of HIEs. An enterprise HIE typically serves a hospital or a health system that can comprise multiple hospitals, related clinics, and other specialized healthcare facilities. A service area HIE usually means all of the physicians and practices in some geographic area around a large hospital or health system. Often referred to as the health system's catchment or referral area, it is the region from which the hospital or health system gets patients. The term HIE by itself usually means something geographically more extensive. It might be statewide, or it might even be a regional grouping of multiple states. As was mentioned earlier, the federal government has developed the term eHealth Exchange for the national health information network, which is actually a network of networks based on standards that will connect state- or regional-level information exchanges that meet certain technical criteria. Within those there might be service area HIEs, and within those, there might be enterprise HIEs.

One reality in health information exchange is that economic sustainability is generally harder with increased size and scope. This is the reverse of the situation in many other businesses where large organizations are typically thought of as being more efficient and more able to sustain themselves than smaller organizations.

This unusual inverse relationship between size and sustainability of HIEs is based on another reality that represents the complex adaptive system in action. Health systems often want to "own" their patients, so they are not necessarily interested in sharing their health data with other health systems, particularly not if they view them as potential competitors. Moreover, the vendors that supply enterprise software solutions to healthcare enterprises want their clients to buy a "total solution" from them, so historically they too have not always been open to facilitating data exchange with outside systems (interoperability). That may be changing in the face of federal pressure and industry dynamics. Seven major health information technology (HIT) vendors (Cerner, McKesson, Allscripts, athenahealth, Greenway, RelayHealth, and Sunquest) created the CommonWell Health Alliance. The stated goal is interoperability among their systems, and the alliance says it is open to other vendors that wish to participate.

Finally, most healthcare is actually local. People usually seek care close to where they live, and physicians usually refer patients to specialists who are close to them geographically, unless the patient requires care not locally available or the patient or their provider prefers a provider located elsewhere. So the advantage of having a HIE that extends beyond a local hospital or health system diminishes rapidly with distance.

Enterprise Health Information Exchange

A health system is usually more than one hospital. There has been a recent strong trend for health systems to acquire physician practices in their service area, which may now stretch out for quite a distance into surrounding rural areas. This is driven in large part by the desire of health systems to be at the center of their regional ACO and the resulting need to be able to deliver care, primary care in particular, in that area. As a result of this strategy, many physicians are now working for their local hospital or health system. Beyond accountable care, these systems strive to "capture" their patients and grow their revenue by making care more convenient and easy to access because it is delivered within the system. For example, they want the patient to be able to go from any part of their system to any other part of their system without being presented with a clipboard at each stop and asked for their name, address, and insurance card numbers. They also want to improve the efficiency of their care by eliminating duplicative or unnecessary tests and procedures in preparation for the new financial incentives that are on the horizon. Unless the entire system is using technology from a single vendor (this can be an expensive strategy but many larger systems are implementing it), some form of third party HIE is needed to make that happen.

Under ACOs or other outcome-based reimbursement systems, errors and inefficiency can be the financial responsibility of the health system. HIE is essential for coordinating, measuring, and managing quality across all the providers that are involved in the care of the patients within a health system. For example, as discussed in chapter 2, chronic disease will usually account for most of the cost within a health system. These patients, particularly those with multiple chronic diseases, will receive care from many providers. Gaining a complete understanding of that care requires bringing together data from all of those providers into a tool that can analyze and present that data in a form that is useful for measuring quality against the contractual commitments the health system has made to its payers.

Population health management tools can complement and take advantage of HIE in such an environment. This will be discussed in more detail in chapter 8, but in essence, they aggregate, normalize, analyze, and present key clinical data from each of the discrete systems within a health enterprise (or even within a group of providers who are not under common ownership or management but have banded together to contract with payers who offer pay-for-performance or outcome-based contracts).

All this has the positive effect of creating a community-wide patient care network, where there is improved coordination and a reduced chance of errors, duplicate tests, or unnecessary procedures. It is most likely essential to success under outcome-based contracting, such as an ACO, which is almost certainly going to extend beyond the physical facilities owned by an individual hospital or even a health system.

Beyond an Enterprise

Wide-area HIEs are beyond enterprise scale. It is certainly true that some care requires referrals from further away than a local community or an enterprise health system's service area, particularly to treat a rare disease, such as Acromegaly (in which the anterior pituitary gland produces excess growth hormone), or a very serious disease, such as cancer. These patients may want to travel some distance to seek highly specialized or expert care. That is one justification for a wide-area HIE covering a state or region. However, as stated earlier, this is a relatively small part of healthcare. Perhaps an even more important reason for wide area HIE is the ability to aggregate data for public health. Every state has a public state agency with the mission of aggregating and analyzing data for the entire state. Additionally, research studies may need to draw subjects from a wide area even beyond the state where they are located. Finally, there is the case of an out-of-town medical emergency, in which a patient shows up in an emergency room in an unfamiliar city. To provide optimal care, the physicians may need to access the patient's remote medical record. This is yet another relatively uncommon, but potentially very serious, event.

Status of HIEs

eHI is a broadly based, collaborative, not-for-profit organization focused on improving healthcare quality and efficiency. Among its numerous projects is support of HIE. eHI has developed a seven-stage classification to track the status of the exchanges across the United States.

- Stage 1: HIEs are just getting started. The need has been recognized and multiple community stakeholders are engaged in discussions.
- Stage 2: HIEs are getting organized, including defining goals and objectives.
- Stage 3: HIEs are actual planning their businesses.
- Stage 4: HIEs are piloting their approaches.
- Stage 5: HIEs are in operation.
- Stage 6: HIEs have made the often difficult transition to a sustainable business model.
- Stage 7: HIEs have moved beyond sustainability and are innovating.

Figure 3.2 presents the latest data from the 2012 eHI HIE survey (eHealth Initiative 2012), showing the number of HIEs in each stage across the United States. The figure shows a clear migration toward more mature and sustainable HIEs. Another key finding is that the environment is right for new organizations to form and to hopefully persevere (eHealth Initiative 2012). As a result, HIE is playing an increasingly key role in healthcare reform.

Figure 3.2   HIEs are becoming more advanced according to the eHealth Initiative.

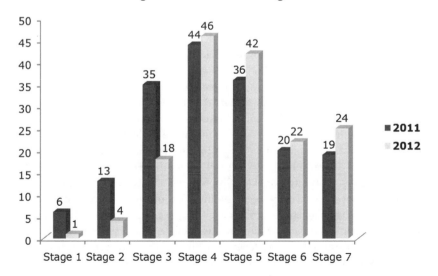

An alternate financial model is being tried. "Private HIEs" are typically sponsored by local healthcare organizations from the private sector, and they raise capital from participants to implement a narrow set of services in a relatively short period of time. As incentives change to reward care coordination, this model may well spread.

Perhaps the most common services deployed by private HIEs are for care delivered in the emergency department (ED). The ED, by the very nature of the care delivered there, is highly likely to serve patients that will often be unknown to the physicians caring for them and whose medical records may exist, at least in part, outside of the organization providing the emergency care. The need for ED-based HIE was confirmed by the results of a survey study of ED physicians by New York Clinical Information Exchange (NYCLIX), a not-for-profit organization with a mission to implement HIE in the New York City metropolitan region:

> Although 63% said more than one quarter of their patients would benefit from external health information, the barriers to obtain it without HIE are too high—85% said it was difficult or very difficult to obtain external data, taking an average of 66 minutes, 72% said that their attempts fail half of the time, and 56% currently attempt to obtain external data less than 10% of the time. (Shapiro et al. 2007)

Carolina eHealth Alliance (CeHA) is an example of a private HIE focused on ED care. It is also an example of competing systems collaborating to improve patient care, albeit on the narrow basis of ED care. It links 11 EDs at four main hospital organizations and has published a pilot study obtained via a voluntary physician survey that was completed for 105 cases using patients' records available through the HIE (Carr et al. 2014). Key results of the study included savings of $283,477.69 over four months ($850,000 annualized) that were typically derived by avoiding duplication of services that had been performed previously, since the results could now be obtained in the ED:

- Laboratory/microbiology: 30.5 percent of visits (32 studies avoided) saved $462.85
- Radiologic studies: 47.6 percent of visits (50 studies avoided) saved $160,893.00
- Consultations: 19 percent of visits (20 consultations avoided) saved $3,990.00
- Hospital Admissions: 11.4 percent of visits (12 admissions avoided) saved $118,131.84

In addition the physicians reported time savings of 121 minutes for patients with records in the HIE (Carr et al. 2014). Another ED-based study from Vanderbilt University showed that HIE resulted in reduced hospital admissions, reduced radiology tests, and an annual cost savings of nearly $2 million (Frisse et al. 2011).

Also of interest from the eHI survey is the doubling of support for Direct information exchange from 2011 to 2012 (eHealth Initiative 2012). Direct is a new federated approach to HIE based on the use of standard email-based technologies to both simplify and lower the cost of information exchange. This will be discussed in detail later in this chapter.

Finally, HIEs have grown in number such that some markets are actually seeing competition among them (eHealth Initiative 2012). Despite these encouraging results, there are still ample challenges. At the top of every list is developing a sustainable business model. Often the second concern is privacy, security, and trust of health data. The third challenge is usually funding, which closely relates to developing a sustainable business model. In this context, it is important to remember the substantial federal investment in HIE and to consider what may happen to HIEs that depend on this funding when it ends if they have not been able to develop an alternate, sustainable model.

Architecture of HIEs

HIEs can also be classified into one of three commonly recognized technical architectures: centralized, federated, or hybrid as shown, in figure 3.3.

Centralized Architecture

A centralized HIE, as the name implies, features a master repository where data are stored. To make that data useful, it is typically normalized so that differences in terminology and data definitions can be bridged across the many EMRs that are contributing data. That normalization process can be expensive; however, this challenge can be overcome with sufficient resources and community support. This will be discussed in detail later in this chapter.

Federated HIE

In the federated approach, all of the clinical data stays at the source—it remains in the EMRs, PHRs, and other data sources where it was recorded. It is brought together for exchange as is required for care coordination and other purposes. There are new federated technology approaches to HIE in which there is a minimal, if any, central system. Examples include Direct and Fast Healthcare Interoperability Resources (FHIR), both of which leverage relatively simple and typically more easily implemented technologies that are widely used elsewhere on the Internet, factors that substantially lower the cost.

Hybrid HIE

In the hybrid approach, some data stored is stored centrally. This would typically be a patient index and indexes to where the actual clinical data is stored. As discussed earlier, these are often called a document locator or registry service. For example, there could be a record of all the x-ray images in the HIE with a pointer to the place where each is stored. The same thing could be done for various other types of clinical documents. Alternately, clinical data could be stored in the HIE but in "data lockers," where it remains under the control of each source provider. People often refer to the hybrid model as being similar to Internet search because the familiar search engines create indices and other mechanisms to facilitate rapid retrievals. People have sometimes referred to the federated model as Internet without search because there are no central indices to expedite finding needed data. However, newer distributed query technologies are making it possible to find data in federated EMRs. This will be discussed further in this chapter and in chapter 9.

Functionality of HIEs

The final classification is functionality, the approach used by ONC. One category is directed exchange, which is essentially the federated approach, and it provides the ability to send

Figure 3.3   The key characteristics and an example of each for the three prevalent HIE architecture are summarized in this table.

	Centralized	Hybrid	Federated
Data Storage	Central repository	Some central data storage	All data at the source
Data Curation	Data normalization	Document indexes/locators	All data at the source
Data Access	One click "Virtual" EHR	Source provider retains control	All data at the source
Query	Central query	Similar to Internet Search	Distributed query
Example	IHIE	BioSense 2.0	Current Care

and receive information securely between providers for care coordination. Query-based exchange is the ability to find or request information on a patient from other providers. This would be required in the ED example given earlier when providers have to offer unplanned care. Absent an effective means of query-based exchange, at least at present, the use case of a patient showing up unexpectedly in an ED requires at least a hybrid model, if not a centralized model, of HIE.

ONC also recognizes consumer-mediated exchange where patients aggregate and control health information among their providers. Recall that in Meaningful Use Stage 2 one of the requirements is that providers must actually share health information with their patients. This is the essential first step toward consumer-mediated exchange because it puts clinical data in patients' hands and under their control. The Georgia Tech engineered HIE Challenge Grant project is an example of this that will be discussed later in both this chapter and in chapter 7.

Case Study: The Indiana Health Information Exchange (IHIE)

The Indiana Health Information Exchange (IHIE), launched in 2004, is arguably the premiere example of centralized HIE. It is also the country's largest HIE, with some of its functions available statewide. IHIE highlights what can be done under the centralized model if the sustainability and community-wide cooperation issues can be overcome. IHIE provides a variety of services that will be discussed in some detail, but to support providing them, IHIE has a cost structure that few, if any, other HIEs could sustain. It has a technology licensing agreement in place with the Regenstrief Institute and operates a sustainable business model based on revenue from clients. The major services that IHIE provides include:

- **Docs4Docs®:** A portal (web application) that delivers lab results and clinical reports to physicians via fax, web portal, or HL7 interfaces with practice EHR systems
- **Indiana Network for Patient Care (INPC)™:** A patient-centric community health record
- **Quality Health First®:** A population health management system (discussed further in chapter 8)
- **ImageZoneSM:** A cloud-based diagnostic-quality image sharing service
- **ACO Services:** Analytics and technology tools for managing care under an outcome-based contract

Providing these services requires a robust set of centralized capabilities sitting between the sources of the data and the value-added services that the exchange provides using that data. This is shown in figure 3.4 which provides a very high-level representation of the IHIE technology architecture.

Access to data is strictly governed by a representative panel of participating organizations. IHIE employs a centrally federated exchange model with shared repositories. Under this model the exchange uses a system of interfaces to enable participants to submit data to the repository managed centrally by IHIE. This model allows participating organizations to control their data and even remove it should they withdraw from the exchange, which enables participation and adoption among stakeholders.

Figure 3.4   A high-level overview of the IHIE technical architecture shows the key role that data governance plays in achieving provider comfort in contributing and sharing data.

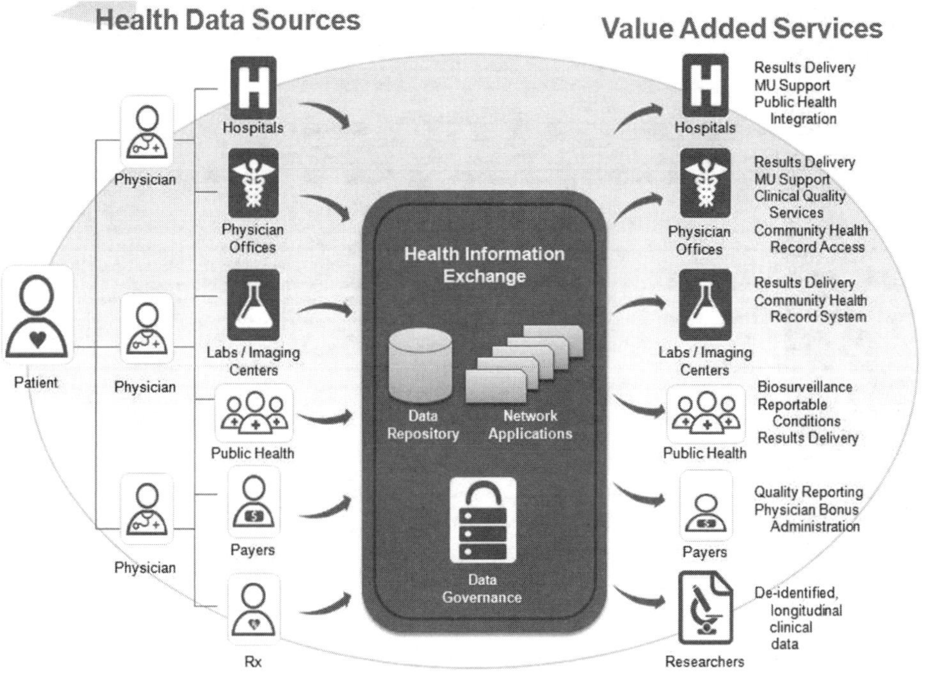

IHIE uses a Global Patient Index to link records from disparate systems. A patient's data is viewed by pulling from all participating repositories. The Global Provider Index regulates the security and privacy of the data delivery to the appropriate point-of-care. The Concept Dictionary is an application layer for data normalization that sits on top of the IT framework.

Docs4Docs

Docs4Docs is a service that provides clinical information (laboratory tests, radiology tests, transcriptions of information they may have recorded, pathology reports, and so on) to physicians from hospitals and other organizations that perform the tests and procedures the physicians have ordered. Docs4Docs results are delivered based on the provider information coded into the message by the originating facility. IHIE has connected more than 25,000 providers around the country to receive clinical results from an originating facility, mainly hospitals, in Indiana. Access to these results is provided in three forms: fax delivery, web portal access, or HL7 message delivery into a practice's EMR system. Figure 3.5 is a screenshot of Docs4Docs and illustrates that the service offers diverse documents and data items across providers. The figure shows several different document types that originated from different hospitals or laboratories, all brought together so they appear in one list, as though they came from a single source. It is important for readers not familiar with

Figure 3.5   A sample screenshot from the IHIE Docs4Docs service illustrates the wide variety of clinical data types that are available from multiple sources.

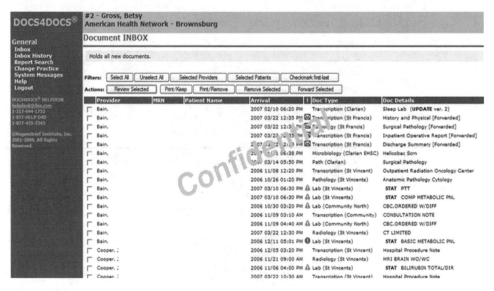

healthcare delivery to understand that this is not a typical scenario. Normally providers can only get data from one particular source at a time. Differences in computing and communications standards are being bridged by IHIE to make this convenient and efficient single page presentation possible.

The Indiana Network for Patient Care (INPC)

The Indiana Network for Patient Care (INPC) provides a single, virtual, community-wide electronic health record (EHR) that includes data from all providers, payers, and public health, as well as pharmaceutical data. It is used primarily in EDs where, as discussed earlier, physicians commonly treat patients with whom they have no prior history. It is also accessible to ambulatory care providers. Keep in mind that primary care providers are often interested in getting as broad a view of each patient as possible. Available statewide, INPC delivers more than a million transactions a day from an immense data warehouse containing five billion pieces of clinical data for over ten million patients. It is accessed via web pages, which look very similar to an EMR that any single provider might use in his or her office, increasing its usability (figure 3.6). For example, it has the same sections that an EMR has, so effectively, data from all the sources across the community are brought together and presented as though there were a single EMR.

The underlying data that is creating this virtual community-wide EHR comes from a multiplicity of EMRs and other sources and from many different organizations. The INPC is the largest interorganizational clinical data repository in the country. It normalizes and maps health data from disparate sources and systems to make healthcare information available to healthcare providers in near real-time. The United States does not yet have anything approaching a comprehensive standard for extracting clinical data from

Figure 3.6   The IHIE Indiana Network for Patient Care service presents integrated data aggregated across providers in a unified EMR-like format.

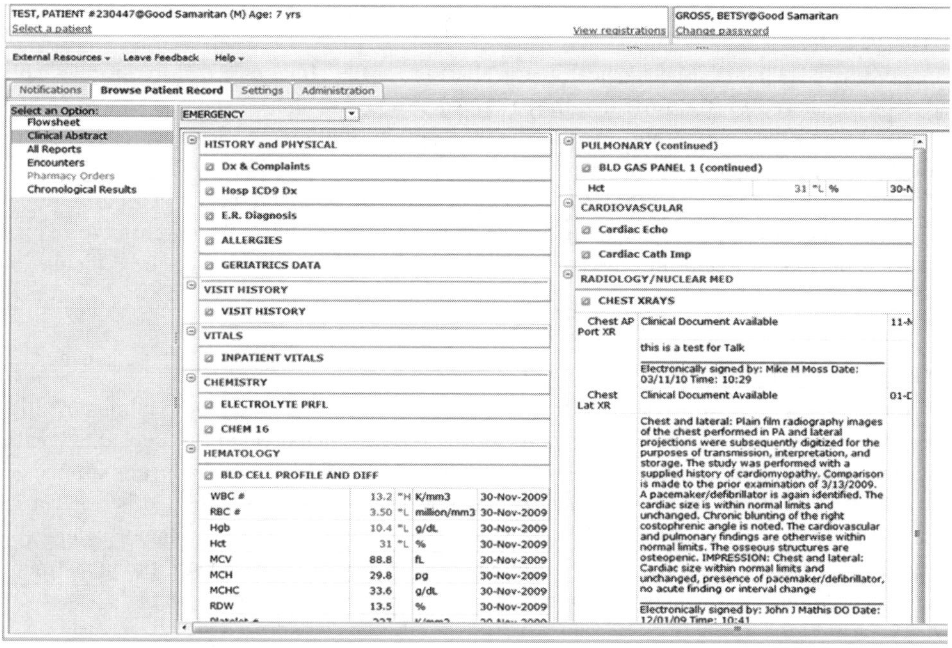

disparate systems. This means that all of the interoperability problems alluded to previously are operative in Indiana. The same data item may be coded in one system but free text in another. It may be coded differently across systems. The quality of the coding will vary from provider to provider. The list of data curation issues goes on, so accomplishing what is done by IHIE requires a sophisticated and specialized infrastructure to bridge these differences and provide a unified and reasonably accurate view of care delivered to the same patient across multiple providers in the community. The Concept Dictionary mentioned earlier is a key part of this infrastructure and facilitates the conversion of the diverse types of clinical data that come into standard representations, such as HL7 and LOINC, which will be covered in detail in chapter 5. INPC shows why organizations pursue the centralized model of HIE.

ACO Services

ACO Services are the newest IHIE offering, and they add the following capabilities:

- Tracking where care has been delivered
- Managing transitions of care
- Following up to ensure care has been delivered as needed

As the reimbursement system is changing, ACOs and hospitals are interested in knowing when and where their patients are receiving care—particularly when it occurs outside their network of providers and facilities. IHIE's ACO services are developed to provide timely, actionable, forward-looking analysis of patients' care.

ImageZone

ImageZone is a cloud-based medical image sharing service. Images are stored for 45 days after being shared by the provider they derived from. The sharing is to a shared image repository and the originating provider has the option of allowing receiving providers to save the image to their personal repository. As a result, for providers using IHIE, it may not matter where the patient had their x-ray or some other image-based procedure done. This can not only make care more timely and efficient, but it also has the potential to reduce ordering of duplicate and often expensive imaging procedures because of the difficulty of obtaining the prior image.

Future Expansion

In April 2013, The Regenstrief Institute licensed the INPC and Docs4Docs clinical results delivery software to a for-profit subsidiary of the IHIE, which created this subsidiary with the clear intent to license and further develop this technology to create a larger connected network of healthcare providers. The specific strategy that will be pursued is not yet in place, but it is clear that IHIE feels it is positioned to provide HIE on a far broader geographic scale than the state of Indiana and, in doing so, leverage the substantial investment that has been made over many years in its software and data curation expertise.

Case Study: CONNECT

CONNECT is the federal government's open source solution for creating a centralized or other models of HIE. Unlike the IHIE, a model of centralized exchange that uses internally developed technology, CONNECT is an open source project through which a community of developers can collaborate.

The CONNECT technology could be used to create an IHIE-type centralized exchange. It also provides a gateway to eHealth Exchange, the proposed national health information network. Think back to the earlier discussion of the tradeoffs between functionality, complexity, and cost in HIE. CONNECT provides sophisticated functionality and capability. The price that is paid is increased complexity and operational and support cost, even if the software itself is free.

CONNECT began in 2007 and first went into live production in 2009 at the Social Security Administration. It is currently in the fourth version, but versions 3.0 and beyond support Meaningful Use. CONNECT can be used within a single organization—a health system for example—as the core of their HIE. Figure 3.7 provides a block diagram of CONNECT and shows there are three primary functional elements:

- Core Services Gateway
- Enterprise Service Components
- Universal Client Framework

Each of these elements consists of software modules or components. Some CONNECT components (as indicated by their shading in the diagram) are mandatory and should be used as delivered. Some components are customizable, while others are completely replaceable. In general, a hospital or health system might already have the components that are

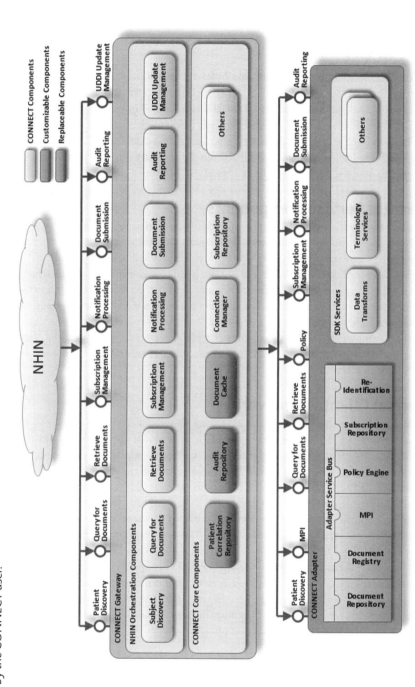

Figure 3.7 The basic architecture of CONNECT illustrates that its components may be required, customizable, or replaceable by similar components selected by the CONNECT user.

Source: Cothren and Westberg 2009

completely replaceable as part of its existing enterprise software solution. A few examples of these have been mentioned earlier, such as the MPI or clinical document repository that are often provided as part of a commercial enterprise software solution. An organization using such a commercial solution, even if they intend to use CONNECT, would not have to replace those components.

Core Services Gateway

The Core Services Gateway provides many of the capabilities covered in the general discussion of the central model of HIE. This includes software that can be used to locate patients at other organizations; to request and receive documents associated with patients; to record those transactions for auditing; and to manage authorization of who can have access to specific clinical data, considering patient preferences about sharing their information. It also includes the interface to eHealth Exchange. Any implementation of CONNECT that uses this interface has the technical ability to become a node in eHealth Exchange.

Enterprise Service Components

The Enterprise Service Components are more focused on capabilities that a particular user of CONNECT might need, including a MPI and a document registry. Another component is an authorization policy engine that allows users of CONNECT to build rules into the HIE that enforce their local policies about such things as who can get to what protected data and when they can access it. Another component is the consumer preferences manager, which stores information about patient specifications as to who can access their data and for what purposes they can use it.

Among some of the HIPAA mandates is a requirement for a log of all accesses to protected clinical data. Another CONNECT component is a HIPAA-compliant audit log to meet this requirement.

Universal Client Framework

The Universal Client Framework (UCF) allows CONNECT sites to create so-called edge systems, typically a place where data is stored for a particular specialized purpose. For example, this might be in support of research. The UCF also supports test and demonstration systems. Finally, it turns CONNECT into a platform for the development of applications that need access to the data that the HIE can access.

CONNECT is implemented as a set of web services (a technical means for exposing computer capabilities over the Internet). Using web services, two computers can interact via an "always on" software function provided at a specific network address. The actual interface is described in an XML-based interface description language called WSDL. This overall approach is called a service-oriented architecture (SOA).

The open source CONNECT approach is an option for health systems to develop their HIE solution instead of purchasing a proprietary HIE technology from a vendor. A number of vendors provide services to assist organizations in the implementation of the open source CONNECT technology.

Federated Architecture: Direct

Direct is a rapidly evolving standard for the federated HIE model, where the clinical data stays within the source EHRs, and there is no central storage of protected clinical data.

Direct is described using the basic technical concepts in this section. This is followed by a second description that focuses on physician workflow as an introduction to where Direct is heading.

Direct Technical Concepts

Health data exchange must be secure, private, and trusted. Encryption assures security—no one but the intended recipient can read the message. Privacy assures that patient permission has been obtained for the transfer and use of the data. Trust is how the sender, Doctor A, knows that the data they are sending to Doctor B is actually going to Doctor B and not, for example, to someone who is going to use the information to submit false healthcare claims.

Direct assures security and trust (privacy is managed externally to Direct at present) while taking advantage of existing and widely used Internet technologies, such as Simplified Mail Transport Protocol (SMTP), Multipurpose Internet Mail Extensions (MIME), and X.509 certificates. Direct transmissions are managed and processed by special server-based software called a health information service provider (Health ISP or HISP). Each provider registers with a HISP and has a special Direct e-mail address assigned for use only with that HISP. A trust process will have taken place before assigning this address to assure the provider is who they say they are. Increasingly patients are also being assigned Direct addresses which can complicate how trust is assured.

SMTP is used to *send* e-mails. MIME defines the formats available for e-mail attachments. MIME is important because Direct stores the patient record in an attachment (many formats are available). Once the sender is ready, the entire message, including the attachment, is addressed to the recipient and transmitted to the sender's HISP using SMTP/S, the secure version of SMTP (typically if using an e-mail client), HTTPS (if using webmail), or other secure communications protocols.

In what follows, the sender and recipient providers are assumed to be using different HISPs (the case where they use the same HISP is actually simpler but describing both situations at the same time is not easy to do clearly). The sender's HISP can find the recipient provider's X.509 certificate (their public key) using the Domain Name System (DNS) or the Lightweight Directory Access Protocol (LDAP), two technologies for managing distributed resources over a network. Once it has the recipient's public key, the HISP uses it to encrypt the message. It then uses SMTP to send the message to the recipient's HISP (having used DNS or LDAP to find it based on the recipient's e-mail address). It is now encrypted so SMTP/S is not needed. The recipient's HISP decrypts the message, using the recipient's private key, which is normally stored in the HISP as a service to its registered providers. The recipient then retrieves the message like any e-mail but using the secure versions of either the Post Office Protocol (POP) or Internet Message Access Protocol (IMAP) e-mail retrieval protocols (if using an e-mail client) or HTTPS (if using webmail).

Confirmation of delivery is available, although currently not very robust, but it is accomplished using encrypted and signed Message Disposition Notification (MDN). Efforts to make MDN more robust are discussed later in this chapter.

The Fax Replacement Use Case

The discussion of centralized HIE emphasized the sophisticated capabilities that are possible under that HIE architecture. However, even Georgia Tech experts were challenged when they implemented CONNECT in the institution's Interoperability and Integration Innovation Lab. If CONNECT is such a complicated, large package that it was difficult for

Georgia Tech experts to install, it is certainly not something a physician practice is going to use in their office (to be fair that was never the intent). Indeed, as mentioned in the prior section, CONNECT adoption has been limited to date to large organizations with significant technical and operational capabilities.

Direct is intended as something physicians can use from their offices without much help. The initial goal was simple, yet secure, exchange of health information between physicians. It was even described initially as a fax machine replacement for small practices. This section will start with the fax machine use case and follow it with a discussion of a number of newer enhancements that are expanding both Direct's reach and its functionality.

To use Direct, each physician must have Internet access and be able to create, send, and receive e-mail securely, something virtually any client e-mail software can do. They must also be registered in a HISP.

A key service that the HISP provides is a special Direct e-mail address only given out after some form of due diligence is done to make sure that the entity that is assigned that e-mail address is the physician or other healthcare practitioner (or even patient) that they say they are. The actual vetting process is designed by each entity that operates a HISP to meet their perceived local trust issues (although, this process is being standardized by Direct trust communities to facilitate trust among HISPs). This introduces the key role that policy plays in Direct. In fact, according to Cerner's Greg Meyer, a leading expert on Direct, as much as 80 percent of Direct is policy while only 20 percent is technology (remember that most of the technology already existed while only has been adopted for use in Direct).

Figure 3.8 presents a diagram of the same HISP shared by two providers. It will be used to illustrate a basic example of using Direct as a fax replacement. This will explain, again in basic terms, how public and private keys (the public key infrastructure, or PKI, will be described in more detail in chapter 4) are used to provide both security and trust. These keys are two special electronic documents that are issued by particular organizations that will also

Figure 3.8   A simple one-HISP illustration of Direct HIE demonstrates the role of PKI in security, as well as the basic e-mail functions of the HISP.

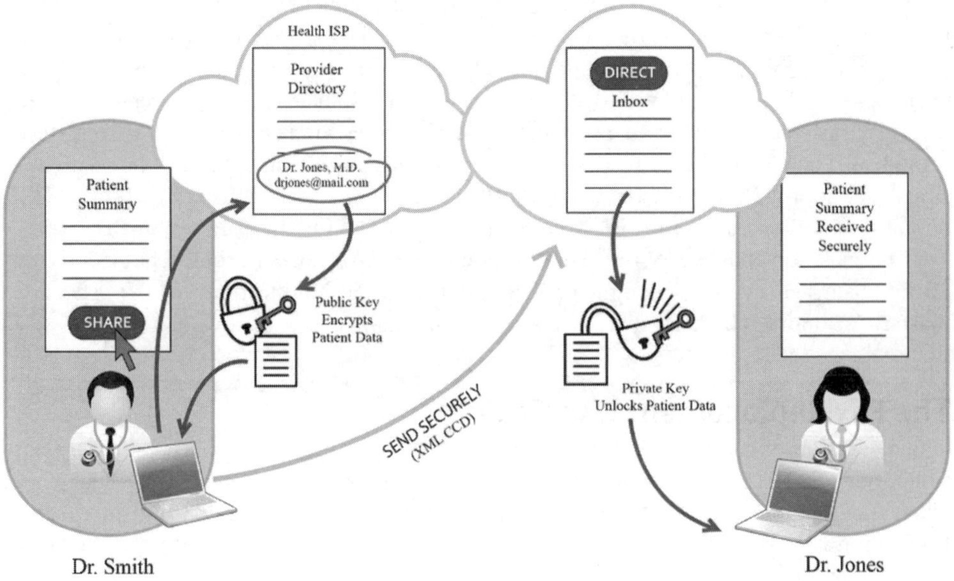

be discussed later. People who have a public key can freely give it out to anyone who needs it. They can even post it on their website because their secret private key is required to reverse (decrypt) the encryption. Therefore a public key can be used to encrypt a message intended only for the owner of that key. That's what happens with Direct. Since only the recipient of a Direct message (more likely their HISP, although this is not a requirement of Direct) has access to the private key that matches their public key, only that person (or their HISP acting as their agent) can decrypt the message providing them access to the information in it.

In figure 3.8, Dr. Smith, a primary care physician, wants to refer his patient to Dr. Jones, a specialist. Dr. Jones will need to refer to the patient's record to provide quality care. Remember, we assume that they are both registered in the same HISP. Given that most healthcare is local, this is not an unlikely scenario. As health systems spread into the areas surrounding cities in order to prepare for managing patient populations under outcome-based contracts, it is becoming more likely. In the scenario where both physicians are using the same HISP and are set up within the same domain within a health enterprise network, PKI may not be required. In the end, whether or not to use PKI in the single HISP scenario is a policy-driven decision.

Direct can be used from both webmail (such as Gmail) and local e-mail software (such as Outlook or Thunderbird). The HISP will provide a directory so Dr. Smith can look up Dr. Jones, find her special Direct e-mail address and have confidence that this is actually the correct Dr. Jones. Dr. Smith uses his preferred e-mail software to compose a message and attaches the patient's record in whatever format he chooses (this could be a PDF, a scan of a paper chart, or an XML formatted CCDA document). He then sends the message as described earlier in this section.

Alternately, Dr. Smith could use his HISP's web-based Direct e-mail (similar to using Gmail) to compose and attach the record and send the message. Here, the record uploads to the HISP using HTTPS (the same secure HTTP used for banking and many other purposes on the Internet).

Dr. Jones has the same two e-mail options. With local e-mail software Dr. Jones uses either IMAP/S (secure IMAP) or POP3/S (secure POP3) to read the incoming message from her inbox on the HISP. The HISP will have first used Dr. Jones' private key to unencrypt the message. With web-based e-mail, Dr. Jones reads the incoming message using a browser and downloads the attachment. Reading and downloading this way are done using HTTPS.

Workflow Issues

This fax replacement scenario for Direct is very simple at both ends, but it still illustrates a workflow problem that derives from using a stand-alone or web-based e-mail program to send and receive Direct messages. Dr. Smith is in the middle of documenting the patient visit in his EMR. The information he wishes to send to Dr. Jones is right there on the screen, so why should he have to go through a process to create the record of care he will transmit as an attachment, then open up his e-mail software or bring up a webmail page to create an e-mail, add the attachment, look up Dr. Jones' e-mail address, and send it on? To facilitate this process it is clear that EMRs need something like a Share button, where users can share webpages they find interesting with the push of a button.

Cerner is one of the major health enterprise software vendors. According to Greg Meyer, Cerner's director and principal architect, the company has built a Direct messaging system into their EMR. If a physician uses it while charting, it will default to the current patient, so they need only click a box to create a patient summary, enter the e-mail address of the intended recipient, add any text comments, and send it on. Cerner also provides the HISP. The specifics of what happens next depend on whether the receiving physician is connected to it or to another HISP.

To facilitate this more broadly, EMR Direct, a new company, has developed phiMail, a stand-alone Direct messaging platform that includes an integrated HISP and an integration application programming interface (API) to facilitate direct incorporation by EHR systems or other health applications. The EMR Direct Certification Authority issues certificates both to phiMail users and to users of other systems for use in Direct exchange. Certificates can be bound to Direct addresses within the user's domain or to dedicated health information domains maintained by EMR Direct.

Other large vendors are likely to develop their own software and many of them are listed on the Direct project website as planning to enable the Direct project to be used as a transport in connection with one or more of their solutions or services (The Direct Project 2013).

Whatever the Direct messaging workflow involved, there is more that could be done to expedite the care process. Understanding that requires looking in a little more detail at what actually goes on in Direct exchange. As stated earlier, the attachment can be virtually anything. For example, the sending physician could copy the chart on a scanner and send that scanned image. It could be an XML abstract of the patient's record created by the EMR. The latest standard for that XML format is called Consolidated Clinical Document Architecture (CCDA) and is designed specifically to support the scenario we described. It would usually be a combination of coded and text-based clinical information about the patient, but it could contain an image or any digital information the providers want to share.

If the document is machine readable (that is, uses CCDA which can be sent using Direct alone or as part of the Blue Button + initiative), it can be parsed. This means a computer can not only read it, but it can also pull apart at least the coded data into its constituent elements, such as the patient's lab results, their medications, and so on. That information could be recorded in the recipient's EMR, a scenario that both saves time and reduces the chance of error. There would typically be some validation process through which the receiving provider decides to accept the data into their EMR.

There are many use cases that can be constructed for Direct. The first is a primary care physician sending a patient to a specialist and the reverse, a specialist sending the results back to the primary care physician. A similar pair of use cases would be a primary care physician referring a patient to the hospital and wanting to send the needed information to the hospital, and the hospital sending discharge information back to the referring provider. Another example is a lab sending results back to the care provider. This would be a good opportunity for parsing, so the lab test results could go right into the receiving EMR's lab profile.

Beyond the Fax Machine

Fax machines do not parse the documents they receive and file them away so Direct can facilitate improved workflow by automating some or all of that process. Beyond workflow, there are other issues that people are working on to improve and expand Direct.

Trust among HISPs

The earlier example assumed that Drs. Smith and Jones were connected to the same HISP. This simplifying assumption allowed us to mostly ignore the issue of trust. It was said that each HISP made sure that each e-mail address actually belonged to the provider to whom it was attached (again via the enforcement of policies). However, suppose the doctors are connected to different HISPs. Will each HISP trust that the other has done this properly? This issue grows exponentially as the number of HISPs increases, since the total number of HISP trust relationships grows exponentially as the number of HISPs involved increases linearly. This happens because each HISP needs to establish trust with all the other HISPs that any of its providers want to communicate with. Since this is not predictable in advance, it means that each HISP would ideally establish a trust agreement with all the other HISPs in the country (or even potentially beyond if Direct spreads further). In the likely scenario that there will be hundreds of HISPs in the United States, the trust that is necessary for cross HISP, Direct exchange quickly becomes unwieldy and expensive, if not impossible in practice, to manage and maintain.

The solution is a trust community, a concept being developed by DirectTrust (and others). In this approach there is community agreement about the policies for critical issues, such as establishing trust. There are also standard agreements so that individual HISP-to-HISP negotiations are not necessary. Using these community approaches and policies, each HISP then assembles its individual provider trust agreements into a trust bundle, and the HISPs exchange those bundles at a website established for this purpose by Direct-Trust. Trust bundles are packaged using cryptographic message syntax formats (specified in the Internet standard RFC 5652). Cryptographic message syntax was identified as the preferred standard by the community because Direct security/transfer agents (STA) are components of HISPs that process, validate, and consume S/MIME messages that are based on the cryptographic message syntax standard.

In addition to the role of HISP, DirectTrust introduces the role of health identity provider (HIDP). An HIDP can be both a registration authority (RA) and a certificate authority (CA). As an RA, it collects information for the purpose of verifying the identity of an individual or organization and produces a certificate request, which is in a standard format for expressing information about an individual or organization. As a CA, it digitally signs certificate requests and issues X.509 digital certificates that tie a public key to attributes of its owner. A single organization can be both an RA and a CA.

DirectTrust is rapidly gaining traction. As of publication, according to the Direct-Trust's president and chief executive officer, David C. Kibbe, MD, MBA, there were nine organizations that had reached full Electronic Healthcare Network Accreditation Commission (EHNAC)—DirectTrust accreditation and audit as HISPs CAs and RAs, 24 HISPs and CAs that had reached candidate accreditation status, with another 17 organizations having applied for accreditation but not yet at candidate stage. A December 2013 year-end letter from Dr. Kibbe reports growth from 40 to over 100 organizational and several individual memberships in DirectTrust (Kibbe 2013). A link to the latest numbers is provided in Recommended Reading and Resources at the end of this chapter.

Patient Involvement

Providers might create a clinical snapshot, reminders, or other information about a recent visit and send it to a patient via Direct. Remember, Meaningful Use Stage 2 says that doctors need to share information with 5 percent of their patients. Direct is an obvious way to send this information. Georgia Tech did the technical development for the HIE Challenge Grant in Rome, Georgia, that provides a current state-of-the-art example. There cancer patients record symptoms using a Microsoft HealthVault PHR app. Then, using GA Direct, Georgia's Health Information Network's Direct HISP, they send the information to their provider. One provider sends a CCDA-based clinical summary back to their patients via Direct.

A PHR is a patient managed repository of health data that can increasingly host apps that can access that data and can upload clinical data into that repository using Direct (as a

CCDA using Direct alone or as part of the Blue Button + initiative). PHRs will be discussed further in chapter 7.

To facilitate patient use of Direct, DirectTrust's Patient and Consumer Participation in Direct Workgroup is developing policy issues related to how consumers and patients can become full participants in Direct exchange with their providers and anyone else they choose to communicate with via Direct. Their HISP Policy already includes nonproviders as end users of HISP services.

A key concern is that the appropriate identity vetting be performed prior to the issuance of a Direct digital certificate to a patient or consumer. The federal government defines four Levels of Assurance (LOAs) for issuing credentials that range from low to very high (Bolten 2003). DirectTrust providers must have a LOA 3 (High Level of Assurance) and there is discussion that patients might have LOA 2 (Some Level of Assurance). Alternately, patients and consumers might be able to make their own choices about the LOA in association with the product or service vendors they choose. Patients and consumers also should be able to acquire stronger credentials, should they desire to do so. This is in keeping with DirectTrust's philosophy that members have the choice of whom they want to trust and exchange personal information with.

Pull (or Triggered Push)

The Direct messages discussed so far are all referred to as "push"—they are initiated at the sending end. Direct would become more valuable in clinical situations, such as an ED patient visit that could not have been anticipated, if messages could be "pulled"—initiated using one of various means by the recipient. There are several proposed mechanisms for this that are both provider and patient facing.

A recent white paper proposes that the health data recorded by patients in their PHR could be viewed as a repository that could be queried by their physician to obtain needed data (figure 3.9) (Project HealthDesign 2013). One of the problems with provider use of patient recorded data (particularly from in home sensors of physiologic measurement devices) is that there may be much more of it than the provider wants, and sifting through it to find what's needed can be time consuming. In essence this proposal suggests that a provider interested in the patient's last three blood pressure readings at home could send a query asking for just that and get it back from their PHR. Both communications would be via Direct.

Much of the interest in Pull centers on its use by patients so that they can easily maintain an up-to-date record of their care. One possible mechanism is that the patients register their Direct e-mail address with the source of their clinical data (for example, their providers' EHRs) and updates are automatically sent to their PHR. The term "triggered Push" is sometimes used to describe this approach. Another approach is illustrated by Growth-tastic! developed by Boston Children's Hospital's ONC-funded Strategic Health IT Advanced Research Projects (SHARP) project. Parents register with their child's pediatrician, and each time Growth-tastic! starts up, it queries the provider's patient-facing system for updates using a REST API (a web service in which HTTP formatted requests are sent by a client—Growth-tastic! in this case—to a server, the provider's portal, or another patient facing system). The result is an updated growth chart that compares the development of a child with the CDC's norms for their age and sex. They key point is that, once this is setup, the parent need only start the app to get the latest information.

Message Delivery Notification

Message delivery notification was mentioned earlier as a core requirement for Direct but, at present, it is incompletely implemented. HISPs that receive and process a message are

Figure 3.9   The Project HealthDesign pull proposal for clinician access to patient data stored in a PHR treats that data as a repository that can be queried via specially formatted attachments to a Direct message.

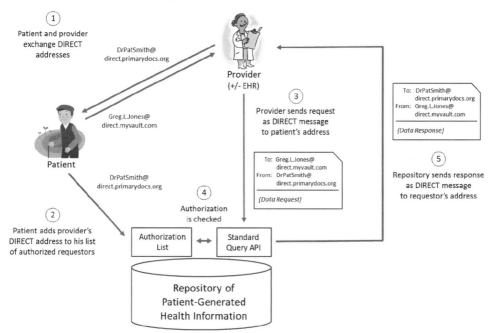

Reprinted with permission from Walter Sujansky, Sujansky & Associates, LLC (www.sujansky.com).

required to send MDN. However, this only covers successful processing of messages. In some cases this is inadequate. A common use case for Direct is clinical labs reporting results back to the ordering provider. These labs are regulated by CMS under the Clinical Laboratory Improvement Amendments (CLIA) program that requires they know for sure that these results were received. It is not hard to understand why. If a critical lab result showing that a patient is in need of immediate treatment were not received, the patient might be at risk.

Full MDN is needed but is not simple to define and implement. For example, suppose that the lab is connected to a HISP, the provider is connected to another HISP, and for some reason, the receiving HISP does not trust the sending HISP. The receiving HISP is prohibited from communicating with a suspect HISP to help avoid attacks. Clearly a mechanism is needed to safely signal any occurrence where the conveyance of a Direct message has failed. Providing the mechanical means to accomplish this is highly technical and is a current ONC-sponsored project, particularly for this lab use case.

Edge Protocols

There are cases where it is desirable for Direct to transmit information encoded in protocols beyond the current scope of Direct. The usual example is the XD* protocols sponsored by IHE:

- Cross-Enterprise Document Sharing (XDS): sharing of documents among healthcare enterprises

- Cross-Enterprise Document Media Interchange (XDM): using a common (zipped) file and directory structure so that patients can carry PHI using physical media (for example, a USB stick) or can use e-mail to convey medical documents
- Cross-Enterprise Document Reliable Interchange (XDR): a means of direct (not Direct) source-to-recipient document exchange (for example, EMR to EMR), even in the absence of an XDS infrastructure

In XD* the PHI is encrypted and metadata (data about the data such as the provider and patient identity) is used to manage the interchange. If Direct were used to convey these messages complexities would arise. In some cases conversion or creation of metadata would be required, a function that HISPs currently do not provide.

Case Study: CurrentCare

CurrentCare is the state of Rhode Island's HIE. It utilizes an opt-in approach to patient consent and involvement. Many HIEs use the opt-out model, where patients are registered in the exchange unless they say they do not want to be. Here it is the reverse. Patients have to specifically say they do want to be registered in the exchange. According to the Rhode Island Quality Institute's website, over 276,000 Rhode Island patients have consented to be connected to the hospitals, labs, pharmacies, and medical practices that are part of the exchange. (Rhode Island Quality Institute 2013) Some of these have high speed point-to-point data feeds, a logical approach for sites like clinical labs that produce a large volume of health information. Most other communications are via the Direct technology, using a HISP operated by CurrentCare. An interesting attribute of this exchange is the approach to obtaining patient consent. There is a consent gateway that is effectively adjoined to the HISP and proposed Direct transactions can only go through it if the patient that the transaction involves is recorded in the gateway as having consented.

Trust has been discussed as the means through which the sender knows that the e-mail address they are using actually goes to the intended recipient. The Rhode Island Quality Institute (RIQI) is the agent to create the trust community, and it takes each provider through a validation process before they are provided with a Direct e-mail address. Once trust is established, the HIE can use Direct to send patient alerts to providers—for example, notification of an ED visit or a hospital admission. Providers subscribe to receive these alerts or patient events and receive them automatically and electronically in their Direct inbox.

REFERENCES

Bolten, J.B. 2003. Executive Office of the President, Office of Management and Budget. E-Authentication Guidance for Federal Agencies. http://www.whitehouse.gov/sites/default/files/omb/memoranda/fy04/m04-04.pdf

Bull, F.C., T.P. Armstrong, T. Dixon, S. Ham, A. Neiman, and M. Pratt. 2004. Physical Inactivity. Chapter 10 in *Comparative Quantification of Health Risks*. Edited by Ezzati, M., A.D. Lopez, A. Rodgers, and C.J.L. Murray. Geneva: World Health Organization. http://www.who.int/healthinfo/global_burden_disease/cra/en/

Carr, C.M., C.S. Gilman, D.M. Krywko, H.E. Moore, B.J. Walker, and S.H. Saef. 2014. Observational study and estimate of cost savings from use of a health information exchange in an academic emergency department. *The Journal of Emergency Medicine*. (46)2:250–256. http://www.jem-journal.com/article/S0736-4679(13)00774-9/fulltext

Cothren, R. and L. Westberg. 2009. CONNECT: Architecture Overview. http://www
.connectopensource.org/sites/connectopensource.org/files/CONNECT_
ArchitectureOverview.pdf

The Direct Project. 2013. http://wiki.directproject.org/

eHealth Initiative. 2013. 2012 Annual HIE Survey Results: Report on Health Information Exchange.
http://www.ehidc.org/policy/pol-resources/view_document/43-survey-2012-annual-hie-survey-
results-report-on-health-information-exchange-supporting-healthcare-reform-data-exchange

Frisse, M.E., K.B. Johnson, H. Nian, C.L. Davison, C.S. Gadd, K.M. Unert, P.A. Turri, and Q. Chen.
2011. The Financial Impact of Health Information Exchange on Emergency Department Care.
http://jamia.bmj.com/content/early/2011/11/03/amiajnl-2011-000394.full.html

HIMSS. 2009. A HIMSS Guide to Participating in a Health Information Exchange. http://www
.himss.org/content/files/HIE/HIE_GuideWhitePaper.pdf

IBM. 2013. Memorial Sloan-Kettering Cancer Center. http://www-03.ibm.com/innovation/us/
watson/pdf/MSK_Case_Study_IMC14794.pdf

IHIE Quality Health First. 2013. Clinical Quality Measures Public Reports. http://mpcms.blob.
core.windows.net/bd985247-f489-435f-a7b4-49df92ec868e/docs/d15a9773-5d71-4e32-b91e-
2dd38b438848/20120930r5-public-reporting.pdf

Kansky, J. 2008. Indiana health information exchange: HIE success in the heartland—Indiana
Network for Patient Care. *Proceedings of the 2008 HIMSS Conference.*

Kibbe, D. 2013 (December). E-mail exchange to author.

Project HealthDesign. 2013. A Standards-Based Model for the Sharing of Patient-Generated
Health Information with Electronic Health Records. Sujansky & Associates. http://www
.projecthealthdesign.org/media/file/Standard-Model-For-Collecting-And-Reporting-PGHI_
SujanskyAssociates_2013-07-18.pdf

Rhode Island Quality Institute. 2013. CurrentCare—Overview. http://www.docehrtalk.org/about-
ri-rec/currentcare/overview.

Schoen, C. and R. Osborne. 2011. The Commonwealth Fund 2011 International Health
Policy Survey of Sicker Adults in Eleven Countries. Commonwealth Fund. http://www
.commonwealthfund.org/Publications/In-the-Literature/2011/Nov/2011-International-
Survey-Of-Patients.aspx

Schuman, S.H., M.L. Braunstein, J.D. James, et al. 1976. A computer-based health communications
network in a rural county: Part 1—Design and Evaluation, *Proc VII World Conf on Fam Med
and General Pract.* Toronto.

Shapiro, J.S., J. Kannry, A.W. Kushniruk, G. Kuperman, and The New York Clinical Information
Exchange (NYCLIX) Clinical Advisory Subcommittee. 2007 (Nov–Dec). Emergency physicians'
perceptions of health information exchange. *J Am Med Inform Assoc.* 14(6):700–705.
http://www.ncbi.nlm.nih.gov/pmc/articles/PMC2213478/

Sujansky & Associates, LLC. 2014. http://www.sujansky.com

Wilcox, A., G. Kuperman, D.A. Dorr, G. Hripcsak, S.P. Narus, S.N. Thornton, and R.S. Evans. 2006.
Architectural strategies and issues with health information exchange. *AMIA Annu Symp Proc.*
2006: 814–818. http://www.ncbi.nlm.nih.gov/pmc/articles/PMC1839562/

RECOMMENDED READING AND RESOURCES

If you have a specific interest in HIE, read the entire eHealth Initiative 2012 Annual Survey
(eHealth Initiative 2012).

HIE Status: For more detail on the current state of HIE across the United States, visit this online
dashboard: http://statehieresources.org/program-measures-dashboard/.

For very detailed information on HIE, read the HIMSS Guide to Participating in a HIE, available at http://www.himss.org/content/files/HIE/HIE_GuideWhitePaper.pdf.

For a more complete discussion of HIE architecture, read *Architectural Strategies and Issues with Health Information Exchange* (Wilcox et al. 2006).

A more detailed discussion of CONNECT is posted on the CONNECT developer website at https://developer.connectopensource.org/display/NHINR24/System+Overview. Many other technical documents are referenced from that page.

CONNECT adopters are listed here: http://www.connectopensource.org/adopters.

To learn more about Direct as it evolves, visit its Wiki (http://wiki.directproject.org/), which is maintained by the Direct project, so you can explore those issues that you find interesting. You will gain a much higher understanding of what is necessary to operate this appealing approach to HIE.

The various transformations that take place for Direct e-mail messages are clearly illustrated on this page: http://api.nhindirect.org/java/site/agent/2.0.2/users-guide/dev-nhindagent.html#Message_Encryption_Stage_Representation.

Vendors planning to use Direct as part of their products or services are listed here: http://wiki.directproject.org/HIT+Vendor.

To learn more about DirectTrust, the independent nonprofit trade association that seeks to establish and maintain a national security and trust framework in support of Direct exchange, visit: http://www.directtrust.org/.

DirectTrust bundles are distributed at this site: Bundles.directtrust.org.

DirectTrust community members are listed here: https://bundles.directtrust.org/transitionalCommunityDetails.html.

This interesting white paper posits both unstructured and structured formats for the query and the response of an approach to using patient recorded data as a repository. http://www.projecthealthdesign.org/media/file/Standard-Model-For-Collecting-And-Reporting-PGHI_SujanskyAssociates_2013-07-18.pdf.

A discussion of e-Authentication policies for the federal government that includes a detailed discussion of levels of assurance: http://www.whitehouse.gov/sites/default/files/omb/memoranda/fy04/m04-04.pdf.

Chapter 4

Privacy, Security, and Trust

Overview

A key goal of contemporary health informatics is the engagement of patients through web, mobile, and consumer-facing new technologies. According to a 2010 national survey done by the California Health Foundation (CHF), patient access to health data does actually improve care (California Health Foundation 2010). People who access personal health records (PHRs) report that they know more about their health; ask more questions; and take better care of themselves. Of course, the people who are more likely to access a PHR may already have been more motivated to manage their health. This may well be a factor to consider, since the use of PHRs has been disappointingly low for a long time. However, that may be changing because, although the CHF survey shows that only 1 in 14 Americans had used one, this represented a doubling from the year earlier (California Health Foundation 2010). Hopefully, this is a trend that will continue. Chapter 2 introduced the Meaningful Use stage 2 VDT requirements that providers actually share records electronically with their patients, which may further increase the use of PHRs for information sharing among patients and their providers in the future.

Patients report that secure, password-protected PHRs give them confidence that they can access their personal health information online and, as a result, they do pay more attention to their health. Indeed, one in three PHR users say they have taken specific action to improve their health as a result (California Health Foundation 2010). Most interestingly of all, particularly considering the focus on chronic disease, is that these benefits seem to be most valued among the people who have been the most difficult for healthcare providers to engage historically, including people with multiple chronic diseases, lower educational levels, and lower incomes (Xerox 2012).

However, security of their data is a significant and legitimate patient concern. Sixty-eight percent of respondents to the CHF foundation survey are very or somewhat concerned about the privacy of their medical records (California Health Foundation 2010). This is not hard to understand since PHRs are housed in the cloud and are accessed via the Internet. In a 2012 survey of over 2,000 adults, only 26 percent said they wanted their medical records to be digital, and this was actually down two points from a similar survey done in 2011. Forty percent of patients believe PHRs will result in better, more efficient healthcare. Fully 85 percent express concern about privacy and security of their digital information (Xerox 2012). It seems that the reticence that many people feel about having digital health records springs from their concern about the privacy and security of their information. The survey also asked about specific concerns patients had. Sixty-three percent of patients were concerned that their information might be stolen by a hacker. Half were worried about their files being lost, damaged, or corrupted; that their information could be misused; or that a power outage or a computer problem might prevent their doctor from accessing their information. Only 15 percent had no concerns about their medical record being digital (Xerox 2012).

There are numerous examples that show that these concerns are legitimate. There have been numerous instances of breach of the HIPAA laws and of illegitimate access to patient health records by public health officials, healthcare professionals, and others. When they occur, these have often been highly publicized (Gorman and Sewell 2013). There have also been instances of worms and other forms of malware getting into hospitals and health systems. In 2009 a worm infected the controllers of MRI machines in the United States (Electricity Forum 2009). In 2011 a hospital in Atlanta was forced to "divert all non-emergency admissions to other medical centers" after shutting down their information systems and reverting to paper records for several days because "unidentified malware" had gotten into those systems (Dunn 2011).

The motivations for stealing health data are clear. First of all, it can be valuable, since it can be used to generate fraudulent claims. For example, the largest Medicare fraud in history was carried out in 2010 by an organized crime syndicate using the stolen identities of thousands of Medicare beneficiaries and many physicians. The criminals generated $163 million in fraudulent billings through 118 phony clinics in 25 states (FBI 2010). Clearly patients do have a reasonable concern about security of their health data.

PHRs are cloud-based services often provided by companies that are unaffiliated with hospitals and health systems. Patients can establish these accounts on their own, and a number of currently unresolved challenges arise from that:

- How can patients who are willing to share health data from their PHR specify the data they wish to share? How can they be confident that only that data will be shared?

- Once the data is shared, how can patients control further access to it?

- When patients share data with their providers, how can the providers trust the validity and the source of data coming from PHR accounts established completely outside of the control of their offices or health systems?

- How does a provider know that the person they are dealing with is actually their patient?

This is an even more significant concern if the physicians are going to facilitate the downloading of protected data back to that PHR. Today, PHRs facilitate the ability for patients to request that their digital records (ideally in a CCDA format that could be parsed by the PHR and stored in appropriate the appropriate sections within it) be downloaded into their PHR using both Direct and Blue Button +, and Stage 2 of Meaningful Use essentially mandates that providers support this access, so these are no longer hypothetical concerns.

These are just a few questions from a very important and substantial part of health informatics: privacy, security, and trust. The terms privacy, security, and trust require separate definitions, which will be provided within a health context, although the technologies have applicability to other domains, such as financial services.

For our purposes, **privacy** means that only authorized people can see health data. Typically, in healthcare, that authorization is provided by the patient.

Security means that data is protected from unauthorized access. This is particularly of concern when the data is being transported, such as from provider to provider, from provider to patient, or from patient to provider. When that transport is taking place over the open Internet, as opposed to within the private network of a clinic, hospital, or health system (a digital "walled garden"), concerns about security grow substantially, as does the difficulty of maintaining it.

A working definition of trust is the means by which the recipient or sender of information knows that people and organizations we are interacting with electronically—who might be physicians, hospitals, or patients—are who they say they are. Again, as with security, this issue gets more difficult the further removed those people are from the other party's specific working environment and organization.

There are, of course, technologic approaches to each of these issues (although assuring trust always involves policies and nontechnical procedures to assure identity). For privacy, there must be some system for prior authorization of use by the owner of the data. In healthcare that usually means the patient. For security, it is most commonly through the use of a public key infrastructure (PKI), which was introduced in chapter 3 and will be discussed at some length later in this chapter. The definition of trust is somewhat circular. It means that some trusted third party confirms the identity of the people or organizations. Once trust is established, PKI can be bound to the trusted entity and used to convey or transport that trust. Most of these are not yet fully mature technologies, and this is a very active research area with some particular challenges being:

- Transparent, situationally aware, access control
- Anomaly detection
- Provenance both for auditing and compliance
- Dynamic detection and resolution of policy conflicts
- Metadata privacy inference attacks
- Identity management: users (providers) and nonusers (patients)
- Digital consent
- Intrusion detection/tolerance, malware analysis and detection

This area is a focus of the Standards and Interoperability (S&I) framework task forces of the Office of the National Coordinator for Health Information Technology (ONC), which sponsors a public-private initiative to promote health information exchange (HIE), and S&I has several active volunteer work groups. Each focuses on a defined list of challenges pertaining to promoting HIE and goes through a process that is shown in figure 4.1. It begins with an environmental scan, looking at the area and the issues. Next a consensus is formed on the list of standards that might help solve the problem. For example, a working group recently published standards to support the Direct approach to HIE (ONC 2013).

In general, the actual standards definition process begins with use cases—the core or related scenarios that lead to the definition of requirements. The next section will discuss a relatively nontechnical and easy-to-understand use case focused on data segmentation, one aspect of the privacy issue.

A very simple use case (figure 4.2) represents a provider who wants to receive test results ordered previously, and the lab sending them to that provider. Starting with that very simple statement, the process leads to a definition of the data flows and what the systems at either end of the processes must do. This includes defining the actors, their roles, and the events they are involved in. This leads directly to the data that needs to be both input and output to or from them in each step of the process. Finally, there must be a description of the data elements involved, divided into segments to facilitate patient

Figure 4.1   The ONC has created this Standards and Interoperability (S&I) work process.

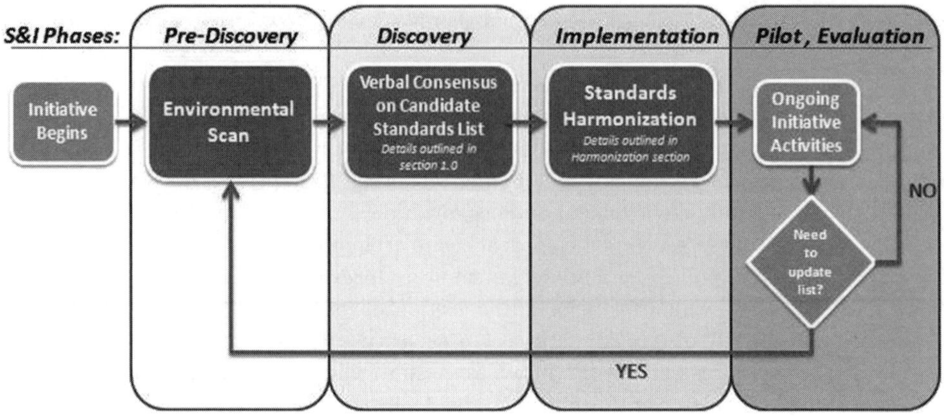

Source: S&I Framework 2014

specification of what can be shared. This patient specification is facilitated by a technology concept called data segmentation and is important, but it turns out to be quite difficult to manage.

Privacy and Data Segmentation

Data segmentation—a key concept within the larger topic of privacy—is the specification by the owner of the data as to what data can be shared and who can see that data. Many patients are willing to share their medical records to one degree of another based on "the type of information being shared, the type of activity being performed, and the respondent's relationship with the selected person" (Zulman 2011). Although there is a low level of patient comfort with having their health data digital in the first place, "patients [are] generally very supportive of research provided safeguards are established to protect the privacy and security of their medical information" (Institute of Medicine 2009). Most favor an opt-in sharing model. In other words, they want to be able to make decisions about who can see their data. There are a number of potential models for obtaining consent from the patient for sharing of their data. There is "no consent," where all health information is automatically included and shared. The patient cannot opt out. This is not a reasonable model for healthcare in most contexts. Another model is "opt-out," where the default is that the patients are sharing their data, but they can choose not to. Some HIEs are using that model. A more sophisticated model would be opt-out with exceptions. Again, the default is the patient's data is included, but the patient can opt-out—either completely or they can allow only selected data to be shared. The final model is "opt-in," where the default is no data sharing, and patients must actively agree if they want their data to be shared. CurrentCare, the Rhode Island HIE discussed in chapter 3, uses this model. A paper by the Massachusetts eHealth Collaborative (MAeHC) suggests that the opt-in model can achieve as much as 90 percent patient acceptance (Tripathi et al. 2009). Opt-in is most often an all-in or an all-out situation. Either all or none of a patient's data is shared. The optimal model, but the most difficult to implement, may well be opt-in with restrictions, since patients are known to be sensitive about sharing certain information, such as care for mental health problems (Zulman 2011). Here, the patient has to opt-in, but they can restrict

Figure 4.2   This diagram of a simple lab test result use case developed by the S&I workgroup illustrates the key information flows involved.

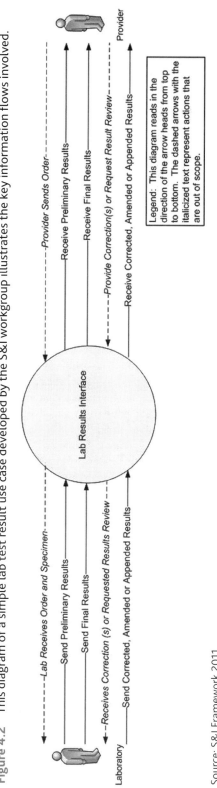

Source: S&I Framework 2011

their permission for sharing to only specific, selected data. The introduction of sharing only selected data leads inevitably to the data segmentation problem.

Data segmentation is defined as the process of sequestering certain data elements that are perceived, in this case by the individual patient, as undesirable to share. The goal of health data segmentation is that individually identifiable health information may be appropriately shared for various purposes. For example, a patient thinks that a clinical drug trial that is ongoing might be worth joining because the patient has not been able to find a satisfactory treatment for their problem. Within their electronic health record (EHR) only part of their data is related to that trial. Logically the patient may want to share only the data that is related to the trial but sequester the data that is unrelated to it. This is a very typical use case, and it sounds very simple, but there are a number of issues:

- Who actually should have access to that data?
- For what purposes should they have access to it and for how long?
- How do patients actually define and describe the data they want to be shared and how do they wish it to be shared? (Goldstein and Rein 2010)

Other issues add additional complexity of this specification problem. If all health data were structured—if it could be presented as a list of choices—then patients might be able to understand how to indicate which data they want to share (such as, by checking the appropriate boxes in that list). However, a great deal of health data is not structured, it is free-text. Within that free-text there could easily be information patients want to share and information they do not want to share. A possible solution to address this is to divide the clinical data into predefined categories, so patients can choose the data they want to share by choosing one or more of those; however, many patients want more granular control than that. Another issue is getting patients engaged in the process, whatever it is, because it can be quite a daunting task to specify what is to be shared and what is not to be shared. Another issue is provider reluctance. Providers typically want all the data and may not want to spend time both convincing patients to share their data after explaining the potential benefits and risks and possibly assisting them to go through a complicated segmentation specification exercise.

There are currently three models for data segmentation: patient-controlled, provider-assisted, and other systems, including organization-controlled models, hybrid models, and innovative tools. Patient-controlled data segmentation is the norm in PHRs, where there is generally no one but the patient to specify what data can be shared. Some approaches have providers talk to the patient and then specify what is to be shared on their behalf. This typically works within a closed health system, where there is a greater degree of control of the information, the information flows, and the information specifications. However, such specifications would rarely extend with any degree of accuracy or consistency beyond that closed health system.

To consider the potential for innovative tools, imagine a scenario where a patient has several medical problems, including hypertension and depression. The clinical trial the patient wants to join only needs information about the patient's hypertension. It would be wonderful if the patient could just check hypertension from a list of their problems and know with confidence that only the information pertinent to that problem is being shared and that nothing else is being shared, particularly not information about depression. Psychiatric problems can be particularly sensitive to patients. What would be required to do that? Figure 4.3 is a design proposal that was created to assist doctors in focusing on clinical data that is pertinent to the problem currently under care, but it illustrates the kind of data structures needed under the surface of today's electronic medical records (EMRs) and PHRs to support the more sophisticated, more consumer-friendly version of data segmentation specification that was just proposed. It illustrates a hypothetical patient with hypertension and depression, among other clinical problems (Conditions). Here, hypertension is selected and the related Interventions and Observations are automatically selected, the ideal scenario for data segmentation just outlined.

This approach would require that EMRs understand clinical relationships among and between data elements. So, in this example, the EMR would know which medications (under Interventions in figure 4.3) and laboratory tests (under Observations in figure 4.3) relate to hypertension. By inference the EMR knows that the other Interventions and Observations are not related to it. So, in the example, the patient checking hypertension is, also by inference, allowing the list of drugs and lab tests that are related to hypertension to be shared but is not consenting to share any other data. It is a key point that the patient need not know which drugs and tests should be included because they are related to the condition under consideration, which is the key advantage to simplify things for the patient. What would be required to support this approach? The normal EMR system in use today does not understand these inferences. It does not understand the interrelationships among and between the various clinical data elements it records. There are coding systems that could support this. Systemized Nomenclature of Medicine (SNOMED) may be the prime example because it has clinical interrelationships among its data elements built into a hierarchical structure. If these coding systems were routinely used to support at least the structured data elements in EMRs, it would be an important start toward the approach to data segmentation support that may ultimately be required. Unfortunately, current technology and approaches are a long way from that. This dependence of an effective approach to patient privacy on sophisticated data standards like SNOMED serves to illustrate how interrelated the core technologies in health information technology are. In fact, sharing of patient data from a PHR is dependent on all three of the core technologies covered in chapters 3 to 5.

A potentially related development is the semantic web that is described by the World Wide Web Consortium (W3C), the main standards organization for the web, as "a common framework that allows data to be shared and reused across application, enterprise, and community boundaries." If, as W3C envisions, it becomes easier to find, share, and combine information more easily on a semantic web, and the standards that support this encompass health related ontologies, such as SNOMED (which W3C envisions), one can imagine new tools that facilitate patient understanding of complex medical terms and a more workable and informed approach to their specification of data-sharing preferences without overly burdening their healthcare providers.

Figure 4.3   Jonathan Nebeker's EMR design exercise visually shows the links between the selected clinical problem and related interventions, observations, and patient specified goals.

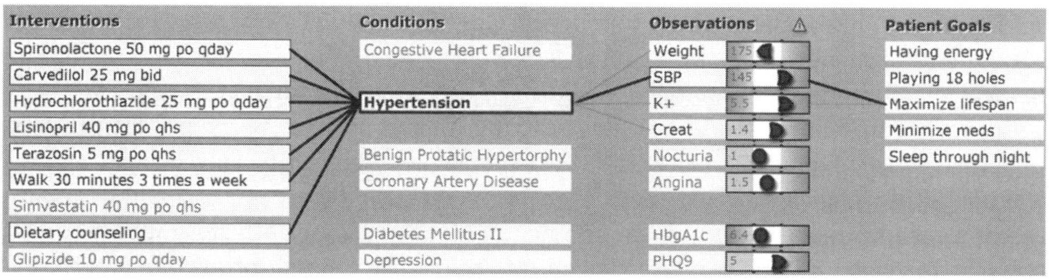

Interventions	Conditions	Observations	⚠	Patient Goals
Spironolactone 50 mg po qday	Congestive Heart Failure	Weight	175	Having energy
Carvedilol 25 mg bid		SBP	145	Playing 18 holes
Hydrochlorothiazide 25 mg po qday	Hypertension	K+	5.5	Maximize lifespan
Lisinopril 40 mg po qhs		Creat	1.4	Minimize meds
Terazosin 5 mg po qhs	Benign Protatic Hypertorphy	Nocturia	1	Sleep through night
Walk 30 minutes 3 times a week	Coronary Artery Disease	Angina	1.5	
Simvastatin 40 mg po qhs				
Dietary counseling	Diabetes Mellitus II	HbgA1c	8.4	
Glipizide 10 mg po qday	Depression	PHQ9	5	

Used with permission from Jonathan Nebeker, MD.

Security and Trust

Security and trust will be discussed together because these topics are interrelated, particularly with respect to the technology that is most commonly used to assure them—Public Key Infrastructure (PKI), a technology that can be confusing. Understanding it in basic terms depends on mastering three key concepts. The first concept is the pair of public and private keys. The second concept is the difference between the message (the sensitive information that is being sent) and an electronic signature that is attached to (and derived from) that message. The third concept is the function of entities that confirm the identity of the people or entities involved in the exchange of information (the registration authority or RA) and that actually sign the digital certificates that are tied to (bound to) that identity (the certificate authority or CA).

It is easiest to discuss these concepts within the context of Direct because it is a particularly simple and clear way to look at them. Moreover, Direct is becoming an increasingly important part of HIE outside of the firewalls (walled gardens) of health systems. It may well be indispensable as HIE extends to patients in their homes.

Public and Private Keys

Public and private keys can be thought of as a pair of numbers, but it is not quite that simple. The pair is mathematically related, and the relationship between them is complex and hard to understand. The specifics are unimportant and too complex for this book. What is important is that determining the *private* key—if you have the *public* key—is prohibitively time consuming and expensive. In fact, the whole notion of public key encryption rests on this principle because the public key really is public. In fact, the public key can be freely distributed. The private key, on the other hand, must be available only to the certificate authority that issued it and to its owner (or, in many cases in Direct, to their health information service provider [HISP]). If the private key becomes public, the security provided by PKI is lost.

An often surprising fact is that information can usefully be encrypted with either the public key or the private key. This is a concept that is a little difficult to grasp at times. Anything encrypted with either one of these keys can be decrypted using the other. The confusion comes about because it is easy to forget that encrypting a message with a private key is different from revealing or losing control of that private key. In fact, encryption with a private key is how digital signatures can be verified as coming from the person or entity claiming to have sent a message.

Figure 4.4 shows the PKI within the context of Direct. Note that there are two data flows shown in order to illustrate both security and trust using PKI. At the top is the security part related to the message (including a message attachment in Direct). This would typically be some part of or a summary of the patient's record. The bottom flow establishes trust via a digital signature.

Figure 2.11 in chapter 2 shows the specific clinical content is use case dependent under Meaningful Use Stage 2. The sender of this PHI encrypts it using the recipient's public key. Remember, the public keys are public, so the sender (or anyone for that matter) can easily get the recipient's public key. The message eventually ends up at the recipient's HISP, which either has or can gain access to the matching private key. Only then can it be unencrypted and read. If this message is being sent over the Internet, and entities that should not have access somehow get it, so long as they do not have the recipient's private key, they cannot read the message. That is the core concept of *security*. Encrypting protected information

Figure 4.4   A simple illustration of Direct shows how PKI can be used to insure both security and trust.

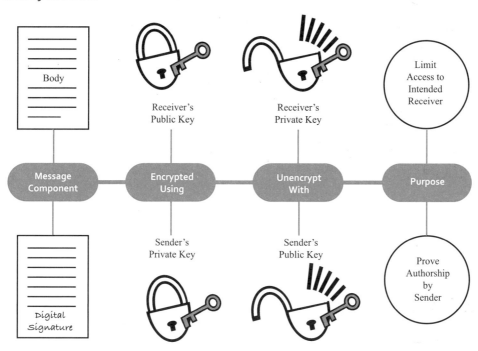

with the receiver's public key means the intended receiver—and only the intended receiver (or, in Direct, their agent, the HISP)—can unencrypt it, using the matching private key.

Trust and Digital Signatures

Trust deals with how that recipient knows that the PHI actually came from the entity that said they sent it. It is particularly an issue when a provider is dealing with an unknown provider at some distance or a patient is sending data to a provider. Here, the concept of a digital signature becomes important.

The digital signature is created by a series of mathematical processes that transform the data being sent into a unique (or virtually unique) "message digest," which is then encrypted with the sender's *private* key. The private key still remains private because the sender is not sending their private key; the sender is using it only to encrypt the digital signature. Only the digital signature encrypted with the private key is sent. The receiver can easily get the sender's *public* key because it is public, so the receiver (or anyone for that matter) can unencrypt the signature. It is important to remember that the signature is not protected health information, it is just something that proves that the message containing the PHI is actually coming from the person who claims to have sent it—the owner of the private key—because only the sender could have encrypted it with his or her private key.

Since the digital signature was generated at the sender's end from the original message, the unencrypted version can be compared to what was received (by regenerating the signature from the decrypted message) to confirm that the message was unaltered in transit. Thus, the digital signature can actually serve two purposes. It verifies that a message was unaltered in transit, and it verifies that the message came from the person or entity claiming to have sent it.

It is now important to recall the role of the RA. Before the certificates were issued, the RA went through a carefully prescribed (and hopefully adequate) process to assure that the people the certificates are being issued to, in fact, are who they say they are. This process can be time consuming and expensive, but it is manageable with providers, particularly since they can already be well-known to the RA (if it has established a relationship with their health system), are publicly licensed, and should have readily available means to establish their identities and credentials.

Policy Issues

Establishing trust is more difficult with PHRs, where thousands and even millions of patients could be involved. Moreover, the health system or HIE may have had no formal relationship with these patients. Policies with respect to establishing trust for patients must take all of this into consideration.

In any case the RA must be able to enforce defined compliance policies within the community of interest. Earlier it was noted that Direct expert, Greg Meyer, says that Direct is 80 percent about policies. There are no hard and fast rules about how to establish that somebody or some entity is who they say they are. It is even possible that a fraudulent HISP could be created. Each health system, HISP, or state HIE could have its own policies. There are, of course, guidelines on this. In fact, there is a large body of literature on this issue publicly available on the Internet. However, as discussed in chapter 3, the Trust Community approach is being used by Direct Trust to lessen the burden by standardizing these policies. At present this extends to HISPs and providers but not to patients.

PKI on the Web

Direct and its HISPs are, to a large degree, walled gardens accessible only to persons or entities that have gone through a careful trust determination process. How does PKI work to insure security (trust is another matter entirely) in the more complex and open environment of the Internet? This is more than a topic of general interest because the secure HIE is not limited to Direct. Cloud-based HIT systems now include EMRs, care coordination systems, and PHRs. All of these typically store PHI, so exchanges between them must be protected.

It is easiest to explain the use of PKI on the web using a very simplified scenario based on Google Mail to send or receive e-mail. Some web pages have a URL that begins with HTTPS,[1] instead of the more common HTTP. Along with banking and financial services sites, mail.google.com is one of these pages.

When you visit the Google Mail server, it sends you (more specifically it sends your browser) Google's *public* key. Remember, the public key is public so anyone can obtain it, in this case by visiting the server where it is stored. Your browser will use the public key to encrypt the messages you send to Google Mail. As with Direct, only Google knows their private key, so only they can decrypt your data and display it on the recipient's Google Mail web page.

---

[1]Technically, HTTPS is not a protocol but is the result of layering the more commonly used Hypertext Transfer Protocol (HTTP) on top of the SSL/TLS protocol, thus adding the security capabilities of SSL/TLS to standard HTTP communications.

But how do you know it is really Google? In Direct, trust is established because an RA has validated that each person is who he or she claimed. Your browser supplier could do the same thing. They could verify that Google Mail is who they say they are. They could then encrypt Google Mail's public key using their *private* key and provide this with their browser. Then, when Google Mail sends you that encrypted public key, your browser could use your browser supplier's *public* key to decrypt and verify Google's key. This verifies the identity, just as the digital signature was verified in Direct.

However, browser suppliers do not want to do this for obvious reasons. There are thousands, if not millions, of websites that would need to be vetted. This is the problem that originally led to the certificate authorities (CAs) discussed with respect to Direct. Their business is to check websites and make sure the company behind them is who they say they are, are legitimate, and actually own the domain name they claim they have. The full due diligence process goes far beyond that, if it is done properly. Once everything is verified, the CA encrypts the public key for each site using their *private* key. The browser suppliers include the *public* keys for all the CAs in their browsers, so they can authenticate that a public key actually comes from one of these authorities.

Again, suppose your *public* key has been encrypted by a CA (such as Verisign or Thawte) using the browser supplier's *private* key. The browser suppliers use the CA's public keys to make sure your public key came from that CA. This is similar to the trust process used in the digital signature case discussed earlier.

So, if Google's server sends Google's public key, it ought to be accessible from a browser. Indeed it is. Depending on the browser, there is usually a clickable icon near the URL. In Firefox it is the closed lock which has been clicked in figure 4.5. Clicking the More Information button, as shown in figure 4.6, shows that the HTTPS site was verified by Thawte.

Clicking the View Certificate button shows Google's public key (figure 4.7), which is a 2,048-bit number called the modulus. The symbol for that is "n". There is a usually small number (24-bits for Google Mail) as well, which is called the exponent (e). These are two

Figure 4.5   This is the first step in viewing Google's public key using Mozilla Firefox.

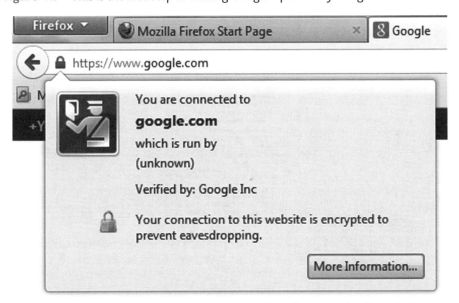

Google and the Google logo are registered trademarks of Google Inc., used with permission.

Figure 4.6   This more detailed view of Google's public key using Mozilla Firefox shows details such as the Certificate Authority that issued the key.

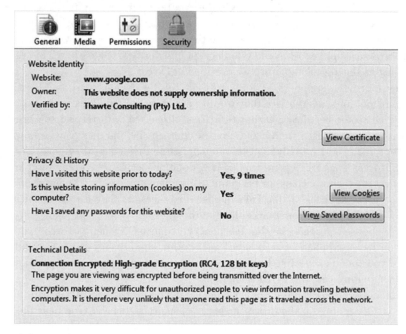

Google and the Google logo are registered trademarks of Google Inc., used with permission.

Figure 4.7   This most detailed view shows Google's public key using Mozilla Firefox, illustrating that the key is truly public.

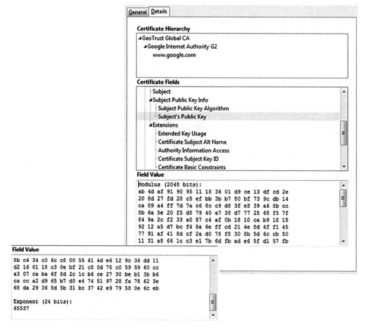

Google and the Google logo are registered trademarks of Google Inc., used with permission.

important numbers. The private key also uses the modulus; its exponent is a much larger 96-bit number called d. The calculation that is involved is very complicated. If you are really mathematically inclined, use your search engine to look for "rsa explained simply," but be forewarned, the term "simply" is relative in this context.

Other PKI Issues

PKI is, as the name implies, a public system for protecting information. This allows it to be used for many purposes: to secure e-mail; for secure browsing for other purposes, such as banking; to secure computer code; to secure a wireless network; or for digital rights management. In that last case, PKI is why when you download legitimate copies of movies, they will not play unless you have met the requirements to be able to view them. PKI is also used to encrypt files on computers, something that is often done in healthcare, particularly for mobile devices that might be lost or stolen.

This has been an intentionally simple explanation of PKI. The reality is more complex. Here is just a small list of some of the additional complexities:

- The validation for the certificate really needs to be more comprehensive than described here to fully trust a certificate. The term for this is extended validation and major CAs do that.

- To simplify things and reduce the computational load, there are some approaches that create a special set of keys just for a particular session when two people are interacting. These are termed hybrid approaches, one of which is called Pretty Good Privacy (PGP). This is probably insufficiently secure for use in healthcare.

- There is also the ever-present concern about advances in computing. You may have read about the potential impact of quantum computing on PKI encryption. It was said at the beginning that, given the public key, it is prohibitively difficult and time consuming to calculate the private key. However, if computers were fast enough, that might change. Quantum computers do not exist yet, but if they do in the future, the PKI might have to be modified to remain useful.

Finally, there is no technology that is completely foolproof. The biggest potential issue with PKI is malware stealing the secure keys. It should be very clear at this point that if the private key is compromised—if a private key becomes public or falls into the wrong hands—then encryption will not protect its owners' data. Healthcare providers must keep this ever in mind and must rigorously and routinely use adequate software defenses. Proper, periodic employee training is equally critical to reinforce proper procedures (for example, USB flash drives from home should never be brought into the medical office unless it is certain there are adequate protections for the home computer and network). Loss of the private key defeats the whole scheme.

It is possible that keys can be attacked. For example, someone can just try all possible keys. They are large numbers to make this as difficult as possible. There is also the potential for what is called a "man in the middle of attack." This is where someone gets between the two people interacting, grabs a public key, substitutes his or her own public key, and can then impersonate one of the parties in the interaction. This is one reason why it is so important that the CA provides a signature authenticating the person you are dealing with.

Data security is a field where technology has gotten very sophisticated. For example, the Georgia Tech Information Security Center (GTISC) has developed MedVault, a set of technologies and approaches to protecting health data against malware, probably the most prevalent threat to security (MedVault 2013). One MedVault approach has clinicians work in a separate, protected virtual machine environment. There is another isolated environment that is separate to protect it from malware and houses monitoring software. Any requests for patient data must go through this environment, where the monitoring system checks to make sure that everything looks as it should before the request is fulfilled. Other research examines the use of an intermediary repository that sits between PHRs and those interested in using clinical data; it obeys patient instructions about release of the data that is housed in an "agent" that enforces those instructions (Bauer et al. 2009) such that, for example, a patient could change his or her mind about sharing data and anyone who has it would no longer be able to access it.

Conclusion

For health information to help with care coordination it must be shared. For it to be used to manage quality over many provider practices it must be aggregated within a provider network. For it to be used for research purposes beyond direct patient care, it must often be aggregated across many providers and many health systems. Patient consent is required for any use beyond direct patient care, practice administration or quality management.

To facilitate sharing and use of health data from many diverse and geographically dispersed systems many of the latest health informatics tools are web based, using the same technologies that are commonly used for many other purposes. However, the Internet was not designed as a secure network; health information is especially sensitive and is protected by laws that impose strict penalties if that data is compromised. Privacy, security, and trust are different aspects of this one grand challenge. Good solutions for all three are critical health informatics challenges. This will therefore remain a dynamic and interesting area of health informatics for many years to come.

REFERENCES

Bauer, D., D.M. Blough, and A. Mohan. 2009. Redactable signatures on data with dependencies and their application to personal health records. *Proceedings of the CCS Workshop on Privacy in the Electronic Society.* http://dl.acm.org/citation.cfm?id=1655201

California Health Foundation. 2010. New National Survey Finds Personal Health Records Motivate Consumers to Improve Their Health. http://www.chcf.org/media/press-releases/2010/new-national-survey-finds-personal-health-records-motivate-consumers-to-improve-their-health

Dunn, J.E. 2011. Hospital Turns Away Patients after "Virus" Disrupts Network. http://www.computerworld.com/s/article/9222656/Hospital_turns_away_patients_after_virus_disrupts_network

Electricity Forum. 2009. Conficker infected critical hospital equipment: Expert. http://www.electricityforum.com/news/apr09/Confickerinfectedcriticalequipment.html

Federal Bureau of Investigation. 2010. Fraud and Organized Crime Intersect: Eurasian Enterprise Targeted. http://www.fbi.gov/news/stories/2010/october/medicare-fraud-organized-crime-bust

Goldstein, M.M. and A.L. Rein. 2010. Data Segmentation in Electronic Health Information Exchange: Policy Considerations and Analysis. http://www.healthit.gov/sites/default/files/privacy-security/gwu-data-segmentation-final-cover-letter.pdf

Google. 2013. "Google's Public." http://www.google.com

Gorman, A. and A. Sewell. 2013. Six people fired from Cedars-Sinai over patient privacy breaches. *Los Angles Times.* http://articles.latimes.com/2013/jul/12/local/la-me-hospital-security-breach-20130713

Institute of Medicine. 2009. Committee on Health Research and the Privacy of Health Information: The HIPAA Privacy Rule; Nass S.J., Levit L.A., and Gostin L.O., editors. *Beyond the HIPAA Privacy Rule: Enhancing Privacy, Improving Health Through Research.* Washington (DC): National Academies Press (US); 2, The Value and Importance of Health Information Privacy. Available from: http://www.ncbi.nlm.nih.gov/books/NBK9579/

Martino, L. and S. Ahuja. 2010. Privacy policies of personal health records: An evaluation of their effectiveness in protecting patient information. *IHI '10 Proceedings of the 1st ACM International Health Informatics Symposium*, 191–200. http://dl.acm.org/citation.cfm?id=1883020&bnc=1

MedVault. 2013. http://medvault.gtisc.gatech.edu

ONC. 2013. Direct: Implementation Guidelines to Assure Security and Interoperability. http://www.healthit.gov/sites/default/files/direct_implementation_guidelines_to_assure_security_and_interoperability.pdf

S&I Framework. 2014. CET - Standards Identification. http://wiki.siframework.org/CET+-+Standards+Identification

S&I Framework. 2011. Use Case and Requirements (UCR) Workgroup. LRI - FINAL Use Case. http://confluence.siframework.org/display/SIF/LRI+-+FINAL+Use+Case

Tripathi, M., D. Delano, B. Lund, and L. Rudolph. 2009. Engaging patients for health information exchange. *Health Affairs* 28(2):435–443. http://content.healthaffairs.org/content/28/2/435.full

Xerox. 2012. Only 26 Percent of Americans Want Electronic Medical Records. http://news.xerox.com/news/Xerox-Surveys-Americans-Electronic-Health-Records

Zulman, D.M. 2011. Patient interest in sharing personal health record information: A web-based survey. *Ann Intern Med.* 155(12):805–810. http://annals.org/article.aspx?articleid=1033219

RECOMMENDED READING AND RESOURCES

For more on data segmentation read *Data Segmentation in Electronic Health Information Exchange: Policy Considerations and Analysis* (Goldstein and Rein 2010).

For more details on protecting patient health records within a PHR environment, read *Privacy Policies of Personal Health Records: An Evaluation of Their Effectiveness in Protecting Patient Information* (Martino and Ahuja 2010).

For more details on security in Direct, read Implementation Guidelines to Assure Security and Interoperability (ONC 2013) at http://www.healthit.gov/sites/default/files/direct_implementation_guidelines_to_assure_security_and_interoperability.pdf.

ONC maintains a webpage devoted to privacy and security at http://www.healthit.gov/policy-researchers-implementers/privacy-security-policy.

Chapter 5

Data and Interoperability Standards

Among the most important goals of health informatics is interoperability—facilitating the meaningful and useful exchange of a patient's data among providers who may care for that patient. Given its potential importance, perhaps it should not be surprising that a recent bipartisan legislative proposal would "require EHRs to be 'interoperable by 2017' and it also would 'prohibit providers from deliberately blocking information sharing with other EHR vendor products.'" (Conn 2014) Secondary goals include the aggregation of data from many patients for purposes from public health surveillance to managing care against agreed-upon quality standards to research aimed at gaining new medical knowledge.

Doing these usually requires standards for the data itself—how it is packaged into electronic documents and how those documents are exchanged. As a result, data and interoperability standards are core technologies that support all modern health informatics systems. This can be a challenging area of technology to master. It is often a complex and rather arcane field, filled with acronyms, abbreviations, and technical jargon. There are many organizations and many standards, and they sometimes overlap. Some of the specific concepts and standards can be challenging to grasp in detail.

To keep this discussion to a manageable length this chapter will focus, for the most part on the key, most widely used standards, but it will look at some other standards in the final section. Even so, this is easily the longest chapter in the book. Given its length, readers should consider their own needs. Healthcare providers should aim for a good overview of what these standards are used for, how they are constructed, and to a reasonable degree, how they work. This should help them gain a better understanding of how important accurate data entry is to the use of the clinical records they create by others and for purposes beyond direct patient care. Health informatics professionals will need a more in-depth knowledge, particularly of those standards that directly pertain to their job function. Potential system developers will need a very firm and detailed understanding of the standards that are applicable to their work and to those standards that may apply to other system components that depend on the software they develop.

Interoperability is the ability of diverse systems and organizations to work together. It is clear why interoperability of health information systems is both essential and challenging, considering healthcare as a complex adaptive system; the overarching goal of care coordination and the critical enabling role health information technology (HIT) plays; and the plethora of systems available in the commercial market.

Figure 5.1   Semantic and syntactic incompatibilities across systems like those illustrated here create the need for standards.

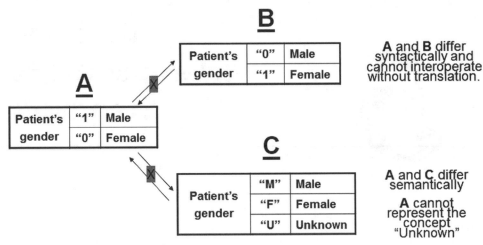

©Health Level Seven International, reprinted with permission from HL7.

Standards have long been viewed as a necessary supporting element to achieve interoperability. Although advances in machine learning and natural language processing may be starting to change this view because of their ability to work with free text, it is likely that standards will play a key role for many years to come.

Standards are also important if electronic records are going to become the basis for intelligent clinical reminders and decision support. This is the idea that electronic medical records (EMRs) should actively intervene to help their users avoid mistakes and make the best possible clinical decisions. Ideally, standardized representations of clinical logic could be linked to the standardized clinical data from patient chart to enable precisely personalized, evidence-based care for each patient. This is a key goal of the Health eDecisions Workgroup, which was chartered in July 2012 within the S&I Framework supported by the Office of the National Coordinator for Health IT (ONC).

If EMRs are going to be a source of maximally useful data for public health and for various research purposes, it is important for that data to have as great a degree of structure and consistency as possible.

Figure 5.1 helps illustrate why standards are important. It shows three hypothetical EMR systems: A, B, and C. In system A, the patient's gender (a simple and straightforward data element) is represented by the number 1, if the patient is male, and by the number 0, if the patient is female. In system B, that is reversed, so 0 means male, and 1 means female. If data from systems A and B were mixed without any thought, individual patient gender would become unclear. These two systems differ in their syntax. System C, on the other hand, uses the letter M to represent male, F to represent female, and U for unknown sex. Thus, A differs semantically from C. A and B cannot represent the concept of unknown. C also differs from A and B in its use of letters instead of numbers to represent sex. This is a very simple illustration of the data incompatibilities that make interoperability a challenge without shared standards.

The Evolution of Standards

Standards have evolved over many years to help prevent syntactic and semantic incompatibilities. This evolution can be divided into three dimensions: structure, purpose, and technology.

Structure

Standards can be a classification, such as a group or a list of similar objects. This might be a list of all the possible infections that people can have, such as an upper respiratory or urinary tract infection. It might be a list of all of the lab tests that could be ordered to diagnose and/or treat an infection, such as urine, sputum, or blood cultures, or a count of the various types of blood cells, some of which are involved in fighting infections. Standards can be structurally more complex if they become ontologies. Ontologies are more than a list of all the possible objects or concepts in a class, they represent relationships among those objects or concepts. For example, a medical ontology might indicate which bacterial cultures are used to diagnose particular infections. In the simple examples given, this would allow the computer to infer that a sputum culture was done to evaluate an upper respiratory infection and not a urinary tract infection. There has been an evolution over the years from classification systems, which is what most of the early standards were, to ontologies.

Purpose

Purpose is the reason(s) for which standards are created. Figure 5.2 is an illustration to give an overview of the various roles that can be played by health standards. There you see a birthday invitation in an envelope. The aggregate pieces of information in that document, the words or the phrases, could be thought of as data, and one would want a standard for that data. International Classification of Disease (ICD), Logical Observation Identifiers Names and Codes (LOINC), and Systematized Nomenclature of Medicine Clinical Terms (SNOMED CT) are important healthcare data standards that will be discussed later in this chapter. There are also standards for the document format. In this document there is a section for the address at the upper right, and that might be an accepted convention for all documents of this type. The standards for clinical documents specify headers, routing areas, and other necessary components. The new consolidated clinical document architecture (CCDA) is the accepted standard for healthcare document formats. It recently replaced, and is a close derivative of, the clinical document architecture (CDA). Finally, once there are standards for the data and the document, how do you actually move the information from one system to another? Health Level 7 (HL7) is the most widely used transport (message) standard.

Process and workflow, the latest and most sophisticated area for standardization, is shown at the left of figure 5.2. The document consists of standardized data that is

Figure 5.2   The major roles of health standards are shown using a birthday party invitation as the illustration.

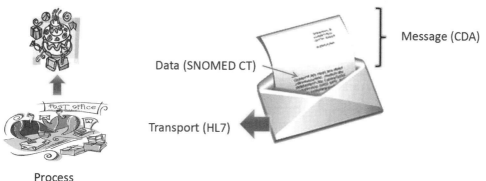

Data (SNOMED CT)

Message (CDA)

Transport (HL7)

Process

organized according to other standards and then put into an envelope representing a transport standard. There is also a process that takes place. The message goes to the post office, it is sorted and transported, and ultimately, it is delivered. Since it is an invitation to a birthday party, receipt triggers yet another sequence of events. Processes may not be as obvious or easily envisioned as the data, the document, or its transport. They are also more complex to represent. As a result this is a newer area, but there are processes interwoven throughout healthcare, and standards are evolving to represent them. As reimbursement changes lead to new care delivery models, understanding process and how to optimize it will become more important, as will these standards, if they prove to be workable.

Figure 5.3 shows many of the major standards and the dates when they began to give a sense that health standards have evolved, beginning with data standards (and, within those, from classifications to ontologies). It also shows the evolution over time from messaging standards to document standards and, more recently, to work flow and process standards.

There are many healthcare standards. There are five that are particularly important: ICD, CPT, LOINC, NDC, SNOMED, and HL7. This section discusses them to illustrate the purposes for which standards have been developed in healthcare. ICD, SNOMED, and HL7 will be discussed briefly here because each will be discussed in detail in separate sections of this chapter.

Introduction to the International Classification of Disease (ICD)

ICD was developed and is supported by the World Health Organization (WHO). It is an almost universally used standard for medical diagnoses. It is also, by far, the oldest standard with direct roots going back into the 1800s and more indirect roots going back centuries before then. It is a requirement for virtually all claims for healthcare payment. ICD is revised every 10 years, and in recent revisions (particularly ICD-10—the current version), it has evolved from a classification to an ontology. ICD is particularly important to clinical records, so it will be looked at it in more detail later on in this chapter.

Current Procedural Terminology (CPT)

CPT was developed, is maintained, and is copyrighted by the American Medical Association (AMA). CPT is updated annually. It is effectively the US standard for coding medical procedures and is used almost universally in this country for billing. Despite that role, because they are so universally available, CPT codes are often used for purposes other than billing including quality reporting and clinical research.

Selection of the appropriate code is the responsibility of the licensed provider caring for the patient (but may be delegated to an employee with special training), and this directly affects the amount that can be billed. CPT coding is therefore important and is also complex.

For example, here is a set of codes for a psychotherapy visit, where the only difference is the length of the visit. The psychiatrist can bill insurance more or less depending on the code that is applicable to each visit:

- **90791:** (diagnostic evaluation without medical services)
- **90832:** (30 minutes)
- **90834:** (45 minutes)
- **90837:** (60 minutes)

Figure 5.3   This illustration of the evolution of health standards over time shows their migration from data to messaging to documents and to workflow and process.

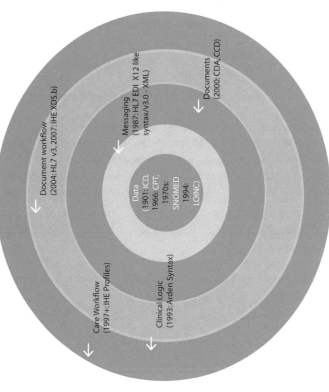

Purpose Evolution

Data (classify, ontology)
Messaging
Document
Workflow/Process

ICD: World Health Organization
CPT: American Medical Association
LOINC: Regenstrief Institute
IHE: Integrating the Healthcare Enterprise
HL7: Health Level Seven International
SNOMED: International Health Terminology Standards Development Organisation

Here are two codes for debriding (removal of dead, damaged, or infected tissue to promote healing):

- **11042**: Debridement, subcutaneous tissue (includes epidermis and dermis, if performed); first 20 square cm or less
- **11045**: Each additional 20 square cm, or part thereof (list separately in addition to code for primary procedure)

In this case, the codes indicate the amount of debridement done and, again, determine the amount that can be billed.

Code selection can be quite a bit more complex than these two relatively straightforward examples. In 2010, the Medicare Learning Network published an 89-page *Evaluation and Management Services Guide* to assist providers in selecting the right CPT codes. Here is a brief excerpt that discusses the proper coding for taking a patient history:

> The levels of evaluation and management services are based on four types of history (Problem Focused, Expanded Problem Focused, Detailed, and Comprehensive). Each type of history includes some or all of the following elements:
>
> - Chief complaint (CC)
> - History of present illness (HPI)
> - Review of systems (ROS)
> - Past, family and/or social history (PFSH)
>
> The extent of history of present illness, review of systems, and past, family and/or social history that is obtained and documented is dependent upon clinical judgment and the nature of the presenting problem(s) (Medicare Learning Network 2010).

Other factors may be the complexity of medical decision making, as shown here:

Decision Making Complexity	Number Of Diagnoses Or Management Options	Amount And/ Or Complexity Of Data To Be Reviewed	Risk Of Significant Complications, Morbidity, And/Or Mortality
Straightforward	Minimal	Minimal or None	Minimal
Low	Limited	Limited	Low
Moderate	Multiple	Moderate	Moderate
High	Extensive	Extensive	High

Source: CMS

Given this complexity, selection of the optimum CPT code to maximize practice revenue has become a skill that is taught and for which various informatics tools have been developed. AHIMA Press publishes *Basic Current Procedural Terminology and HCPCS Coding* annually, and there is an entire industry based on teaching medical and hospital office billing personnel to use the codes correctly and optimally.

There are three categories of CPT codes:

- **Category I:** Procedures that are consistent with contemporary medical practice and are widely performed

- **Category II:** Supplementary tracking codes that can be used for performance measures
- **Category III:** Temporary codes for emerging technology, services, and procedures

CPT provides a description for each code in full, medium, and short form. Here is an example for CPT 90673:

Description	
Full	Influenza virus vaccine, trivalent, derived from recombinant DNA (RIV3), hemagglutinin (HA) protein only, preservative and antibiotic free, for intramuscular use
Medium	Influenza Virus Vaccine Trivalen RIV3 PRSR FR IM
Short	Flu Vacc RIV3 No Preserv

Source: AMA 2013

Category I codes are five digit numbers and are divided into six sections (the codes for each section may not be entirely sequential, as is shown next) in order to better align them with the major medical practice specialty areas: evaluation and management (99201–99499), anesthesiology (00100–01999, 99100–99140), surgery (11021–69990), radiology (0010–79999), pathology and laboratory (80048–89356), and medicine (90281–99199, 99500–99602). Here, as an example, is the Category I CPT code that would be used for a sputum culture to investigate an upper respiratory infection:

87070: Culture, bacterial; any other source except urine, blood or stool, with isolation and presumptive identification of isolates

Category II codes consist of four digits followed by the letter "F" and are intended to facilitate the collection of information about the quality of care delivered by coding for services or test results that support performance measures. Here are two Category II examples that you may recall from our discussion of the criteria for Meaningful Use:

0001F: Blood pressure measured
0002F: Tobacco use, smoking, assessed

Category III codes are four digits followed by the letter "T" and are temporary to allow for data collection and utilization tracking for new procedures or services that may not be performed by many healthcare professionals, may not have FDA approval, or may not have proven clinical efficacy. The coded procedure or service must be involved in ongoing or planned research. The rationale is to help researchers track emerging technology and services to substantiate widespread usage and clinical efficacy without having to go through the lengthy process required to obtain a permanent CPT code.

Logical Observation Identifiers Names and Codes (LOINC)

LOINC was developed and is maintained by the Regenstrief Institute as a standard for laboratory and clinical observations. The codes in this system are currently a simple number that may contain up to seven digits (the last one is separated by a dash and is a check digit that can be used to verify the entire code). There are currently nearly 60,000 codes, but LOINC recommends that system developers anticipate expansion to as many as 10 digits in the future (McDonald et al. 2013).

The codes are simple, but the names associated with them can be complicated. According to the *Logical Observation Identifiers Names and Codes (LOINC®) Users' Guide*, the "fully specified name" of a test result or clinical observation:

> has five or six main parts including: the name of the component or analyte measured (e.g., glucose, propranolol), the property observed (e.g., substance concentration, mass, volume), the timing of the measurement (e.g., is it over time or momentary), the type of sample (e.g., urine, serum), the scale of measurement (e.g., qualitative vs. quantitative), and where relevant, the method of the measurement (e.g., radioimmunoassay, immune blot). These can be described formally with the following syntax:
>
> <Analyte/component>:<kind of property of observation or measurement>:<time aspect>:<system (sample)>:<scale>:<method>
> (McDonald et al. 2013)

The first part of the name can be further divided into three subparts, separated by carats (^). The first subpart can contain multiple levels of increasing taxonomic specification, separated by dots (.). The third and fourth parts of the name (time aspect and system/sample) can also be modified by a second subpart, separated from the first by a carat. In the case of time aspect, the modifier can indicate that the observation is one selected on the basis of the named criterion (maximum, minimum, mean, and so on) in the case of system, the modifier identifies the origin of the specimen, if not the patient (for example, blood donor, fetus, and blood product unit).

Figure 5.4 provides an annotated example of a fully specified LOINC Name.

Here is another example that illustrates the use of the carat (^) to divide the first part of the name (Analyte/component) into subparts:

Glucose^2H post 100 g glucose PO:MCnc:Pt:Ser/Plas:Qn

Here is an explanation of each of the parts of this name:

Part	Example Text	Explanation
Analyte/component	Glucose	The lab test, a blood glucose level determination
Subpart (^)	2H post 100 g glucose PO	The test was performed two hours after the patient consumed 100 grams of glucose by mouth (PO)
Measurement	MCnc	Mass concentration (versus molar concentration)
Time aspect	Pt	Point in time (not measured over time)
System (sample)	Ser/Plas	Serum or plasma (from the patient's blood)
Scale	Qn	Quantitative (numeric) result
Method		Not specified

National Drug Code (NDC)

The National Drug Code (NDC) is maintained by the Food and Drug Administration (FDA) and identifies all medications. Each NDC is a unique 10-digit, 3-segment, numeric identifier that specifies the labeler or vendor, the product (within the scope of the labeler), and the trade package (of this product).

Figure 5.4   This illustration shows the six parts that can potentially be part of a code in the LOINC system.

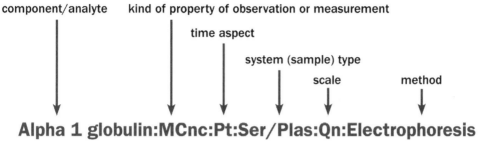

Used by permission of Mayo Foundation for Medical Education and Research. All rights reserved.

Figure 5.5   This illustrates the three subparts of the National Drug Code (NDC).

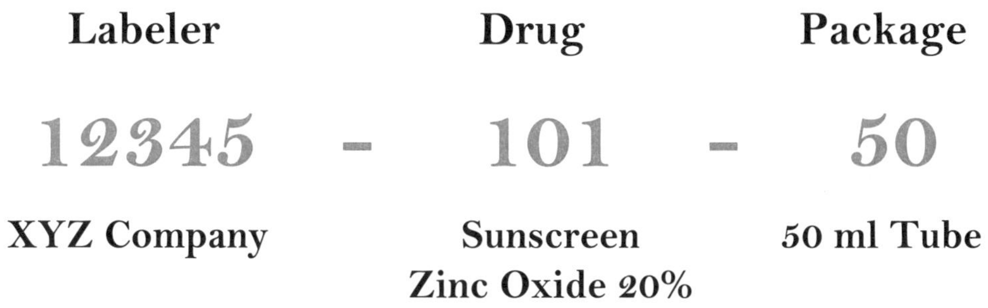

Labeler		Drug		Package
12345	**-**	**101**	**-**	**50**
XYZ Company		Sunscreen Zinc Oxide 20%		50 ml Tube

The first segment, the labeler code, is four or five digits long. A labeler is any firm that manufactures, repacks or distributes drug products. The second segment, the product code, is three or four digits long and identifies a specific strength, dosage form, and formulation for a particular firm. The third segment, the package code, is one or two digits long and identifies package forms and sizes.

In rare cases, product and package segments may contain characters other than digits. The digits in an NDC codes may be grouped as: 4-4-2, 5-3-2, or 5-4-1. Figure 5.5 presents an example of an NDC code.

Introduction to the Systemized Nomenclature for Medicine (SNOMED)

SNOMED is an important major international data standard that was created initially as an ontology. It attempts to include relationships that encompass all of medicine, going well beyond clinical practice. SNOMED CT, which is a main focus in this book, is limited to the concepts and relationships that are used in clinical practice. SNOMED-CT will be discussed in more detail later on in this chapter.

Introduction to Health Level 7 (HL7)

HL7 is the most widely used messaging and document standard. It has gone through a number of revisions and scope expansions, but it began with messaging so that diverse information systems—typically within a hospital—could communicate data with each other to achieve a degree of interoperability.

The latest version, HL7 Version 3, consists of many components and a rich set of standards, each of them quite complex—this is also an area with a great deal of specialized jargon and acronyms. It is therefore particularly important to try to understand the big picture before drilling into detail. HL7 provides ready-to-implement models for messages, documents, and services. With Version 3, HL7 has transitioned from EDI/X12 to Extensible Markup Language (XML) technology. HL7 will be discussed in more detail later on in this chapter.

Standards Technology Evolution

As the structure and purpose of standards has evolved, so has the format through which they are expressed. HL7 will be used to illustrate this trend. Historically, HL7 used Electronic Data Interchange (EDI) formats maintained by ASC X12 (EDI/X12 formats). EDI arose almost as soon as commercial entities started installing computers and is widely used in manufacturing and other industries, including healthcare. More recently the trend in HL7 standards has been toward XML, a technology that was developed for the Internet, in which tags and formats are used to describe data elements within webpages.

These technologies have key differences. In EDI, the structure and the meaning of each data element are implicit, they are not explicitly stated. It is important to know that a particular number or some other type of data element—based on its location within a cryptic string—means the quantity of an item on order, or the name of the company ordering it. The meaning and source of data items in XML is made explicit through the use of tags. Each field of data is explicitly labeled in human readable form. A tag might say that the value which follows it is a diastolic blood pressure or that it is the patient's name. The notion of human readability does not exist in EDI, which was designed only with machine readability and concise expressions in mind in large part because EDI was developed in an era where memory was expensive, so conserving space was essential. XML is both human and machine readable, but relative to EDI, it is quite verbose. A human being looking at an XML document, with some effort, can get a good feel for what it says.

With some effort, EDI-based strings can be converted for display for humans on a webpage. XML documents can be displayed simply by viewing them in a web browser. However, the format is usually not very satisfactory, so people often write software to display an XML clinical document in an easy-to-read and more clinically useful way. Figure 0.1, in the introduction, a patient summary, is an example of this.

EDI is how manufacturers exchange information with their suppliers, including documents such as purchase orders, shipping documents, and invoices. The standards are maintained by ASC X12, a group chartered by the American National Standards Institute (ANSI) for this purpose. It serves many industry sectors, including healthcare. Here is an illustration of EDI used in healthcare—specifically a part of a very important, common, and widely used 837 ANSI X12 transaction, a healthcare claim.

```
ISA|00|  |00|  |ZZ|99999999999 |ZZ|888888888888 |111219|1340|^|00501|000001377
|0|T|>
GS|HC|99999999999|888888888888|20111219|1340|1377|X|005010X222
ST|837|0001|005010X222
BHT|0019|00|565743|20110523|154959|CH
NM1|41|2|SAMPLE INC|||||46|496103
PER|IC|EDI DEPT|EM|FEEDBACK@1EDISOURCE.COM|TE|3305551212
NM1|40|2|PPO BLUE|||||46|54771
HL|1||20|1
PRV|BI|PXC|333600000X
```

```
NM1|85|2|EDI SPECIALTY SAMPLE|||||XX|123456789
N3|1212 DEPOT DRIVE
N4|CHICAGO|IL|606930159
REF|EI|300123456
HL|2|1|22|1
SBR|P|||||||BL
NM1|IL|1|CUSTOMER|KAREN||||MI|YYX123456789
N3|228 PINEAPPLE CIRCLE
N4|CORA|PA|15108
DMG|D8|19630625|M
NM1|PR|2|PPO BLUE|||||PI|54771
N3|PO BOX 12345
N4|CAMP HILL|PA|17089
HL|3|2|23|0
PAT|19 …
```

(1edisource.com 2013)

Most healthcare providers get paid by using 837 EDI claims like this example. As already stated, EDI documents are quite cryptic but also quite compact. This is almost certainly an inevitable trade-off, something that is more readable by humans is going to be more verbose, since it has to provide humans with information so they understand—as they view the document. This might include the context in which fields of data are presented; if they are codes, what coding system they derive from; and, ideally, their name.

Each line in EDI begins with a segment name, typically a series of letters, for example, the line that begins with PER in the above illustration. After PER this line contains various items of data separated with the pipe character – | – that is commonly used to separate fields in an EDI document. It is not obvious what the data fields in this line represent. The last field is a phone number, but to really understand much of the data, a reference guide is needed, as shown in figure 5.6. The guide shows that the PER (PER*IC) segment has fields for the contact information for the organization that is submitting the claim: their name, their contact number, their telephone number, and so on.

A more complex example is shown next; it shows four lines from a lab test result EDI transaction: the MSH segment, which is the header; the PID segment, which is the patient identification; the OBR segment, which is the observation request; and the OBX segment, which is the observation result.

```
MSH|^~\&|GHH LAB|ELAB-3|GHH OE|BLDG4|200202150930||ORU^R01|CNTRL-3456|P|2.4
PID|||555-44-4444||EVERYWOMAN^EVE^E^^^^L|JONES|19620320|F|||153 FERNWOOD
DR.^ ^STATESVILLE^OH^35292||(206)3345232|(206)752-121||||AC555444444||67-
A4335^OH^20030520
OBR|1|845439^GHH OE|1045813^GHH LAB|15545^GLUCOSE|||200202150730|||||||||
555-55-5555^PRIMARY^PATRICIA P^^^^MD^^|||||||||F|||||444-44-
4444^HIPPOCRATES^HOWARD H^^^^MD
OBX|1|SN|1554-5^GLUCOSE^POST 12H CFST:MCNC:PT:SER/PLAS:QN||^182|mg/
dl|70_105|H|||F
```

(HL7 2013)

The MSH message header segment contains the sender, the receiver, when it was sent, and the message type. There can also be a trigger event, something that requires a response. The next segment, PID, is the patient ID that contains the name of the patient, when they were born, their address, their phone number, and so on. The OBR, observation request segment, contains the ordering physician, who is going to perform the test, and the test that has been ordered, in this case a glucose level. Next to it is the number 15545. As you will see later in this chapter, if this were an XML document, there would be a tag that explains the coding

Figure 5.6 An example of an ANSI 837 (healthcare claim) Reference Guide illustrates the need for detailed explanation of cryptic EDI/X12 formatted documents.

ANSI 837 Reference

Default View | Segment Index

- Introduction
- ⊞ Loop 0000A - INTERCHANGE CONTROL HEADER
- ⊞ Loop 0000B - FUNCTIONAL GROUP HEADER
- ⊞ Loop 0000D - TRANSACTION HEADER
- ⊞ Loop 0000E - TRANSACTION HEADER
- ⊟ Loop 1000A - SUBMITTER NAME
  - ⊞ NM1*41 - Submitter Name
  - ⊟ PER*IC - Submitter EDI Contact Information
    - PER02 - Submitter Name
    - PER03 - Submitter Contact Number Qualifier
    - PER04 - Submitter Telephone Number
- ⊞ Loop 1000B - RECEIVER NAME
- ⊞ Loop 2000A - BILLING/PAY-TO PROVIDER
- ⊞ Loop 2000B - SUBSCRIBER HIERARCHICAL LEVEL
- ⊞ Loop 2000C - PATIENT HIERARCHICAL LEVEL
- ⊞ Loop 2010AA - BILLING PROVIDER NAME
- ⊞ Loop 2010AB - PAY-TO PROVIDER NAME
- ⊞ Loop 2010BA - SUBSCRIBER NAME
- ⊞ Loop 2010BB - PAYER NAME

Used with permission of EZClaim, Medical Coding and Billing Software.

system from which this number derives. Since this is an EDI/X12 document, there must be some external knowledge that this is the LOINC code for the glucose test. This illustrates again that EDI/X12 is compact but, as a result, is also quite cryptic. The OBX segment is the result of the test, including a detailed test description explaining that this is a postprandial 12 hour (done 12 hours after the patient's last meal) glucose test done using certain techniques. The result is 182 milligrams per deciliter. There is also a normal range for this test (70 to 105), and a flag that indicates the result is high, since 182 is well above the normal range. This transaction presents a lot of useful information in a cryptic, compact form.

XML is much more descriptive and verbose. It is a general purpose meta-language—a language used for describing other languages—now widely used on the web. For example, you may have visited a website and filled out a form and wondered how your browser is smart enough to know what your address is when you just type a small part of it in. There are XML tags in the webpage code saying that this field is city, this one is state, and so on.

As shown on the first line in the example here, the basic format constructs within XML are the name of some element; element specific content; and the element name repeated but preceded by a slash indicating the end of that element. It can also begin with the element name, a specific attribute name, and an attribute value, as shown on the second line.

```
<ElementName>element specific content</ElementName>
<ElementName AttributeName="attribute value">element specific content</
ElementName>
```

HL7 Version 3, the most recent and sophisticated version of HL7, uses XML. This chapter will look at several parts of a complex HL7 V3 document to see how this works in practice and to further explore XML syntax in the health domain.

What follows is the transmission wrapper for an HL7 V3 message. It specifies the message type, the trigger event, and the receiver's responsibilities, illustrating how, in HL7 V3, process and workflow is becoming part of the standard. The receiver section of this part of the message is indented and colored. Even in XML, it is quite cryptic.

```
<POLB_IN224200 ITSVersion="XML_1.0" xmlns="urn:hl7-org:v3"
xmlns:xsi="http://www.w3.org/2001/XMLSchema-instance">
<id root="2.16.840.1.113883.19.1122.7" extension="CNTRL-3456"/>
<creationTime value="200202150930-0400"/>
<!-- The version of the datatypes/RIM/vocabulary used is that of May 2006 -->
<versionCode code="2006-05"/>
<!-- interaction id= Observation Event Complete, w/o Receiver Responsibilities -->
<interactionId root="2.16.840.1.113883.1.6" extension="POLB_IN224200"/>
<processingCode code="P"/>
<processingModeCode nullFlavor="OTH"/>
<acceptAckCode code="ER"/>
   <receiver typeCode="RCV">
   <device classCode="DEV" determinerCode="INSTANCE">
   <id extension="GHH LAB" root="2.16.840.1.113883.19.1122.1"/>
   <asLocatedEntity classCode="LOCE">
   <location classCode="PLC" determinerCode="INSTANCE">
   <id root="2.16.840.1.113883.19.1122.2" extension="ELAB-3"/>
   </location>
   </asLocatedEntity>
   </device>
   </receiver>
<sender typeCode="SND">
<device classCode="DEV" determinerCode="INSTANCE">
<id root="2.16.840.1.113883.19.1122.1" extension="GHH OE"/>
<asLocatedEntity classCode="LOCE">
<location classCode="PLC" determinerCode="INSTANCE">
<id root="2.16.840.1.113883.19.1122.2" extension="BLDG24"/>
</location>
</asLocatedEntity>
</device>
</sender>
<! -- Trigger Event Control Act & Domain Content -- >
</POLB_IN224200>
```

(HL7 2013a)

Here is the Trigger Event Control Act Wrapper (a wrapper within a wrapper in this context):

```
<controlActProcess classCode="CACT" moodCode="EVN">
<code code="POLB_TE224200" codeSystem="2.16.840.1.113883.1.18"/>
<subject typeCode="SUBJ" contextConductionInd="false">
<!-- domain content -->
</subject>
</controlActProcess>
```

(HL7 2013a)

The ISO Object Identifier (OID) code is yellow in this example. The International Standards Organization (ISO) describes OIDs as "paths in a tree structure, with the left-most number representing the root and the right-most number representing a leaf. The leaf may represent a registration authority (in which case the OID identifies the authority), or an instance of an object" (HL7 2013b). This particular OID—2.16.840.1.113883.1.18—codes for a leaf: the trigger event.

The trigger event is optional and is used when information about the interaction that led to the creation of a message needs to be communicated to the receiver along with the message. Examples include a query or a request to a master patient index, both of which require a response. The date and time the trigger event occurred, as well as the responsible parties for the trigger event are not present in this example but can be included in the trigger event wrapper.

Here is the same lab test we looked at earlier:

```
<observationEvent>
<id root="2.16.840.1.113883.19.1122.4" extension="1045813"
assigningAuthorityName="GHH LAB Filler Orders"/>
<code code="1554-5" codeSystemName="LN"
   codeSystem="2.16.840.1.113883.6.1"
displayName="GLUCOSE^POST 12H CFST:MCNC:PT:SER/PLAS:QN"/>
<statusCode code="completed"/>
<effectiveTime value="200202150730"/>
<priorityCode code="R"/>
<confidentialityCode code="N"
codeSystem="2.16.840.1.113883.5.25"/>
<value xsi:type="PQ" value="182" unit="mg/dL"/>
   <interpretationCode code="H"/>
<referenceRange>
<interpretationRange>
<value xsi:type="IVL_PQ">
   <low value="70" unit="mg/dL"/>
   <high value="105" unit="mg/dL"/>
</value>
<interpretationCode code="N"/>
</interpretationRange>
</referenceRange>
```

(HL7 2013a)

In this XML version, not only is the code (1554-5) specified (and identified as a code) but the coding system is also specified since 2.16.840.1.113883.6.1 is the OID designation for LOINC, the coding system for lab tests from which 1554-5 derives. The test and the results are described as in the EDI version, but in EDI, there was just an H that had to be interpreted as meaning the results are high. Here, <interpretationCode code="H"/> explicitly indicates that H is an interpretation of the result and the normal range follows, which is a much more human readable and useful form than in the EDI. For example, the high and low numbers are specified along with their specific units (<low value="70" unit="mg/dL"/>).

International Classification of Diseases (ICD)

The ICD is the oldest of the data standards. In fact, its history can be traced back to the mid-fifteenth century in northern Italy, a period where there had been a great plague. For the first time, death certificates from the victims of the plague were used as a source of data for analysis. In the mid-1600s, John Graunt, one of the first demographers, published *Natural and Political Observations Made Upon the Bills of Mortality* (Graunt 1662), an analysis of bills of mortality in London for the purpose of determining why children died. This was essentially the same idea: using mortality data to gain knowledge about health, at least at a population level, the precursor to today's public health. The 1700s saw the beginning of the first national registration systems for births, deaths, and certain diseases. England passed a national registration act in 1837. Massachusetts was the first state in the United States to do the same in 1842. Not long thereafter, with this data becoming available, people saw the need to classify the information, to achieve a degree of consistency, and to organize it into a more manageable form. One long list would be unwieldy to work with, so there needed to be some internal classification of the information. William Farr first proposed this in 1844:

> The advantages of a uniform nomenclature, however imperfect, are so obvious, that it is surprising no attention has been paid to its enforcement in Bills of Mortality. Each disease has, in many instances, been denoted by three or four terms, and each term has been applied to as many different diseases: vague, inconvenient names have been employed, or complications have been registered instead of primary diseases. The nomenclature is of as much importance in this department of enquiry as weights and measures in the physical sciences, and should be settled without delay. (Farr 1844)

Surprisingly, his well-reasoned idea received scant attention at the time. From today's perspective, this is the foundation of the interoperability problem we are still dealing with 175 year later. Interestingly enough, the triggering event to making this happen was the Great Exposition of 1851, where various countries presented displays that could be compared, if comparable data was provided. This led to discussion of the need for standards for cross-country statistical comparison. This led to the idea of meeting internationally to create a uniform classification of diseases. The first meeting was in 1853, with a second in 1855, where the issue of how this data could be grouped was a topic. Marc d'Espine proposed a grouping according to the nature of diseases: gouty, herpetic, hematic, and so on (WHO 1997). These are not terms we use to group diseases today (or, in most cases, use at all). William Farr proposed using five groups, according to the cause of diseases: epidemic diseases, constitutional (general) diseases, local diseases arranged according to anatomical site, developmental diseases, and diseases directly resulting from violence (Farr 1856). In 1893, Alphonse Bertillon proposed the first reasonably clinically correct grouping:

- General diseases
- Diseases of nervous system and sense organs
- Diseases of circulatory system
- Diseases of respiratory system
- Diseases of digestive system
- Diseases of genitourinary system
- Puerperal diseases
- Diseases of skin and annexes
- Diseases of locomotor organs

- Malformations
- Diseases of early infancy
- Diseases of old age
- Effects of external causes
- Ill-defined diseases (American Public Health Association 1899)

The categorical organization of the list of diseases in use today is not remarkably different from this list. In 1899 the decision was made to revisit disease categorization every ten years so that advances in knowledge and understanding could be incorporated. This led to the decennial cycle for revising the ICDs organized by WHO, the group that maintains and revises them.

The most recent revision, done in 1994, is ICD-10, the 10th revision. The 11th revision of the classification has started and will continue until 2015. ICD-10 is remarkable in being much more detailed than any of the prior versions. It has expanded to about 8,000 categories, compared with approximately 5,000 in ICD–9, showing more information for many types and sites of disease. This allows for a much more detailed specification of medical problems and their sites.

ICD-10-CM consists of more than 68,000 diagnosis codes and will be the United States' clinical modification of WHO's ICD-10. According to the AMA, the term "clinical" is used to

> emphasize the modification's intent: to serve as a useful tool in the area of classification of morbidity data for indexing of health records, medical care review, and ambulatory and other health care programs, as well as for basic health statistics. To describe the clinical picture of the patient the codes must be more precise than those needed only for statistical groupings and trend analysis. (Buck 2013)

ICD-10-CM provides code titles and language that compliment accepted clinical practice in the United States. WHO Collaborating Center for the Family of International Classifications in North America is housed at the National Center for Health Statistics (NCHS) belonging to the Centers for Disease Control and Prevention (CDC), and it is responsible for the implementation of ICD and serves as the US liaison to the WHO.

Here are the top-level disease categories from ICD-10. The entries that most closely correspond to Bertillon's proposal are bolded to show the similarities:

- A00–B99 Certain infectious and parasitic diseases
- C00–D49 Neoplasms
- D50–D89 Diseases of the blood and blood-forming organs and certain disorders involving the immune mechanism
- E00–E89 Endocrine, nutritional and metabolic diseases
- F01–F99 Mental, Behavioral and Neurodevelopmental disorders
- G00–G99 **Diseases of the nervous system**
- H00–H59 Diseases of the eye and adnexa
- H60–H95 Diseases of the ear and mastoid process
- I00–I99 **Diseases of the circulatory system**
- J00–J99 **Diseases of the respiratory system**
- K00–K95 **Diseases of the digestive system**
- L00–L99 **Diseases of the skin and subcutaneous tissue**

- M00–M99 **Diseases of the musculoskeletal system and connective tissue**
- N00–N99 **Diseases of the genitourinary system**
- O00–O9A Pregnancy, childbirth and the puerperium
- P00–P96 Certain conditions originating in the perinatal period
- Q00–Q99 **Congenital malformations, deformations and chromosomal abnormalities**
- R00–R99 Symptoms, signs and abnormal clinical and laboratory findings, not elsewhere classified
- S00–T88 Injury, poisoning and certain other consequences of external causes
- V00–Y99 **External causes of morbidity**
- Z00–Z99 Factors influencing health status and contact with health services

However, the ICD-10 code structure is quite different from any prior versions. As shown in figure 5.7, there is now up to a seven character code for each item that allows for the specification of a great deal of detail not available in prior versions of ICD. All codes require the first three characters, and many have four, five, six, or even seven characters. The first three characters specify the category, the next three provide clinical detail, and the last character can be used for various purposes depending on the category.

Figure 5.7   This illustration shows the structure and subparts of an ICD-10 code.

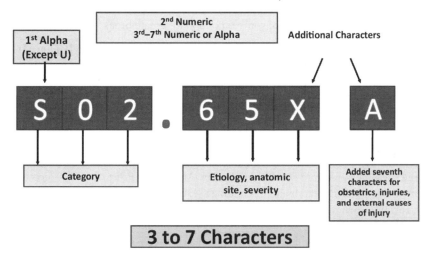

Here is an example of how a code becomes more specific with the additional characters:

Code	Description	Purpose
M1A	Ideopathic Chronic Gout	Category
M1A.06	Knee	Anatomical site
M1A.061	Right Knee	Laterality
M1A.0611	With Tophus	Clinical detail

This example illustrates the coding and shows that ICD-10-CM has become an ontology representing clinical relationships:

M1A.0611—Ideopathic chronic gout of the right knee with tophus (tophi)

The first three characters (M1A) is the "Category" (in this case "idiopathic chronic gout"); the fourth and fifth characters ("0" and "6") represent the clinical detail and anatomic site (in this case "knee"); the sixth character ("1") indicates the right or left side (in this case the right knee); and the seventh character ("1") provides the additional information (in this case there is also a tophus—a deposit of monosodium urate crystals that forms in people with long standing gout).

A key difference from ICD-9-CM is that in ICD-10-CM laterality can be expressed. In ICD-9-CM, there was no designation for a malignant neoplasm of the central portion of the right breast versus the left breast. These ICD-10-CM codes show how this is now provided:

- C50 Malignant neoplasm of breast
- C50.1 Malignant neoplasm of central portion of breast
- C50.111 Malignant neoplasm of central portion of right female breast
- C50.112 Malignant neoplasm of central portion of left female breast

The equivalent section of ICD-9-CM is shown here for comparison and provides no way to code for which breast is affected:

- 174 Malignant neoplasm of female breast
- 174.1 Malignant neoplasm of central portion of female breast

Most of the world is in the process of converting or has converted to ICD-10. It is in 43 languages, and more than 100 countries use it to report their mortality data. Approximately 70 percent of global health payments are done using ICD-10 (WHO 2013). The US deadline for conversion was pushed out a year from October 1, 2013, to October 1, 2014 (the beginning of federal fiscal year, when the annual Medicare financial cycle starts).

SNOMED CT

SNOMED was derived from work done by Dr. Arnold W. Pratt, the first director of the Division of Computer Research and Technology (DCRT), which is now the Center for Information Technology at the National Institutes of Health in Washington, DC. Dr. Pratt was a pathologist, and his goal was for his colleagues to be able to dictate their reports and a computer (in the early 1970s) could recognize the clinical concepts in the reports and encode them so they would be much more useful for research purposes. It was originally implemented on an IBM 7094, a powerful mainframe computer of that era. Since it was limited to pathology, it was called the Systematized Nomenclature of Pathology (SNOP) but, over the years, it evolved substantially into SNOMED. Drs. Roger A. Côte of the University of Sherbrooke and David Rothwell of the Medical College of Wisconsin (and the American College of Pathology) were the key people in nurturing SNOP into SNOMED over a period of many years.

As opposed to a classification system, SNOMED is an ontology, encompassing concepts and their attributes, which consist of relationships to other concepts. SNOMED CT is limited to terms and relationships used in clinical practice, each of which is represented as a triplet of concept, attribute, and concept.

Concepts, a basic unit of SNOMED CT, have clinical meaning and have a unique numeric identifier (ConceptId) that never changes and a unique human-readable, fully

Figure 5.8   An illustration showing that SNOMED-CT can code at various levels of clinical detail.

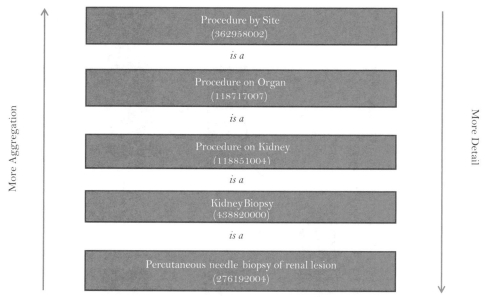

Source: Adapted from IHTSDO 2013.

specified name (FSN). They can be coded at many levels of granularity, as illustrated in figure 5.8. A second basic unit called Relationships links SNOMED CT concepts as defining, qualifying, historical, or additional. These relationships are expressed as "| is a |" as illustrated in this example:

Fracture of tarsal bone (disorder) | is defined as:
```
    | is a | subtype of | Fracture of foot (disorder) |
    and has | finding site | | Bone structure of tarsus (body structure) | ;
    and has | associated morphology | | Fracture (morphologic abnormality)
```
(IHTSDO 2013b)

A third basic unit is Attribute Relationships, associations between two concepts that specify a defining characteristic of one of the concepts (the source of the relationship). Each Attribute Relationship has a name (the type of relationship) and a value (the destination of the relationship). Here is an example:

Definition of |Pneumonia (disorder)|
```
| is a | = | infectious disease of lung |
    , | is a | = | pneumonia |
    , | pathological process | = | infectious process |
    , { | associated morphology | = | inflammation |
    , | associated morphology | = | consolidation |
    , | finding site | = | lung structure | }
```
(IHTSDO 2013b)

Figure 5.9 illustrates SNOMED relationships using bacterial pneumonia as the use case. Keep in mind that | is a | Relationships relate a concept to more general concepts of

Figure 5.9   An illustration showing that different SNOMED-CT clinical concepts representing body structures, clinical findings, and organisms can be combined to illustrate a medical process. In this case bacteria triggers an inflammatory reaction affecting both kidneys of a patient.

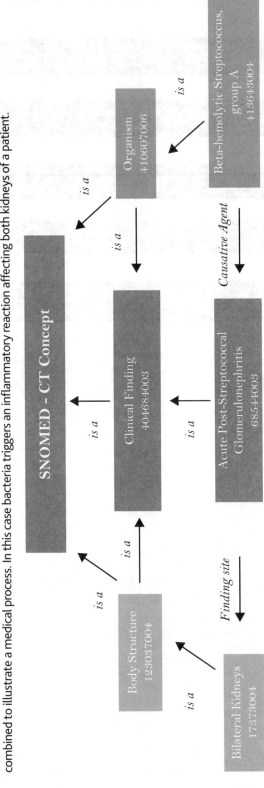

the same type. In contrast, Attribute Relationships (such as | Finding site | and | Causative agent |) relate a concept to relevant values in other branches of the subtype hierarchy.

While it may be only a subset of SNOMED, SNOMED CT is still very large and consists of 311,000 concepts connected by over 1.3 million relationships (IHTSDO 2013a). Given its complexity, exploring SNOMED CT requires a specialized browser, several of which are freely available on the Internet. Figure 5.10 shows a screenshot from a browser searching the concept of "bacterial pneumonia" (a disorder with SNOMED concept ID 53084003 and a FSN of "Bacterial pneumonia [disorder]").

This is a disorder, and above it the browser indicates that its "parents" (further up the granularity tree) are "Bacterial lower respiratory infection (disorder)" and "Infective pneumonia (disorder)." It lists eight "children" (further down the granularity tree); the first of which is "Bacterial pneumonia associated with AIDS (disorder)."

To the right are a number of defining relationships (remember this is the first of the four types of Relationships). From these one can gain an understanding of where this disorder fits within the broader framework of SNOMED and medicine. For example, it is an "Infectious Process" of the "Lung Structure" associated with "Consolidation" and "Inflammation." This indicates the power of this information to support sophisticated queries and retrievals in a computer-stored clinical database.

HL7 Version 3 is reasonably interoperable with SNOMED, since it incorporates many of the same attributes and concepts, and there is a similar interoperability between SNOMED and ICD-10-CM. As shown in figure 5.11, there are mapping tools that can link these ontologies. However, as shown in the figure, there are cases where additional data is required for billing that is not a part of SNOMED CT.

Ontologies find a natural home within the evolving semantic web in which representations of relationships among data elements is a key goal. For example, one group has developed an XML representation of ICD-10 (Hoelzer et al. 2002). The semantic web community wants to incorporate healthcare into its evolving framework. Eric Gordon Prud'hommeaux of the World Wide Web Consortium (W3C), an international effort to develop web standards, says that much of the new Consolidated CDA (CCDA or CDA® Release 2) has been mapped into Resource Description Framework (RDF), a standard model for data interchange on the web (New Health Project 2013).

There could be a convergence of these major coding systems in the future. Such a system could become an essential component of a new semantic web for healthcare. However, it may yet be quite some time before this is sorted out.

Health Level 7 (HL7)

HL7 was discussed earlier to illustrate the technologic evolution of standards. This section will go into much more detail, but HL7 is an immensely complex topic that can only be covered at a high level in this text.

HL7 was founded in 1987 with the objective of creating a reasonably integrated hospital information system from independently developed sub-systems. In those early days hospitals bought systems from many different vendors because, for the most part, no company had solid solutions for all the various departments of the hospital. Hospitals still buy modular software solutions but, to a much larger degree, they buy their core systems from a single company. These modern enterprise systems are developed by (or at least marketed and supported by) a single vendor, and generally their sub-systems integrate at least reasonably well with each other, but that was not true years ago. Back then there was an enormous problem with how to make a lab system which supported the area of the hospital

Figure 5.10   A SNOMED-CT browser shows bacterial pneumonia parents, children, and relationships.

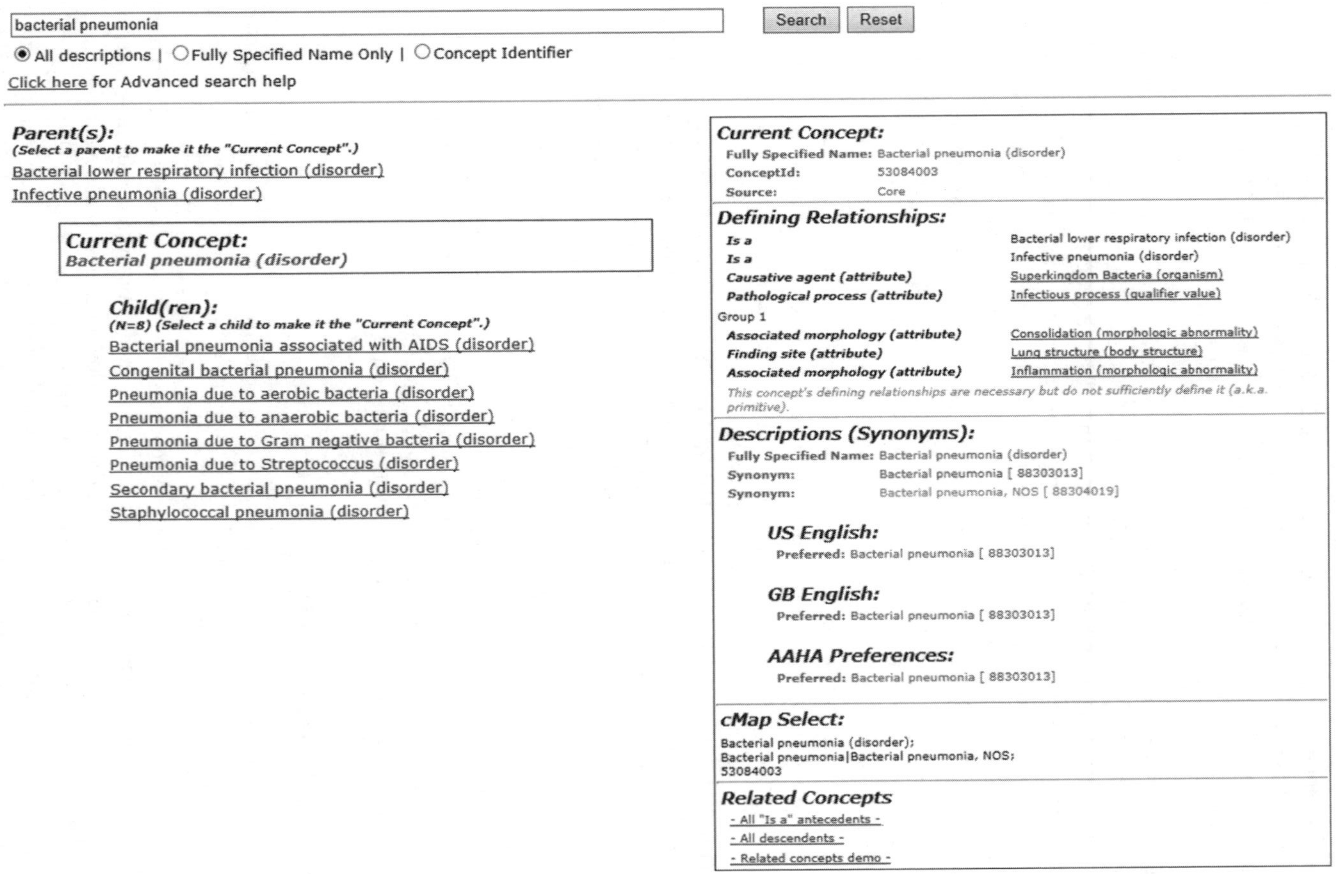

bacterial pneumonia

[Search] [Reset]

● All descriptions | ○ Fully Specified Name Only | ○ Concept Identifier

Click here for Advanced search help

Parent(s):
(Select a parent to make it the "Current Concept".)
Bacterial lower respiratory infection (disorder)
Infective pneumonia (disorder)

Current Concept:
Bacterial pneumonia (disorder)

Child(ren):
(N=8) (Select a child to make it the "Current Concept".)
Bacterial pneumonia associated with AIDS (disorder)
Congenital bacterial pneumonia (disorder)
Pneumonia due to aerobic bacteria (disorder)
Pneumonia due to anaerobic bacteria (disorder)
Pneumonia due to Gram negative bacteria (disorder)
Pneumonia due to Streptococcus (disorder)
Secondary bacterial pneumonia (disorder)
Staphylococcal pneumonia (disorder)

Current Concept:
Fully Specified Name: Bacterial pneumonia (disorder)
ConceptId: 53084003
Source: Core

Defining Relationships:
Is a   Bacterial lower respiratory infection (disorder)
Is a   Infective pneumonia (disorder)
Causative agent (attribute)   Superkingdom Bacteria (organism)
Pathological process (attribute)   Infectious process (qualifier value)
Group 1
Associated morphology (attribute)   Consolidation (morphologic abnormality)
Finding site (attribute)   Lung structure (body structure)
Associated morphology (attribute)   Inflammation (morphologic abnormality)
This concept's defining relationships are necessary but do not sufficiently define it (a.k.a. primitive).

Descriptions (Synonyms):
Fully Specified Name: Bacterial pneumonia (disorder)
Synonym: Bacterial pneumonia [88303013]
Synonym: Bacterial pneumonia, NOS [883040019]

   US English:
   Preferred: Bacterial pneumonia [88303013]

   GB English:
   Preferred: Bacterial pneumonia [88303013]

   AAHA Preferences:
   Preferred: Bacterial pneumonia [88303013]

cMap Select:
Bacterial pneumonia (disorder):
Bacterial pneumonia|Bacterial pneumonia, NOS:
53084003

Related Concepts
- All "is a" antecedents -
- All descendents -
- Related concepts demo -

Used with permission from VTSL, a division of the Veterinary Medical Informatics Laboratory at the Virginia-Maryland Regional College of Veterinary Medicine.

Figure 5.11   An example of an ICD-10 to SNOMED mapping tool illustrates that, for billing purposes, additional ICD codes may be required.

SNOMED-CT	ICD-10-CM Code	ICD-10-CM Name
Diabetes mellitus type 2 (44054006)		
	E11.9	Type 2 diabetes mellitus without complications

ICD notes for "Type 2 diabetes mellitus"

Use additional code to identify any insulin use (Z79.4)

Source: NLM 2013

that did clinical tests, licensed from one company, communicate with a nursing station–based physician-order entry system where the test would actually be ordered and licensed from another company, and how to make them both talk to a billing system that would charge for the test and was licensed from yet a third company. Beyond the separate corporate origins, these systems would typically utilize different technologies that packaged data in different formats and used different representations for the same or similar data elements.

The original concept for HL7 was to develop messaging standards to solve this problem. Today it is an international organization with affiliates in some 40 countries. While it historically charged a fee, the standards are now freely available. The name derives from the open systems interconnection model, which is used in networks and virtually any situation where technologies have to interoperate with other technologies. The model exists at seven layers and the top layer—level seven—is where the data is presented in usable form to the end user. HL7 is named for that top layer, an indication that its focus is on the end users—clinical, financial, and administrative employees of a health enterprise.

HL7 Development Framework

The HL7 Development Framework (HDF) is the architecture within which the HL7 standards are developed. In essence HDF is a standard for developing standards. HDF is intended to specify information models, data types, and vocabularies; messaging, clinical documents, and context management specification; and implementation technology, profile, and conformance specifications. The Unified Modeling Language (UML) is the preferred syntax. The UML is a graphical language for visualizing, specifying, constructing, and documenting the artifacts of a software-intensive system.

Figure 5.12 shows the HDF—the process through which these standards are developed—involves collaboration among the many people involved. It defines a process of initiation, analysis, design, peer review, and hopefully, implementation and testing.

Reference Implementation Model (RIM)

The Reference Implementation Model (RIM) is an HL7 component that seeks to provide a conceptual model of healthcare. It provides diagrammatic representations of the clinical domains in which HL7 operates. With Version 3, HL7 is now moving toward the definition of standards and ways of representing processes and workflow. To accomplish this, it is important to have a representation of those processes and workflows in order to

Figure 5.12   This illustration presents a diagrammatic representation of the HL7 Development Framework (HDF).

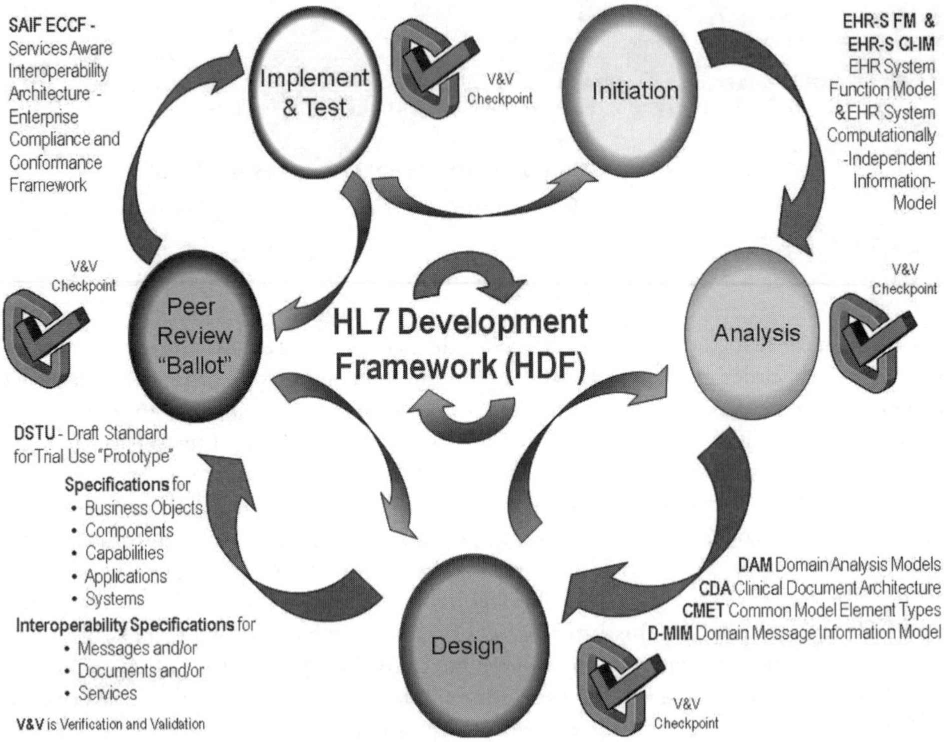

©Health Level Seven International, reprinted with permission from HL7.

understand the data that is needed and the required flows of that data among and between those involved. This is a principle goal of the RIM.

The RIM guides the data content needed in a specific clinical or administrative context or use cases. It includes an explicit representation of the semantic interconnections between the information that will be carried in the HL7 messages and the documents and services associated with them. The development framework documents the processes, the tools, the actors, and the rules involved in processes and work flow.

The RIM is built from six core classes:

- **Act:** actions in care delivery (for example, appendectomy, serum sodium measurement)
  - ○ **ActRelationship:** relationship between two Acts (for example, causality, indication)
- **Participation:** who performed an Act, for whom it was done, where it was done (for example, attending physician)
- **Role**: the roles that entities play as they participate in healthcare acts (for example, patient, family member)
  - ○ **RoleLink:** dependency between two Roles (for example, one role has authority over another role).
- **Entity:** the physical things and beings that are of interest to and take part in healthcare (for example, person, organization)

These classes are intended to be the basis upon which processes are described. They are, of course, interrelated. Every happening is an Act (procedures, observations, medications orders). Acts are related through an ActRelationship (composition, preconditions, revisions, support). Participation defines the context for an Act (author, performer, subject, location). The participants have Roles (patient, provider, practitioner, specimen, employee), which can have dependencies (RoleLink). Roles are played by Entities (persons, organizations, material, places, devices).

Three of the six classes—acts, entities, and roles—can have further specifications assigned to them. Acts are at the center of things so they are the focus here. Acts are divided into classes, such as:

- **ENC**—Encounter
- **OBS**—Observation (lab)
- **SBADM**—Substance Administration (pharmacy admin)
- **SPLY**—Supply (pharmacy dispense)
- **CLINDOC**—Document

Acts have codes that can be from an external coding system, so that, for example, an OBS Act might be a lab test with a LOINC code.

An Act can have a "mood" defined as "specifying whether the Act is an activity that has happened, can happen, is happening, is intended to happen, or is requested/demanded to happen" (Beeler 2011).

Principle Act Moods include:

- **definition (DEF)**—definition of an act
- **intent (INT)**—an intention to plan or perform an act
- **request (RQO)**—a request or order for a service from a request "placer" to a request "fulfiller"
- **promise (PRMS)**—intent to perform that has the strength of a commitment
- **confirmation (CNF)**—promise that has been solicited via an order **event (EVN)**—an Act that actually happens, includes the documentation (report) of the event (Beeler 2011)

Acts have relationships (ActRelationship), such as:

COMP—has component	**ARR**—arrived by
PERT—has pertinent info	**SUCC**—succeeds
SEQL—is sequel	**RPLC**—replaces
OPTN—has option	**OCCR**—occurrence
FLFS—fulfills	**REFV**—has reference values
RSON—has reason	**AUTH**—authorized by
INST—instantiates	**COST**—has cost
PRCN—has precondition	**GOAL**—has goal
OUTC—has outcome	**PREV**—has previous instance

(Beeler 2011)

Figure 5.13   This illustration presents a small part of a larger example of the HL7 Reference Information Model (RIM).

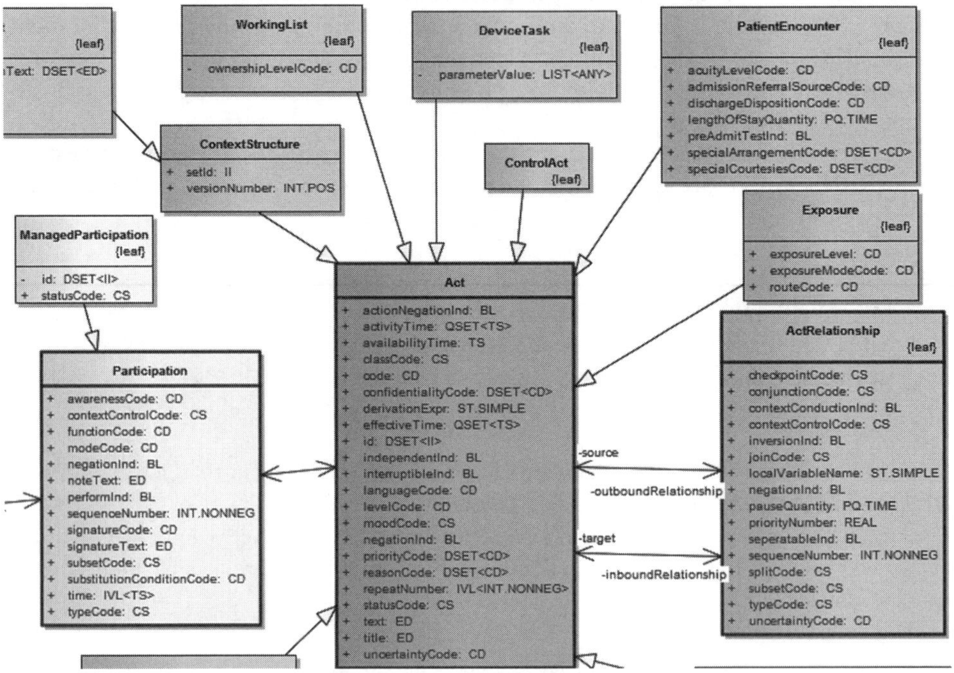

Source: ©Health Level Seven International, reprinted with permission from HL7.

Figure 5.13 is a small example of the RIM. At the top of some of these boxes, one of these six core classes is specified. This is a framework for diagramming complex clinical processes.

Consolidated Clinical Document Architecture (CCDA)

HL7 provides specific standards for messages, documents, and services. The CCDA is the key electronic format for sharing of clinical documents. The Continuity of Care Document (CCD) is a CCDA architected document that is the key for transitions of care and for care coordination to manage chronic disease.

CCDA documents are developed based on the RIM. Here is a simple example of patient demographic data used to illustrate this:

Patient	Isabella Jones	Language	English
Date of birth	1-May-47	Sex	Female
Race	White	Ethnicity	Not Hispanic or Latino
Contact info	1122 Mystical Route 3 Beaverton, OR 97005, US Tel: 555-444-5555	Patient IDs	2.1

Source: Prud'hommeaux 2013

Here some of the information is represented within the RIM framework for a Role:

RecordTarget
[a rim:Participation ;
rim:Participation.typeCode [hl7:coding [dt:CDCoding.code "RCT" ; dt:CDCoding.codeSystem "???"]] ;
rim:Participation.act _:ClinicalDoc ;
rim:Participation.role _:ClinicalDoc_recordTarget0
] .
_:ClinicalDoc_recordTarget0 a rim:Role ;
rim:Role.id [a dt:DSET_II ;
dt:COLL.item [dt:II.root "2.100"]
] ;
rim:Role.player _:ClinicalDoc_recordTarget0_player ;
rim:Role.scoper _:ClinicalDoc_recordTarget0_scoper ;
rim:Role.classCode [hl7:coding [dt:**CDCoding.code "PAT"** ; dt:CDCoding.codeSystem "???"]] ;
rim:Role.telecom [a dt:COLL_TEL ; dt:COLL.item [a dt:TEL ; dt:URL.address "tel: **555-444-5555**" ; dt:TEL.use "HP" ;]];
rim:Role.addr [a dt:COLL_AD ;
err:streetAddressLine "**1122 Mystical Route 3**" ;
err:city "**Beaverton**" ;
err:state "**OR**" ;
err:postalCode "**97005**" ;
err:country "**US**" ;
] ;

Source: Prud'hommeaux 2013

PAT code is bolded indicating that the role is patient as well as the actual demographic data that has been brought into RIM and coded according to each data type.

Finally, here is the XML from the corresponding CCD:

```
# RecordTarget <xsl:apply-templates select="."mode="typedParticipation">
<xsl:with-param select="$actLabel"name="parttnLabel"/>
<xsl:with-param select="'RCT'"name="typeCode"/>
<xsl:with-param select="'patientRole'"name="roleTag"/>
<xsl:with-param select="'PAT'" name="roleCode"/>
<xsl:with-param select="'patient'" name="player1Tag"/>
<xsl:with-param select="'rim:Person'" name="player1Type"/>
<xsl:with-param select="'providerOrganization'" name="scoperTag"/>
<xsl:with-param select="'rim:Organization'" name="scoperType"/>
</xsl:apply-templates>
```

(Prud' hommeaux 2013)

HL7 Messages: HL7 Version 3 messages cover a large number of domains. Each of these is an identifiable and specialized part of a hospital or a healthcare delivery system, such as the lab, the pharmacy, the blood bank, patient scheduling, or of course, billing. The HL7 messages are in the EDI/X12 format we discussed previously with letter codes (which are in color here) indicating what is on each line (segment). Here is an example of a relatively simple HL7 ADT A04 Patient Registration message that would be sent to systems around a hospital when a new patient is admitted (so that, in the example given earlier, the laboratory, CPOE, and billing systems all have the same demographic data):

```
MSH|^~\&|ADT1|MCM|LABADT|MCM|198808181126|SECURITY|ADT^A01|MSG00001|P|2.4
EVN|A01-|198808181123
PID|||PATID1234^5^M11||JONES^WILLIAM^A^III||1961061
5|M-||2106-3|1200 N ELM STREET^^GREENSBORO^NC^27401-
1020|GL|(919)379-1212|(919)271-3434~(919)277-3114||S||PATID12345001^
2^M10|123456789|9-87654^NC
NK1|1|JONES^BARBARA^K|SPO|||||20011105
NK1|1|JONES^MICHAEL^A|FTH
PV1|1|I|2000^2012^01||||004777^LEBAUER^SIDNEY^J.|||SUR||-||1|A0-
AL1|1||^PENICILLIN||PRODUCES HIVES~RASH
AL1|2||^CAT DANDER
DG1|001|I9|1550|MAL NEO LIVER, PRIMARY|19880501103005|F||
PR1|2234|M11|111^CODE151|COMMON PROCEDURES|198809081123
ROL|45^RECORDER^ROLE MASTER LIST|AD|CP|KATE^SMITH^ELLEN|199505011201
GT1|1122|1519|BILL^GATES^A
IN1|001|A357|1234|BCMD|||||132987
IN2|ID1551001|SSN12345678
```

(HL7 2013a)

The MSH segment is the Message Header, containing information such as the sending and receiving facilities and the date and time of the message. It is always the first segment in an HL7 message. The EVN or Event Type segment indicates that this is an HL7 A01—Admit/visit notification—message.

HL7 includes the important concept of Medical Document Management Trigger Events: When was a document created? When did its status change? When was it edited? When was it replaced? When was it cancelled? The event codes are shown here along with the associated message type:

Document Event	Notice	Notice & Content
Creation	T01	T02
Status Change	T03	T04
Addendum	T05	T06
Editing	T07	T08
Replacement	T09	T10
Cancellation	T11	

Here is an example of a T01 Document Creation message:

```
MSH|^~\&|MedOne|FACILITY A|CARECENTER^HL7NOTES|HFH|20060105180000|
D61AFEF1-B10E-11D5-8666-0004ACD80749|MDM^T01|20060105180000999999|T|2.3
EVN|T01|20060105180000
PID|1||1112388^BS||ESPARZA^MARIA
PV1|1|O|BS^15^15
TXA|1|GENNOTES|TX|200601051800|50041^SMITH^CHRIS^M|
200601051800|200601051800|200601051800|||SC^ROBINSON^JESSICA^A|1234567890||
||FILE0001.TXT|PR
```

(HL7 2013a)

One should easily be able to verify that this message concerns the creation of a transcription document (File0001.TXT as indicated in the TXA segment) related to a visit (PV1) by Maria Esparza (PID) who saw Chris M. Smith on January 5, 2006. One can do this by reviewing the following table, which brings together the description of the fields in a TXA segment with the matching data from this example:

Field Name	Data from this Example
Set ID - TXA	1
Document Type	GENNOTES
Document Content Presentation	TX
Activity Date/Time	200601051800 (6PM on January 5, 2006)
Primary Activity Provider Code/Name	50041/Chris M Smith
Origination Date/Time	200601051800 (6PM on January 5, 2006)
Transcription Date/Time	200601051800 (6PM on January 5, 2006)
Edit Date/Time repeating	200601051800 (6PM on January 5, 2006)
Originator Code/Name	
Assigned Document Authenticator	
Transcriptionist Code/Name	SC/Jessica A Robinson
Unique Document Number	1234567890
Parent Document Number	
Place Order Number	
Filler Order Number	
Unique Document File Name	FILE0001.TXT
Document Completion Status	PR
Document Confidentiality Status	
Document Availability Status	
Document St(OR)age Status	
Document Change Reason	
Authentication Person, Time Stamp	
Distributed Copies (Code and Name of Recipients)	

FHIR: The future of interoperability (and HL7 messaging) may well be defined by the Fast Health Interoperable Resources (FHIR®) initiative. This effort is intended to harness the latest web standards (such as RESTful APIs) combined with a defined set of resources that derive from the RIM to facilitate and substantially simplify the implementation of interoperability solutions. FHIR is being made available as a Draft Standard for Trial Use and, based on the results of the trial, HL7 expects to release a full specification by 2015. Interested readers should keep up with this effort at the FHIR site (http://www.hl7.org/implement/standards/fhir/) and may well even wish to become trial users. Recommended

Readings at the end of this chapter provides links to sites with more about FHIR for more technically inclined readers.

Integrating the Healthcare Enterprise (IHE)

Integrating the Healthcare Enterprise (IHE) is focused on healthcare process and workflow. IHE is not a standard setting organization or a certifying authority. Its goal is to create a nomenclature and use it to represent processes and workflows in order to integrate heterogeneous information systems. At present IHE covers the following domains:

Anatomic Pathology (ANAPATH)   Patient Care Coordination (PCC)

Cardiology (CARD)   Patient Care Device (PCD)

Dental (DENT)   Pharmacy (PHARM)

Endoscopy (ENDO)   Quality, Research and Public Health (QRPH)

Eye Care (EYECARE)   Radiation Oncology (RO)

IT Infrastructure (ITI)   Radiology (RAD)

Laboratory (LAB)

(IHE 2012)

Integration profiles are a key concept within IHE and are described in the IHE IT Infrastructure Technical Framework document as follows:

> IHE IT Infrastructure Integration Profiles offer a common language that healthcare professionals and vendors can use to discuss integration needs of healthcare enterprises and the integration capabilities of information systems in precise terms. Integration Profiles specify implementations of standards that are designed to meet identified clinical needs. They enable users and vendors to state which IHE capabilities they require or provide, by reference to the detailed specifications of the IHE IT Infrastructure Technical Framework.
>
> Integration profiles are defined in terms of IHE Actors and transactions. Actors are information systems or components of information systems that produce, manage, or act on information associated with clinical and operational activities in the enterprise.
>
> Transactions are interactions between actors that communicate the required information through standards-based messages. Vendor products support an Integration Profile by implementing the appropriate actor(s) and transactions. A given product may implement more than one actor and more than one integration profile. (IHE 2012)

Each IHE Integration Profile is defined by the IHE actors involved and the specific set of IHE transactions exchanged by each IHE actor. An actor can be a person (for example, the physician) or a system (for example, the EMR). The requirements are presented in the form of a table of transactions required for each actor supporting the Integration Profile. A very simple example involving a profile in which a user is requesting a series of electronic documents (IHE 2012).

Figure 5.14 is the transaction process flow diagram of a cardiac care scenario that spans about 3 weeks of a patient's cardiac episode. The patient presents to their primary

Figure 5.14   This illustration presents an example of an IHE process flow diagram using a cardiac care example.

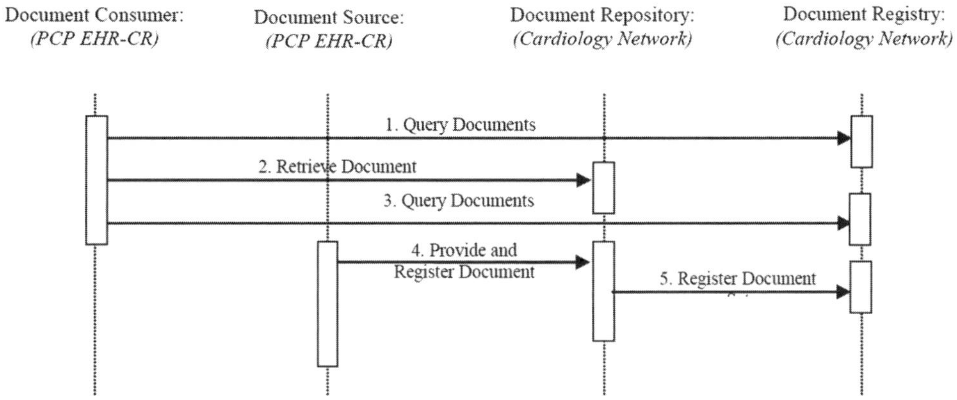

Document Consumer: *(PCP EHR-CR)*	Document Source: *(PCP EHR-CR)*	Document Repository: *(Cardiology Network)*	Document Registry: *(Cardiology Network)*

care provider (PCP) with complaints of shortness of breath, nausea, tiredness, and chest pains. This doctor works closely with a local hospital that has recently established a cardiac care network that allows PCPs, cardiologists, laboratories, and two local hospitals to share clinical documents to improve patient care. This cardiac network is part of a local care data exchange community that has been set up and to which the care plan to which this patient belongs has encouraged patients to subscribe. The patient has been provided a health record account number.

During the patient examination, the PCP records the complaint and determines that he should perform an ECG. The process for doing this might be as follows:

> He queries the cardiac care network to find any prior ECG reports (step 1 in figure 5.14), using a coded document class "report" and a coded practice setting "cardiology" established by the cardiac care network for ECG reports.
>
> Among the matching documents he locates a prior ECG report that is then retrieved (step 2 in figure 5.14). He compares the two results and determines that the patient should be referred to a cardiologist.
>
> He searches for additional reports in the cardiac care network for this patient, but finds none (step 3 in figure 5.14).
>
> Using the ambulatory EHR system, he creates a submission request for a "PCP office visit" that includes a submission set consisting of three new documents (visit note, referral letter, new ECG report) and of one reference to the prior ECG report (step 4 in figure 5.14). Following the Cardiology Network Cross Enterprise Document Exchange (XDS) Affinity Domain policy, he creates a "cardiac assessment" folder to contain all four documents in order to facilitate collaboration with the cardiologist.
>
> The repository used by the ambulatory EHR system will then register the documents that are part of this submission request (step 5 in figure 5.14). (Integrating the Healthcare Enterprise 2012)

These are simple examples, but they illustrate that IHE profiles have the concept of actors and transactions and IHE has developed their own schema for representing them.

The representation and, ultimately, modeling of process and workflow is of interest to many groups and organizations and in many respects is one of the new frontiers for standards and interoperability.

Document Standards

The CCDA specifies the general format of digital health documents for electronic exchange. The specific content of those documents is up to their designers, but the format is specified by CCDA, is encoded in XML, and is further defined by templates.

Templates are a critical component of CCDA. They are intended to provide reusable building blocks facilitating quicker implementation. Since they are modular, templates (such as blood pressure, discharge diagnosis) can be repackaged with other templates in any number of CCDA documents. Finally, templates provide for what HL7 calls "incremental interoperability," in that one can begin with a simple CCDA document and then add templates as needed.

Templates can be defined at three levels in a CCDA document:

- **Document-Level Templates**, such as CCD or Discharge Summary, can be utilized to define a template for the document as a whole.
- **Section-Level Templates**, such as Allergies or Medications, can be utilized to define what specific information will be included in each section of the document.
- **Entry-Level Templates**, such as specific Observations or Procedures, can be utilized to define how the information is encoded within each section.

CCDA is a successor to an earlier CDA standard. A review of eight existing CDA documents and their accompanying use cases (in general the documents were developed by different working groups each with the requisite domain knowledge) identified template inconsistencies and led to an effort to create a single, more consistent set of templates at all three levels. Introduced as CDA, Release 2.0 became the standard in May 2005, and it is now widely referred to as Consolidated CDA or CCDA (Dolin et al. 2006). It provides unified document-level templates, such as these (a complete list can be found at hl7.org):

- Continuity of Care Document
- Consultation Note
- Diagnostic Imaging Report
- Discharge Summary
- History and Physical (H&P) Note
- Operative Note
- Procedure Note
- Progress Note
- Unstructured Document

The major components of a CCDA specification are shown here and include the header and the body.

```
<ClinicalDocument>
    ... CDA Header ...
    <structuredBody>
```

```
          <section>
          <text> (a.k.a. "narrative block") </text>
          <observation> … </observation>
          <substanceAdministration>
             <supply> … </supply>
          </substanceAdministration>
          <observation>
             <externalObservation> … </externalObservation>
          </observation>
          </section>
          <section>
             <section> … </section>
          </section>
       <structuredBody>
     <ClinicalDocument>
```

(Dolin et al. 2006)

The header contains information about the patient, the author of the document, the creation of the document, and so on. The body contains the detailed clinical information. The contents of the document can be defined at three levels of structure:

- Unstructured data (PDF, Word files, or even a scanned image)
- XML with sections each identified with a code
- Entries encoded in ICD, LOINC, SNOMED CT, CPT, or other systems using the RIM

Thus the CCDA architecture encompasses everything from unstructured text to the most precisely coded clinical data. A single CCDA document could use all three levels of structure. An example might be an unstructured list of problems, expressed as free text by the provider. Above that, there might be an XML entry specifying that this section of the CDA document is an active problem list using the coding system LOINC (11450-4 is the LOINC code for a Problem List). A specific data-level example might be a specific coded piece of clinical data, such as an ICD-9 code for essential unspecified hypertension (401). So, diverse approaches to representing data and different coding systems can coexist in one CCDA document.

A CCDA *section-level* template for an objective finding on physical exam is shown here. This illustrates the use of both coded data—61149-1 is the LOINC code for objective data in narrative form—and the corresponding narrative data:

```
<section>
<templateId root="2.16.840.1.113883.10.20.21.2.1"/>
<codecode="61149-1" codeSystem="2.16.840.1.113883.6.1"
codeSystemName="LOINC"
displayName="OBJECTIVE DATA"/>
<title>OBJECTIVE DATA</title>
<text>
<list listType="ordered">
<item>Chest: clear to ausc. No rales, normal breath sounds</item>
<item>Heart: RR, PMI in normal location and no heave or evidence of
cardiomegaly,normal heart sounds, no murm or gallop</item>
</list>
</text>
</section>
```

(Confluence 2013)

Here is a CCDA *entry-level* template for recoding a patient's age:

```
<observation classCode="OBS" moodCode="EVN">
<templateId root="2.16.840.1.113883.10.20.22.4.31"/>
<!-- Age observation template -->
<code code="397659008" codeSystem="2.16.840.1.113883.6.96"
displayName="Age"/>
<statusCode code="completed"/>
<value xsi:type="PQ" value="57" unit="a"/>
</observation>
```

(ONC 2012. PHRI CDA Specification Version 0.2)

Here 397659008 is the SNOMED CT code for patient age and 2.16.840.1.113883.6.96 is the OID code for SNOMED CT. Type "PQ" indicates numeric data, and unit="a" indicates the number represents years, so you should easily be able to verify that this patient is 57 years old.

The goals are to promote the electronic exchange of clinical information while minimizing as much as possible the interoperability issues brought about by differences in data representation among the systems that produced the documents (or at least the information) being exchanged. XML encoded CCDA documents are machine readable, which can lead to machine parsing and, ultimately, use of the specific data elements as if they had been collected initially by the receiving system.

CCDA is compatible with the HL7 RIM process and with the Version 3 data types. CCDA is also intended to facilitate the use of data standards such as SNOMED and LOINC.

The Continuity of Care Document (CCD) is a key CCDA document. As the name implies, it is intended as a basic electronic summary record for use in patient referrals from one provider to the next or in transitions of care from one venue (for example, a hospital) to another (for example, a rehabilitation facility or home). As a result it is often referred to as a Patient Summary, rather than the CCD. The predecessor to the CCD was the Continuity of Care Record (CCR). The major difference between the CCR and CCD is that the CCR predated CDA. When the CDA architecture and the CCD came out, it was recognized that CCR and the CDA needed to be reconciled. This reconciliation was accomplished by collaborating on the design of the CCD, which became an ANSI standard in 2007. In essence the CCD can be thought of as the CCR redefined within the broader context of CDA. It is possible to convert a CCR to a CCD but it is generally a one-way conversion because the CCD supports functionality that is not represented in the CCR specification.

The CCD R2 Implementation Guide specifies the overall format of the CCD within the context of the CCDA and HL7, as shown in figure 5.15.

Like any standard within HL7 V3, the CCD is defined through the use of reusable templates:

Header	Encounters
Purpose	Plan of care
Problems	Payers
Procedures	Advance directives
Family history	Alerts
Social history	Medications
Vital signs	Immunizations
Functional stats	Medical equipment
Results	

Figure 5.15   The CCD is implemented using the CCDA (CDA R2) structure which, in turn, rests on other HL7 standards.

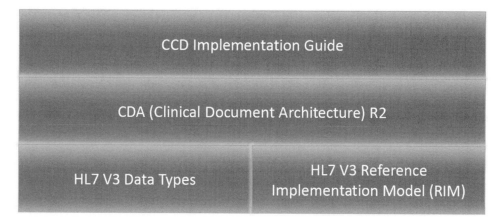

Structural format of the data   Data types, relationships,
                                         state transition model

Here are the first few lines of a template example for vital signs within a CCD:

```
<component>
<section>
<templateId root="2.16.840.1.113883.10.20.1.16" />
<!-- Vital signs section template -->
<code code="8716-3" codeSystem="2.16.840.1.113883.6.1"/>
<title>Vital Signs</title>
```

Vital signs are the basic physiologic measures taken when patients are seen by a provider and include temperature, pulse, respiration rate, blood pressure, and weight. This is in XML, so each code is specified as being part of a particular coding system via the OID number for that coding system. In the systolic blood pressure example shown here, two coding systems are used: LOINC (OID 2.16.840.1.113883.6.1) to specify that this is the Vital Signs section (8716-3), and then, in what follows, SNOMED CT (OID 2.16.840.1.113883.6.96) is used to specify that a specific item of data is the systolic blood pressure (SNOMED CT code 271649006). Note that the display name for "Systolic BP" is explicitly stated.

```
<observation classCode="OBS" moodCode="EVN">
<templateId root="2.16.840.1.113883.10.20.1.31" />
<!-- Result observation template -->
<id root="c6f88323-67ad-11db-bd13-0800200c9a66" />
<code code="271649006" codeSystem="2.16.840.1.113883.6.96"
displayName="Systolic BP" />
<statusCode code="completed" />
<effectiveTime value="19991114" />
<value xsi:type="PQ" value="132" unit="mm[Hg]" />
</observation>
```

(HL7 2009)

In discussing the difference between EDI/X12 and XML, it was said that XML is more verbose, but also much clearer. Both are illustrated here. The example uses a lot of characters to provide a simple systolic blood pressure reading. A human being can easily recognize that what follows the codes is the actual measurement—132 mm—of the systolic blood pressure.

It is worth repeating the CCD is an XML document that supports multiple data formats and is compatible with many existing applications browsers, EMRs, and even legacy systems. It can be explicitly rendered in HTML or as a PDF, so the CCD is a very versatile document. Of course it is also structurally similar to other clinical documents done within the CCDA architecture.

Case Study: Transitions of Care

It will be illustrative to look at how CCD documents can be used at a common source of medical errors—transitions of care. The importance of this is illustrated by this quote:

> Patients admitted to a hospital commonly receive new medications or have changes made to their existing medications. Hospital-based clinicians also may not be able to easily access patients' complete medication lists, or may be unaware of recent medication changes. As a result, the new medication regimen prescribed at the time of discharge may inadvertently omit needed medications, unnecessarily duplicate existing therapies, or contain incorrect dosages. (Cornish et al. 2005)

The authors of another paper propose medication reconciliation as the potential solution:

> Overall, 60% of patients had at least one unintended variance and 18% at least one clinically important unintended variance. None of the variances had been detected by usual clinical practice before reconciliation was conducted. Of the 20 clinically important variances, 75% were intercepted by medication reconciliation before patients were harmed. (Vira et al. 2006)

Medication reconciliation was previously discussed as the potential solution to these problems but now we have the background to consider how structured electronic clinical documents might be used to facilitate it. Discharge from the hospital will be used as our "use case." Standards are developed around use cases—the practical issues faced in healthcare delivery. Transitions of care and hospital discharge in particular are well understood to be potentially problematic so, unsurprisingly, this has been the focus of the Transition of Care (ToC) Initiative, a part of the ONC sponsored Standards & Interoperability Workshops. It recommends the following documents at discharge from the hospital:

- **Discharge Summary**: Reason for admission
- **Discharge Information**: Discharge instructions that also contains a dataset relevant to the discharge summary/discharge instructions context, which includes follow-up/plan of care
- **Referral Request Clinical Summary**: Clinical summary contains a variable data set relevant to the context of the request
- **Clinical Summary Including Consultation Request**: PCP-selected referral-specific variable dataset (S&I Framework 2013)

Key clinical data included in these documents are demographic information, an active reconciled medication list (with doses and instructions) and allergy and problem lists. As we discussed earlier, the CCDA specifies documents through templates at the document, section, and entry levels. Documents are built of sections, and sections are built of entries. Templates are numbered using a long hierarchal string called the templateID.

The key templates for our purposes are at all three levels and note that the hierarchy in the string corresponds to the document, section, entry hierarchy of the templates:

```
2.16.840.1.113883.10.20.21 Root Template ID
2.16.840.1.113883.10.20.21.1.2 CCD
2.16.840.1.113883.10.20.21.1.8 Discharge Summary
2.16.840.1.113883.10.20.21.2.1.1 Medications Section with Entries
```

cdatools.org is a very well organized site where you can search for templateIDs and look at their XML. The XML for the Medications Section with Entries includes this specification of the information to be provided about each medication:

```
<th>Medication</th><th>Directions</th><th>Startdate</th>
<th>Status</th><th>Indications</th><th>Fill Instructions</th>
```

This is the key information that should provide sufficient data to help resolve or even automate the medication reconciliation issue as patients move from one care venue to another. Here's a specific example that illustrates this:

```
<section>
  <text>Take captopril 25mg PO every 12 hours.</text>
  <entry>
    <substanceAdministration classCode="SBADM" moodCode="RQO">
      <effectiveTime xsi:type="PIVL_TS">
        <period value="12" unit="h"/>
      </effectiveTime>
      <routeCode code="PO" codeSystem="2.16.840.1.113883.5.112"
      codeSystemName="RouteOfAdministration"/>
      <doseQuantity value="1"/>
      <consumable>
      <manufacturedProduct>
      <manufacturedLabeledDrug>
        <code code="318821008" codeSystem="2.16.840.1.113883.6.96"
        codeSystemName=SNOMED CT"
        displayName="Captopril 25mg tablet"/>
      </manufacturedLabeledDrug>
    </manufacturedProduct>
  </consumable>
</substanceAdministration>
</entry>
</section>
<section>
<text>Take captopril 25mg PO every 12 hours.</text>
<entry>
<substanceAdministration classCode="SBADM" moodCode="RQO">
<effectiveTime xsi:type="PIVL_TS">
<period value="12" unit="h"/>
</effectiveTime>
<routeCode code="PO" codeSystem="2.16.840.1.113883.5.112"
codeSystemName="RouteOfAdministration"/>
```

```
<doseQuantity value="1"/>
<consumable>
<manufacturedProduct>
<manufacturedLabeledDrug>
<code code="318821008" codeSystem="2.16.840.1.113883.6.96"
codeSystemName="SNOMED CT"
displayName="Captopril 25mg tablet"/>
</manufacturedLabeledDrug>
</manufacturedProduct>
</consumable>
</substanceAdministration>
</entry>
</section>
```

(Dolin et al. 2006)

This single example brings together many of the standards and concepts covered in this chapter. For example, classCode="SBADM" moodCode="RQO" is a reference to the RIM. There is one new concept to point out. This XML includes the use of "PO" the standard abbreviation (taken from the Latin) for a medication to be taken by mouth. The codeSyst emName="RouteOfAdministration"/> is not something that has been referred to previously. There are many examples of lists of terms that are used in medicine and need to be

Figure 5.16   Medication and diagnosis data from a CCD and from the provider's EMR are presented in a format that makes it easy for the provider to reconcile differences and file new data from external practices into their EMR.

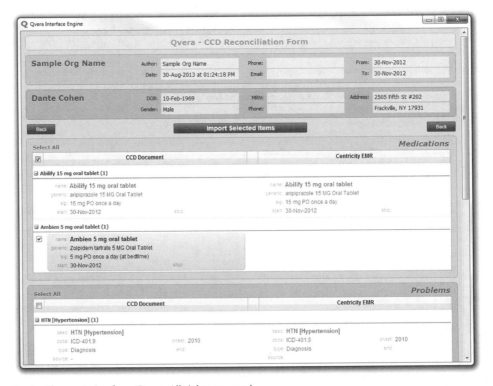

incorporated into CCDA documents. Fast Healthcare Interoperability Resources (FHIR, pronounced "Fire,") is the interesting group within HL7 mentioned earlier that is seeking to redefine the technical approach to interoperability in an effort to simplify things. The Resources section of the FHIR website provides a useful tool for exploring HL7's granular clinical concepts (HL7 2013). There you should be able to find the possible values for RouteOfAdministration. You should also be able to find out that, in the RIM reference cited earlier, SBADM means "substance administration" and RQO means a "request." This illustrates what the RIM is trying to do. These two codes, taken together, describe the process of writing a prescription, which is, after all, a request (but not a guarantee) that the patient administer a substance. Read the rest of this XML carefully to learn more about that prescription and you'll see what a computer should be able to infer correctly from this XML string and how that could be used in transitions of care and for other clinical purposes.

In fact, this is already happening, and it is not limited to reconciling medications. Figure 5.16 presents the physician with the patient's medications, problems, and other clinical data taken from a CCD she has received from another physician, along with the similar data from her EMR. The physician can simply click on data she wants added to the EMR, and it is imported into the proper place within the patient's chart. This both helps prevent errors by eliminating manual data entry. It also helps avoid waste due to data mishandling at transitions of care. Finally it expedites workflow when patients are seen by physicians to whom they have been referred.

Advanced Standards Initiatives

There are three advanced standards initiatives that point the way toward the future and may help deal with many of the limitations of current non-interoperable systems and the usability issues of EMRs that we will discuss in detail in chapter 6. The oldest and most fully developed is The Arden Syntax. The newest are the Clinical Information Modeling Initiative (CIMI) and the Clinical Context Object Workshop (CCOW).

The standards discussed so far are in wide use and largely focused on data elements, assembling them into documents, and messaging. The following section addresses a distinctly different kind of standard that has not yet met with wide acceptance but may gain it as the focus shifts from deploying and adopting electronic records to using the data within them to improve clinical outcomes, the focus of Meaningful Use Stage 3. In fact components of the Arden Syntax are proposed by the Health eDecisions workgroup as the standard to represent clinical logic.

Clinical Decision Support and the Arden Syntax

The mission of the Arden Syntax is to provide a standard approach to describing medical logic in a way that it can be shared across EMRs to support Clinical Decision Support (CDS). This discussion of Arden will be used to also look at the critical issue of CDS. In essence Arden Syntax seeks to help providers avoid medical errors by encoding medical research and the medical knowledge derived from it in a standard form. The goal is that it can be used in diverse EMR and clinical decision support systems to alert providers to errors *before* they occur. It is abundantly clear that medical errors are more common than we would want them to be. Around 3 to 4 percent of hospital admissions lead to an adverse event (Classen and Metzger 2003). Of these, over half are felt to be preventable. Medication errors are among the most common adverse events and can lead to a problem that can potentially injure or even kill a patient. And at least half of these events are thought to be preventable if an effective alerting system were in use (Classen and Metzger 2003).

Clinical decision support is a key concept for preventing errors before they happen. It is not a new idea, and there are a number of ways of supporting improved clinical decision making. Perhaps the simplest is a checklist. It is often pointed out that most people would not get on an airplane if they knew the pilot lacked a checklist to make sure the plane was safe before they took off. Yet most of us go to healthcare providers that do not use a similar checklist approach. A widely quoted study showed that a surgical safety checklist could reduce mortality by nearly 50 percent and reduce post-surgical complications from 11 percent to 7 percent (Haynes et al. 2009).

An initial automated approach, first used in the 1970s, is the stand-alone expert system. MYCIN was an early system that assisted in proper antibiotic use (Shortliffe and Buchanan 1975). More recent efforts help with correctly prescribing many types of medications and providing optimal cancer chemotherapy (Botsman 1995; Gaglio et al. 1987). There are expert systems that are designed to assist physicians in making the right medical diagnosis. An early example of that was AI/RHEUM, which was intended to help unspecialized physicians make the correct diagnosis of rheumatologic problems (joint, soft tissue, and related diseases) (Kingsland et al. 1983). However, the father of this field is undoubtedly the late, legendary Dr. Homer Warner, who began working on using computers for clinical decision support for cardiology in the mid-1950s (Weber 2012) and eventually developed Health Evaluation through Logical Processing (HELP), a system that is still in use today. His early book *Computer-Assisted Medical Decision-Making* was foundational for the field (Warner 1979).

These systems often work. A 2005 survey of the literature on clinical decision support concluded that "Of the 97 controlled trials assessing practitioner performance, the majority (64%) improved diagnosis, preventive care, disease management, drug dosing, or drug prescribing" (Garg et al. 2005). These are the major clinical functions performed by providers, so the results strongly suggest that clinical decision support can improve outcomes and patient safety.

Today, with the availability of large stores of digital health data and extremely fast computers, researchers are increasing mining data repositories to discover new evidence to guide physicians to make the best possible decisions. These repositories need not even be EMRs. A recent example that received widespread attention (including a report in the *NY Times*[1]) was an article by researchers at Microsoft and two universities that they had found previously unrecognized drug interactions by mining the logs of major search engines (White 2013).

Whatever the approach, the ideal way to provide clinical decision support is to integrate it into the clinical workflow. This is a goal of the Health eDecision work group that proposes to use web services to send clinical data to expert systems and provide their advice back to practicing physicians, all within the context of charting in an EHR. Through integration a provider using an EMR would be provided context as they make clinical decisions, and they could receive any applicable guidance based on the best available medical evidence and research. The goal of the Arden Syntax was to facilitate this integration and sharing of the evidence and decision rules across EMR systems and technologies using a standardized formal procedural language that represents medical knowledge in discrete, technology independent units called Medical Logic Modules or MLMs.

Development of Arden began in 1989 under George Hripscak of Columbia University, another leading figure in health informatics (Pryor and Hripscak 1993). There have been

---

[1]Markoff, J. 2013 (March 6). Unreported Side Effects of Drugs Are Found Using Internet Search Data, Study Finds. *New York Times.* http://www.nytimes.com/2013/03/07/science/unreported-side-effects-of-drugs-found-using-internet-data-study-finds.html.

a number of versions released since then. It has been supported by HL7 since 1999, and with the release of HL7 V3, the effort to migrate it to XML is under way. Unsurprisingly, Arden is technically complex, since medical knowledge and medical decision making is inherently more complicated and, hence, harder to represent than simpler concepts, such as a diagnosis or medication. The MLMs consist of production rules about what people do and procedural formalisms, a representation of medical knowledge. Both are required to provide useful clinical decision support. Since much of clinical medicine is about trends or changes in the patient, time is also important—this must occur before that or after this— so temporal operators are an important component of MLMs. The net result is that each MLM is self-contained and sufficient to make a single clinical decision and can generate alerts or reminders to be used by the clinician. Ideally, MLMs would be represented in a way that they could be written by, read by, and verified by clinicians, but this has proven to be a challenge.

Figure 5.17 is a high-level representation of a group of five MLMs designed to help optimize the management of the drug Warfarin, a commonly used but powerful, tricky, and potentially dangerous blood-thinning medication. You can see at the upper left of figure 5.17 that Warfarin is prescribed and the series of five MLMs deals with various situations. The first deals with the start of the therapy. There can be serious consequences if patients take too much or too little of the drug, so blood levels are very critical. Therefore, the second MLM deals with obtaining blood tests that are used to monitor the degree to which the patient's blood has been thinned, and the third deals with the situation where the patient is taking either too much or too little of the drug.

Figure 5.17   An Arden Syntax Warfarin flowchart uses five MLMs (each of which deals with one clinical decision).

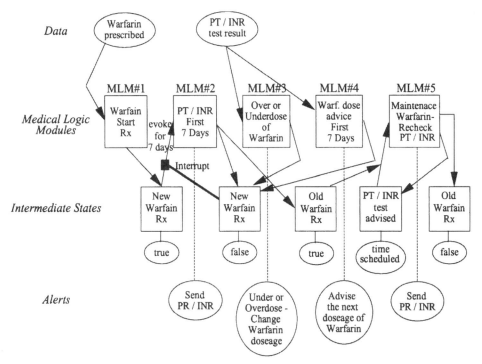

The structure of a MLM at a very high level is:

```
maintenance:
slotname: slot-body;;
slotname: slot-body;;
...
library:
slotname: slot-body;;
...
knowledge:
slotname: slot-body;;
...
end:
```
(Jenders 2013)

As you can see, there are maintenance, library, and knowledge categories. The maintenance category, shown next, deals with administrative matters, such as the title of the MLM, who created it, where it was created, the current version, the date, and where it is in the whole process of development, validation testing, and use. From the title we can see that this MLM deals with imaging the kidneys, using a contrast agent (a chemical that is opaque to x-rays). While these agents facilitate a much better definition of renal (kidney) function, they must be cleared from the body by the kidney and can further damage an already sick kidney. It is therefore important to consider the patient's current renal function before performing such a study.

```
title: Contrast CT study in patient with renal failure;;
mlmname: ct_contr.mlm;;
arden: Version 2;;
version: 1.00;;
institution: Arden Medical Center;;
author: John Doe, MD;;
specialist: Jane Doe, MD;;
date: 1995-09-11;;
validation: testing;;
```
(Jenders 2013)

The library category explains the purpose of the module. The example that follows alerts a provider to a new or worsening serum creatinine level. Serum creatinine is a lab test that is very commonly used as a measure of renal function. A patient whose serum creatinine is above a certain level may have to be looked at carefully before performing the contrast study because they could already be going into renal failure and that could be worsened by the study. The purpose of this module is to recognize those situations and to alert the physician before a mistake is made.

```
purpose: To alert the health care provider of new or worsening serum
creatinine level.;;
explanation: If the creatinine is at or above a threshold (1.35 mg/dl), then
an alert... ;;
keywords: renal insufficiency; renal failure ;;
citations: Proceedings of the Fifteenth Annual Symposium on Computer
Applications in Medical Care; 1991 Nov 17-20; Washington, D.C. New York:
IEEE Computer Society Press, 1991.
links: URL "NLM Web Page", http://www.nlm.nih.gov/ ;;
```
(Jenders 2013)

Knowledge is represented in seven "slots": type, data, priority, evoke, logic, action, and urgency. Here, a data slot is the representational notation used to read the serum creatinine and compare it to the last creatinine:

```
creatinine := read {'dam'="PDQRES2"};
last_creat := read last {select "OBSRV_VALUE"
from "LCR" where qualifier in
("CREATININE",
"QUERY_OBSRV_ALL")};
```
(Jenders 2013)

The evoke slot is used to trigger events.

```
data:
creatinine_storage := event {'32506','32752„};
evoke: 3 days after time of creatinine_storage;
evoke: every 1 day for 7 days starting at time of creatinine_storage;
evoke: every 1 day starting at time of K_storage until K>=3;
```
(Jenders 2013)

Based on this, three days after the time of creatinine storage is an event. Each day for seven days, starting at the time of creatinine storage, is another event. Any creatinine value equal to or above three is an event. Here is the corresponding example of the logic slot:

```
logic:
if last_creat is not present then
alert_text := "No recent creatinine available. Consider ordering creatinine
before giving IV contrast.";
conclude true;
elseif last_creat > 1.5 then
alert_text := "This patient has an elevated creatinine.
Giving IV contrast may worsen renal function.";
conclude true;
else conclude false;
endif;
```
(Jenders 2013)

The logic provides for an action if the last creatinine is not present. It includes alert text and a suggested action. Note the alternate alert text if the last creatinine is present and is greater than 1.5. It warns that "this patient has an elevated creatinine" and "Giving IV contrast may worsen renal function." As you can see, this is a logic rule using the same if, then, and else instructions that are very common in computer programming. However, unlike some computer languages, it is represented at a level high enough that the developers hoped most clinicians could read and understand it.

There is also a messaging function that, for example, deals with a cascading series of actions if the alert is generated and the target physician, presumably the physician responsible for the care of the patient, is unavailable. However, Arden does not explicitly define notification mechanisms for alerts and reminders so this is left to the local implementation. Explicit notification mechanisms may be a part of a future edition.

There are other Arden limitations. Database architectures, clinical vocabulary, and data access methods vary widely so the high-level encoding of clinical knowledge in the MLM must be interpreted and executed in locally executable computer code in order to access the needed data in the local clinical repository. This complicates knowledge sharing and it also adds complexity to implementing Arden.

To appreciate this, look back again at the example of an MLM and you'll see expressions such as "**read {'dam'="PDQRES2"}**," which is colored in the example to make it easier to find. In Arden references to a data source, such as an EHR, are enclosed in curly braces ("{}"). "dam" stands for a Data Access Module. Originally, at Columbia, a PL/I program (PL/1 is an interpretive programming language dating from the 1960s that is still in use today) would actually fetch the data from the local repository as described in an early Arden paper (Jenders et al. 1995). To explain just how localized this can be, look again at the example MLM. At Columbia the creatinine value can be measured as a single test or as part of a battery of tests called a Chem 20. A bit later in the sample MLM you will find "**creatinine_storage := event {'32506','32752,,};**"; this text has also been colored to make it easier to find. The number "32506" is sufficient to find creatinine values from a single test while "32752" will find values done as part of a Chem 20. None of this would make sense at another institution. This has even been dubbed the "curly braces problem" (Choi 2003).

One proposed solution involves the use of yet another HL7 component, GELLO, which is intended to be a standardized interface and query language for accessing data in health information systems, particularly for clinical decision support (Samwald et al. 2012; Kawamoto et al. 2012). Another group has demonstrated an approach to executing MLMs using Drools, a JAVA-based cross platform business rule management system (Jung et al. 2012). A third group has developed Arden2ByteCode, open source code that runs on Java Virtual Machines (JVM) and translates Arden Syntax directly to Java bytecode (JBC) executable on JVMs (Gietzelt et al. 2010). It also serves as runtime environment for execution of the compiled bytecode.

A more contemporary and interesting approach is to provide clinical decision support under a service oriented architecture (SOA). One article describes how Arden-based SOA architecture permits easier integration into existing hospital environments because it is a web service application (Fehre and Adlassnig 2011). Web services are widely used open-web standards that are intended to facilitate interaction between different systems. As a key part of their approach, they provide an Arden Syntax compiler and an Arden Syntax engine, both written in Java.

The web services approach has been adopted by the Health eDecisions workgroup that is charged with developing a standard approach to the provision of clinical decision support services across EHRs. The specific web services protocol used initially is Simple Object Access Protocol (SOAP) but the even simpler RESTful API approach is being added. It is worth noting that FHIR has also adopted RESTful APIs. Web services and RESTful APIs in particular may be the future standard for many aspects of interoperability.

Even though it was a goal that Arden could be read and written by physicians in native form, it is sufficiently technical that most cannot do that. There was one early effort to provide a Microsoft Windows-based "integrated system for generating, maintaining, compiling, and executing Arden Syntax-based knowledge bases," but it does not seem to have gained traction (Sailors 1997). New high-level GUI interface efforts are now underway to create an environment that would allow physicians to develop rules and look at rules in a much more user-friendly form.

Despite these issues, Arden is arguably the most widely used CDS platform and has been adopted by a number of major health information system vendors, including Eclipsys (now part of Allscripts), McKesson, and Siemens. It is also used by MICROMEDEX, a widely used provider of evidence-based data about medications and clinical practice. However, this is a small part of the HIT universe. Its adoption, at least in part, by Health eDecisions could make Arden the de facto standard for the representation of clinical logic.

There are other clinical decision support architectures, including Sebastian and SAGE. An interesting paper suggests a framework for evaluating these systems and proposes four elements to do this:

- **Feature determination:** the ability to provide a set of desirable features (based on a literature review and expert opinion)
- **Existence and use:** from theoretical discussion to widespread adoption and use
- **Utility:** the ability to implement a wide range of decision support use cases
- **Coverage:** ability to cover a large knowledge base of decision support content (Wright and Sittig 2008)

As pointed out at the beginning of this section, the necessary underlying infrastructure of electronic records and the resultant digital clinical data are becoming much more commonly available in clinical practice and should facilitate progress in wider adoption of clinical decision support. Also, both Meaningful Use Stage 3 and new outcome-based contracts will create a focus on improved clinical outcomes and further suggest that CDS will come into more common use in clinical practice. The Health eDecisions workgroup's choice of relatively simple and approachable web services as the transport and knowledge sharing mechanism may provide the glue to link together all the elements needed for more ubiquitous CDS in time for Meaningful Use, Stage 3 (MU3). Among other advantages, this approach should make evidence-based recommendations from research or medical centers with particular expertise and experience in a clinical problems more widely, readily, and inexpensively available thereby facilitating support for CDS in community hospitals and physician practices. Moreover, to the extent that the approach is embraced by EHR vendors and built into their systems the "curly braces problem" could be resolved if those vendors provide full integration with their own clinical databases as a part of their standards-based CDS offering. The proposed CDS standard is designed so that existing CDS frameworks can be mapped to it allowing sites with existing CDS implementations to maintain them while adapting to the standard. Finally, the Arden Syntax was used as a basis for this new CDS standard's expression language which incorporates some aspects of the Arden syntax.

Clinical Information Modeling Initiative (CIMI)

CIMI began in 2011 and is described on the websites of its participating members as "an international collaboration that is dedicated to providing a common format for detailed specifications for the representation of health information content so that semantically interoperable information may be created and shared in health records, messages and documents" (AMIA 2012). It was authorized by the HL7 board in April 2011.

CIMI seeks to provide a conceptual definition of the discrete structured clinical information that is used in a clinical context. The model defines the data elements, attributes, possible values, and types of attributes that are needed to convey the clinical perspective in a manner that is understandable to a variety of stakeholders, including functional and technical experts.

Context Management Specification

The Context Management Specification is another apparently visionary HL7 effort, began independently at Duke University as the CCOW, and the acronym is still associated with it, despite the name change once it became part of HL7. It is developing standards that would allow diverse applications to integrate so that data from different applications could be presented to a clinician or some other healthcare worker as if it is all from one integrated system. This is being done by creating a Context Management Architecture (CMA). Context Management is a computer science concept that uses "subjects" of data in one application to point to data resident in a separate application also containing the same subject(s). Once a user chooses a subject in one application, all other Context Management Specification compliant applications containing information on that same subject "tune" to the data they contain, obviating the need for the user to select the same subject in other applications. Given its mission, Context Management Specification is often combined with the Single Sign On (SSO), a concept that enables applications across a health enterprise to share the same user logging and access directory structures.

The HL7 Context Management Specification defines a means for the automatic coordination and synchronization of disparate healthcare applications that coreside on the same clinical desktop. For example, a provider having already logged on and having specified a particular patient, diagnosis, and reason for their interaction with the record (the "context") would not have to respecify this information as they move from one clinical application to another. Moreover, the applications could, at least in theory, retrieve the related information in advance, significantly speeding things up. Also in theory, all the compliant applications could both retrieve the information and present it to some central program, which could then provide an integrated view, obviating the need for the provider to traverse multiple applications.

However, while Context Management Specification is very precise in prescribing how applications should interact, developers can still interpret how to implement the specifics differently, leading to unavoidable inconsistencies in application behavior at the end-user level.

Conclusion

If there is one theme that weaves throughout this long chapter, it is complexity. Standards are at one and the same time an essential component of contemporary health informatics but one that often adds a great deal of complexity to the development of practical HIT systems. Given that, developers often chose to implement standards in limited and often incompatible ways, actually contributing to the interoperability problem that standards were developed to remedy.

This is illustrated by a recent article by Anthony Brino of HIEWatch about the ONC's HIT Standards Committee's Clinical Quality Workgroup. In it, Brino comments that "the "overarching goal [of the workgroup] remains to help streamline standards" (Brino 2013). Keith W. Boone, a nationally well-respected and self-described "standards geek" at GE Healthcare and a member of the Workgroup, was interviewed by Brino and said "it's important that your standard be able to work, not just with itself, but with other standards" (Boone 2013). Boone lists the key goals of the workgroup and, among them are:

- Ease of implementation
- Ease of use and understandability
- Explainable to MDs
- Use of existing technologies
- Stop reinventing the wheel (Boone 2013)

The article goes on to say that Boone estimates that an online web conference relies on about 20 different standards. "The idea is that there's actually an architecture; there's a plan for how all of these pieces will work together" (Boone 2013).

The United States lacks such a plan in healthcare. Weaving the many standards discussed in this chapter together into a logical, seamless, well-integrated, and practical framework is a clear and rapidly approaching challenge. That may never be fully possible using the standards in their entirety, given their complexity. Efforts such as FHIR and Health eDecisions may be pointing the way to a workable compromise. In a well-known blog post, Grahame Grieve, an active HL7 participant and the father of FHIR, says that it "is intended to address the most common (80%) interoperability needs of implementers, and consciously delegates the remaining 20% to extensions which must still fit within the structure of the standard, but which will not be addressed in the core parts of the standard. After getting rid of the stuff that deals with all the exceptional cases, it turns out that the core can be much simpler (some have estimated that it is 20% of the original, fully encompassed modeling that we currently do in HL7)." (Grieve 2012) In the end a focus on simplicity may provide the long needed path to interoperability.

REFERENCES

1edisource.com. 2013. EDI 837 Health Care Claim. http://www.1edisource.com/learn-about-edi/transaction-sets/tset/837#axzz2kN1f7DqKwww.ezclaim.com 2013. http://support.ezclaim.com/ANSIRef/ANSI837Reference.aspx

American Medical Association. 2013. CPT® Category I Vaccine Codes. http://www.ama-assn.org//ama/pub/physician-resources/solutions-managing-your-practice/coding-billing-insurance/cpt/about-cpt/category-i-vaccine-codes.page

American Public Health Association. 1899. *The Bertillon Classification of Causes of Death* (first English translation from the French). Lansing, MI: Robert Smith Printing Company.

AMIA. 2012. The Clinical Information Modeling Initiative. http://www.amia.org/the-standards-standard/2012-volume3-edition1/clinical-information-modeling-initiative

Beeler, G.W. 2011. Introduction to HL7 Reference Information Model (RIM) ANSI/HL7 RIM R3-2010 and ISO. http://www.hl7.org/documentcenter/public_temp_DC1ECF9F-1C23-BA17-0C200395FDACE896/calendarofevents/himss/2011/HL7%20Reference%20Information%20Model.pdf

Boone, Keith W. 2013. HealthcareITNews. http://www.healthcareitnews.com/blog/author/26431.

Botsman, K.J. 1995. An expert system as a clinical aid in the administration and dosage adjustment of some commonly prescribed therapeutic drugs and antibiotics. http://hdl.cqu.edu.au/10018/25453

Brino, A. 2013. ONC workgroup walks tightrope of standards principles. *HealthcareITNews—HIEWatch*. http://www.hiewatch.com/news/onc-workgroup-walks-tightrope-standards-principles-0

Buck, C.J. 2013. 2014 ICD-9-CM. American Medical Association.

Choi, J. 2003. Adapting current Arden Syntax knowledge for an object oriented event monitor. *AMIA Annu Symp Proc* 2003, 814. http://www.ncbi.nlm.nih.gov/pmc/articles/PMC1479901/

Classen, D.C. and J. Metzger 2003. Improving medication safety: The measurement conundrum and where to start. *Int J Qual Health Care* 15 (suppl 1):i41–i47. http://intqhc.oxfordjournals.org/content/15/suppl_1/i41.full

Confluence. 2013. http://confluence.siframework.org/plugins/viewsource/viewpagesrc.action?pageId=28214182

Conn, J. 2014 (February). Proposed SGR overhaul would affect EHR incentive program. *Modern Healthcare*. http://www.modernhealthcare.com/article/20140206/NEWS/302069958

Cornish, P.L., S.R. Knowles, R. Marchesano, V. Tam, S. Shadowitz, D.N. Juurlink, and E.E. Etchells. 2005. Unintended medication discrepancies at the time of hospital admission. *Arch Intern Med.* 165:424–429

Dolin, R.H., L. Alschuler, S. Boyer, C. Beebe, F.M Behlen, P.V Biron, and A.S. Shvo. 2006. HL7 clinical document architecture, release 2. *J Am Med Inform Assoc* 13:30–39. http://171.67.114.118/content/13/1/30.full

Farr, W. 1856. *Report on the Nomenclature and Statistical Classification of Diseases for Statistical Returns.* London: George E. Eyre and William Spottiswoode.

Farr, W. 1844. The fifth annual report of the registrar general on births, deaths and marriages in England. *The Medico-Chirurgical Review* 41:72.

Fehre, K. and K. Adlassnig. 2011. Service-oriented Arden-Syntax-based clinical decision support. *Proceedings of eHealth2011*, 123–128.

Gaglio, S., M. Genovesi, C. Ruggiero, G. Spinelli, C. Nicolini, G. Bonadonna, and P. Valagussa. 1987. Expert systems for cancer chemotherapy. *Computers & Mathematics with Applications* 14(9–12):793–802. http://www.sciencedirect.com/science/article/pii/0898122187902288

Garg, A.X., N.K.J. Adhikari, H. McDonald, M.P. Rosas-Arellano, P.J. Devereaux, J. Beyene, J. Sam, and R.B. Haynes. 2005. Effects of computerized clinical decision support systems on practitioner performance and patient outcomes: A systematic review. *JAMA.* 293(10):1223–1238. http://jama.jamanetwork.com/article.aspx?articleid=200503

Gietzelt, M., U. Goltz, D. Grunwald, M. Lochau, M. Marschollek, B. Song, and K.H. Wolf. 2012. Arden2ByteCode: A one-pass Arden Syntax compiler for service-oriented decision support systems based on the OSGi platform. *Comput Methods Programs Biomed* 106(2):114–125. http://www.cmpbjournal.com/article/S0169-2607(11)00308-7/abstract
    This group also maintains an Arden2ByteCode site at http://arden2bytecode.sourceforge.net/

Graunt, J. 1662, *Natural and Political Observations Made Upon The Bills of Mortality,* London. http://www.edstephan.org/Graunt/bills.html

Grieve, G. 2012. "Starting a FHIR under HL7." Healthcare Standards, May 14. http://motorcycleguy.blogspot.com/2012/05/starting-fhir-under-hl7.html

Haynes, A.B., T.G. Weiser, W.R. Berry, S.R. Lipsitz, A.S. Breizat, E.P. Dellinger, T. Herbosa, S. Joseph, P.L. Kibatala, M.C.M. Lapitan, A.F. Merry, K. Moorthy, R.K. Reznick, B. Taylor, and A.A. Gawande. 2009. A surgical safety checklist to reduce morbidity and mortality in a global population. *N Engl J Med* 360:491–499. http://www.nejm.org/doi/full/10.1056/NEJMsa0810119

HL7. 2013a. HL7 v3 Guide. http://wiki.hl7.org/index.php?title=Category:V3Guide

HL7. 2013b. OID Registry. http://www.hl7.org/oid/index.cfm

HL7. 2012. https://hssp.wikispaces.com/Harmonization+Framework+and+Exchange+Architecture

HL7 International. 2013. FHIR Resource Index. http://www.hl7.org/implement/standards/fhir/resourcelist.html

HL7 International. 2009. CDA R2 Errata. http://wiki.hl7.org/index.php?title=CDA_R2_Errata

Hoelzer, S., R.K. Schweiger, R. Liu, D. Rudolfe, J. Riegerl, and J. Dudeck. 2002. XML representation of hierarchical classification systems: From conceptual models to real applications. *Proc AMIA Symp*, 330–334. http://www.ncbi.nlm.nih.gov/pmc/articles/PMC2244386/pdf/procamiasymp00001-0371.pdf

Integrating the Healthcare Enterprise. 2012. IHE IT Infrastructure (ITI) Technical Framework. http://www.ihe.net/Technical_Framework/upload/IHE_ITI_TF_Vol1.pdf

International Health Terminology Standards Development (IHTSDO). 2013a. http://www.ihtsdo.org/snomed-ct/

International Health Terminology Standards Development (IHTSDO). 2013b. SNOMED CT® User Guide (US English). http://ihtsdo.org/fileadmin/user_upload/doc/download/doc_UserGuide_Current-en-US_INT_20130731.pdf

Jenders, R.A. 2013. Personal communication with author.

Jenders, R.A., G. Hripcsak, R.V. Sideli, W. DuMouchel, H. Zhang, J.J. Cimino, S.B. Johnson, E.H. Sherman, and P.D. Clayton. 1995. Medical decision support: Experience with implementing the Arden Syntax at the Columbia-Presbyterian Medical Center. *Proc Annu Symp Comput Appl Med Care* 1995:169–173. http://www.ncbi.nlm.nih.gov/pmc/articles/PMC2579077/

Jung, C.Y., K.A Sward, and P.J Haug. 2012 (Jul–Aug). Executing medical logic modules expressed in ArdenML using Drools. *J Am Med Inform Assoc*, 19(4):533–536. http://www.ncbi.nlm.nih.gov/pmc/articles/PMC3384109/

Kawamoto, K., P.R. Tattam, D.E. Shields, and P. Scott. 2012. Virtual Medical Record for Clinical Decision Support (vMR-CDS) for GELLO, Release 1. HIMSS. http://www.hl7.org/documentcenter/public_temp_873BC02B-1C23-BA17-0CF1510A3ACCA173/standards/dstu/V3IG_CDS_VMR_GELLO_DSTU_R1_2012APR.pdf

Kingsland, L.C., D.A. Lindberg, and G.C. Sharp. 1983. AI/RHEUM. A consultant system for rheumatology. *J Med Syst* [Internet]. http://www.ncbi.nlm.nih.gov/pubmed/6352842/

Libery Management Group Ltd. 2013. NDC Labeler Code Assignment. http://www.fdahelp.us/fda-labeler-code.html

McDonald, C., S. Huff, J. Deckard, K. Holck, and D.J. Vreeman. 2013. Logical Observation Identifiers Names and Codes (LOINC®) Users' Guide. http://loinc.org/downloads/files/LOINCManual.pdf

Mead, C.M., N. Orvis and S. Hufnagel. 2010. Health Level Seven®, Inc. Project Scope Statement. Harmonization Framework and Exchange Architecture (HF&EA). https://hssp.wikispaces.com/Harmonization+Framework+and+Exchange+Architecture

Medicare Learning Network. 2010. *Evaluation and Management Services Guide.* http://www.cms.gov/Outreach-and-Education/Medicare-Learning-Network-MLN/MLNProducts/downloads/eval_mgmt_serv_guide-ICN006764.pdf

National Library of Medicine. 2013. I-Magic. http://imagic.nlm.nih.gov/imagic/code/map.

New Health Project. 2013. Notes on the MIT Semantic Health Workshop. http://www.new-health-project.net/wp-content/uploads/2013/06/2013-MIT-Semantic-Health-Workshop-19-Apr-2103.pdf

ONC. 2012. PHRI CDA Specification Version 0.2.

Prud'hommeaux, E.G. 2013. Semantic Interpretation of Health Care Data. SemTech. http://www.w3.org/2013/Talks/0507-HCLS-egp/#(1)

Pryor, TA and Hripcsak, G. 1993. The Arden syntax for medical logic modules. Int J Clin Monit Comput. Nov;10(4):215-24.

Rosenblatt, J. 2012. What is LOINC and Why Does it Matter? Mayo Clinic: *Communique.* http://www.mayomedicallaboratories.com/articles/communique/2012/11.html

Sailors, R.M. 1997. MLM builder: An integrated suite for development and maintenance of Arden Syntax medical logic modules. *Proc AMIA Annu Fall Symp*, 996.

Samwald, M., K. Fehre, J. de Bruin, and K.P. Adlassnig. 2012 (Aug). The Arden Syntax standard for clinical decision support: Experiences and directions. *J Biomed Inform* 45(4):711–718. http://www.ncbi.nlm.nih.gov/pubmed/22342733

Sherman, E.H., G. Hripcsak, J. Starren, R.A. Jenders, and P. Clayton. 1995. Using Intermediate States to Improve the Ability of the Arden Syntax to Implement Care Plans and Reuse Knowledge. JAMIA. http://www.ncbi.nlm.nih.gov/pmc/articles/PMC2579091/pdf/procascamc00009-0268.pdf

Shortliffe, E. and B. Buchanan. 1975. A model of inexact reasoning in medicine. *Mathematical Biosciences* 23(3–4):351–379.

S&I Framework. 2013. Transitions of Care (ToC) Initiative. http://wiki.siframework.org/Transitions+of+Care+(ToC)+Initiative

Vira, T., M Colquhoun, and E Etchells. 2006 (April). Reconcilable differences: Correcting medication errors at hospital admission and discharge. *Int J Qual Saf Health Care* 15(2):122–126. http://www.ncbi.nlm.nih.gov/pmc/articles/PMC2464829/

VTSL. 2013. VTSL Terminology Browser. http://vtsl.vetmed.vt.edu/

Warner, H.R. 1979. *Computer-Assisted Medical Decision-Making.* Academic Press.

Weber, B. 2012. Homer R. Warner, a pioneer of using computers in patient care, dies at 90. New *York Times.* http://www.nytimes.com/2012/12/11/us/homer-r-warner-a-pioneer-of-using-computers-in-patient-care-dies-at-90.html

White, R.W. 2013. Web-scale pharmacovigilance: Listening to signals from the crowd. *J Am Med Inform Assoc.* (web only). http://jamia.bmj.com/content/early/2013/02/05/amiajnl-2012-001482.abstract

Wood, G. 2013. HL7 Ambassador Presentation—Basic Overview. HL7. http://www.hl7.org/documentcenter/public_temp_BD5DFE97-1C23-BA17-0C1ED01C9F6DA016/calendarofevents/himss/2013/2013%20HIMSS%20HL7%20Basic%20Overview.pdf

World Health Organization. 2013. International Classification of Diseases (ICD) Information Sheet. http://www.who.int/classifications/icd/factsheet/en/

World Health Organization. 1997. *Application of the International Classification of Diseases to Neurology.* Volume 3.

Wright, A. and D.F. Sittig. 2008. A framework and model for evaluating clinical decision support architectures. *J Biomed Inform* 41(6):982–990. http://www.ncbi.nlm.nih.gov/pmc/articles/PMC2638589/#!po=65.0000

Wood, G. 2013. (January 30). HL7 Ambassador Webinar: An HL7 Overview.

RECOMMENDED READING AND RESOURCES

A detailed comparison of ICD 9 and ICD 10 is available here: http://www.ama-assn.org/ama1/pub/upload/mm/399/icd10-icd9-differences-fact-sheet.pdf.

An HL7 online tutorial is available here: http://www.hl7.org/documentcenter/public_temp_3D171E93-1C23-BA17-0C7A77E7CA743935/training/IntroToHL7/player.html.

EDIdEv provides an extensive discussion and comparison of the differences between XML and EDI: http://www.edidev.com/XMLvsEDI.html.

The AMA provides a free, public CPT code lookup page, but use of it is limited, as is specified in the agreement that governs its use: https://ocm.ama-assn.org/OCM/CPTRelativeValueSearch.do.

There is a public NDC code searchable database: http://www.accessdata.fda.gov/scripts/cder/ndc/default.cfm.

There is a public LOINC search engine. Try visiting it and typing in some examples (such as "sputum culture") to see the clinical detail available within LOINC: http://search.loinc.org/

A tool for looking up OID codes: http://www.hl7.org/oid/index.cfm.

The templateIDs developed by ONC's Harmonization Workgroup are posted here: http://confluence.siframework.org/display/SIF/TemplateIds.

A useful site listing the CCDA templates: http://ccda.sitenv.org/C-CDA.

A site that provides CCDA template information, including sample XML: http://cdatools.org/infocenter/index.jsp.

A discussion of why standardizing templates can be hard: http://motorcycleguy.blogspot.com/2009/09/template-identifiers-business-rules-and.html.

An excellent overview of the details involved in standards development and the difficulty of reaching a true consensus, in this case the medications section of the CDA: http://wiki .siframework.org/CDA+-+Medications+Section.

The CIMI wiki is located at: http://informatics.mayo.edu/CIMI/index.php/Main_Page.

Standards Implementation and Testing Environment (SITE) information is available here: http:// sitenv.org/.

This site will validate a CCDA document: http://ccda-scorecard.smartplatforms.org/static/ ccdaScorecard/#/.

Fast Healthcare Interoperability Resources (FHIR) namespaces are located at: http://www.hl7.org/ implement/standards/fhir/terminologies-v3.htm.

The Context Management Specifications (CCOW) site is at: http://www.hl7.org/implement/ standards/product_brief.cfm?product_id=1.

HL7 Clinical Document Architecture, Release 2 (Dolin et al. 2006) provides a detailed description of the CCDA including other good examples of XML.

The SNOMED-CT browser used in this chapter: http://vtsl.vetmed.vt.edu/.

Another good SNOMED-CT browser in which each entry has a unique URL, is available here: http://bioportal.bioontology.org/ontologies/SNOMEDCT.

An ICD-10 to SNOMED-CT mapping tool: http://imagic.nlm.nih.gov/imagic/code/map.

Two sites for more information about FHIR which may turn out to be an important effort to expedite interoperability: http://blog.interfaceware.com/hl7/what-is-fhir-and-why-should-you-care/ and http://www.j4jayant.com/articles/fhir.

The VA's VistA Novo project is investigating the feasibility of an open source VistA development toolkit including a FHIR implementation to make VistA test data more easily available: http:// www.osehra.org/content/vista-novo-project-overview.

Part

III

Real World Applications

Chapter

6

Clinical Data Collection and Visualization Challenges

A Brief Review

This chapter will explore the challenges of real world deployment and use of the systems developed based on the technologies covered in the last three chapters. It will also look at some innovative approaches that may have the potential to help solve some of the remaining difficult, long-time problems in provider-facing health informatics.

This chapter will begin with electronic records in medical practice and with the rationale for their use. Among the key goals of these systems are improving care quality, increasing efficiency, and reducing medical errors by making sure the right information is available at the right time and place and to help providers make the right diagnostic and treatment decisions. A second overriding goal is collaboration, including with patients, to facilitate a coordinated care system that can more optimally provide long-term management of chronic disease. The third major goal is to create useful digital health data that can be aggregated, analyzed, visualized, and ultimately, used to help improve care by increasing our understanding of what works in real world practice; what does not work or is not cost effective; and to discover new medical knowledge. Healthcare data analytics will be covered in depth in chapters 9 and 10. A final, but equally important, goal is supporting enhanced public health surveillance and understanding healthcare at the population level, the topic of chapter 8.

Physicians Are in the Data Business

Physicians are in the data business. Despite this, medical records and record keeping often receive minimal attention in medical training and most medical schools offer no training in health informatics beyond the requirement to learn to use whatever electronic record systems are installed in their hospitals and clinics. Physician use of electronic medical records (EMRs) and its impact on patient interaction is also typically not formally taught as a part of medical education (AMA 2012). With or without training, except for surgeons and other interventional physicians whose main jobs are to remove or fix problems or do invasive tests, physicians primarily work by collecting and analyzing data. They begin this by interviewing the patient. Typically they start by asking for a chief complaint, the reason for the current encounter. They then ask about other problems the patient may have and obtain the history of those problems and the current chief complaint. To further explore the chief complaint, they ask the patient about their symptoms and they examine the patient. Based on this classic "history and physical," they make a preliminary diagnosis, if possible, and then order laboratory, imaging, and other tests to obtain as much objective data as possible.

From this aggregated database of subjective and objective clinical data, they make decisions about what is wrong with each patient, and they develop a plan for managing the problem(s). In subsequent visits, they follow up to understand the effectiveness of the treatments (most commonly medications) they have prescribed and make adjustments accordingly. The treatment plan may involve referral to specialists, which, in turn, requires coordination of care among a few or possibly many providers working at different care venues and possibly in different communities and health systems.

This entire care process is driven by data. Many providers do not recognize this as explicitly as they should, and this has been one of the reasons so many providers continued to use paper record systems for such a long period of time after digital approaches have been adopted by other industries.

Medicine is complex and therefore error prone, so another aspect of the data problem is looking at why physicians make these errors. The University of Washington School of Medicine lists three principle reasons and data management is central to them:

- An incomplete knowledge base
- An error in perception or judgment
- A lapse in attention (UWSOM 1998)

An incomplete knowledge base means not having all the information at the right time and in the right place and not necessarily having all of the most current thinking about how best to use that data to treat patients. The other two are errors in perception, judgment, or lapse in attention. A capable EMR system that brings together and usefully presents the relevant and current medical knowledge and complete information about the patient and also provides both reminders and clinical decision support should help avoid all three of these sources of error.

Physicians also need to collaborate. In the United States patients with multiple chronic conditions drive half the cost of Medicare and usually receive care from many providers. Surveys of both providers and patients have shown that distributed care can be more effectively managed when there is information sharing, so that everybody knows what everybody else is doing (Deloitte 2013; Commonwealth Fund 2011).

Paper records are problematic if for no other reason than they are not readily shareable. Of course, they are also passive and cannot issue alerts or help physicians make the best clinical decisions (Wilcox et al. 2005). Physicians seeing long time multiple chronic disease patients can have to deal with thick paper charts that can be an impediment to proper care given the limited time available to review them. Moreover, paper charts may not even be available when they were needed. Studies show that specialists see patients referred to them 20 percent of the time without have the record of that patient's prior care (Commonwealth Fund 2008).

Some History

The case for electronic records may have been first effectively made, and was certainly first described in detail, by Dr. Lawrence Weed in his seminal book *Medical Records, Medical Education, and Patient Care* (Weed 1969). In it Dr. Weed said that medicine needs a systematic approach to documentation, and that this could lead to a more systematic way of delivering care. He proposed an approach that is now commonly used under the acronym SOAP charting. The acronym derives from his view that physicians notes should be rigorously divided into Subjective and Objective data followed by an Assessment and a Plan to aid the physician in decision making and so that the clinical logic used would be clear to all subsequent physicians seeing the patient. At the end of the book, he linked his systematic approach to documentation to the potential for computerized medical records. This was at the very beginning of the time when actually developing such systems was technically feasible and starting to become barely economically viable.

It is also important to acknowledge the insight of Florence Nightingale. While her greatest healthcare achievement was to make nursing a respectable profession for women, her extensive writings on hospital planning and organization had a profound effect in England and across the world. She published over 200 books, reports, and pamphlets. In one of these she stated that

> In attempting to arrive at the truth, I have applied everywhere for information, but in scarcely an instance have I been able to obtain hospital records fit for any purpose of comparison. If they could be obtained . . . they would show subscribers how their money was being spent, what amount of good was really being done with it, or whether the money was not doing mischief rather than good. . . . (Nightingale 1863, 176)

That this quote is largely relevant 150 years later goes a long way toward making the point that healthcare providers are insufficiently aware of the key role that data plays in their profession.

Recognition of these ideas has advanced to the point that the United States now has a national strategy for health informatics. It calls for electronic health records (EHRs) interconnected through health information exchange (HIE) creating clinical databases that can be used to increase medical knowledge and produce the quality and efficiency gains the need for which needed to create a high quality and sustainable healthcare system. The hope is that this informatics framework will provide key tools to solve the many problems that have been identified. EHRs equipped with well designed visualizations and with clinical decision support could go a long way toward improving the quality of care, both by bringing the required clinical data together as decisions are made; by providing the best available medical evidence and by spotting mistakes before they occur. But this goes beyond providers. Inappropriate patient behavior and poor compliance with prescribed treatments can lead to the development of chronic disease and reduce or even defeat the effectiveness of the provider's care plan for the patient, once they have developed chronic disease. The key informatics tools here are personal health records, mobile devices and apps, and other forms of ubiquitous computing that can help monitor and inform patients as they attempt to manage or even prevent chronic diseases. Finally, the episodic and poorly coordinated healthcare delivery system can be unified to a large degree through health information exchange (HIE). The available evidence suggests that this national program is achieving widespread adoption of these technologies. Some of the new approaches discussed in chapter 5 may provide a framework for widespread clinical decision support.

Despite this coordinated national effort, health informatics still faces a number of largely unresolved and difficult problems. Perhaps the key problem is data quality. This further subdivides into the accuracy and completeness of the data and substantial incompatibilities in data representation across health systems and individual providers. These are old problems, as we saw in the quote from Florence Nightingale. In an ideal world, the adoption of EHR technologies would substantially resolve them, but to date, that has not been the case. The central problems are data representation and quality, which in large part lead to the lack of interoperability among EHR systems.

It can be argued that interoperability is a classic problem of the chicken and the egg: Which should come first, the development and implementation of standards that assure interoperability of electronic records or their widespread adoption, after which, it is hoped, market pressures will force interoperability? The recent bipartisan legislative proposal, mentioned in chapter 5, that mandates EHR interoperability by 2017 is a new development that may create an overriding "market force". David Brailer, the first director of ONC, makes it clear that this is a dilemma in a brief paper (Brailer 2005), but he does not reach a conclusion with respect to the direction that should be taken. Driven by political and arguably practical considerations, we have chosen a middle road with the certification of electronic records mandating some degree of interoperability followed by rapid deployment. An economic value can be placed on deploying fully interoperable systems and

> based on our analysis of those elements of interoperability for which we can assign dollar values, net savings from national implementation of fully stand-ardized interoperability between providers and five other types of organizations could yield $77.8 billion annually, or approximately 5 percent of the projected $1.661 trillion spent on US health care in 2003.

The paper then goes on to speculate that:

> the clinical payoff in improved patient safety and quality of care could dwarf the financial benefits projected from our model, which are derived from redundan-cies that are avoided and administrative time saved. Giving clinicians access to data about their patients' care from providers outside their organizations would likely result in fewer medical errors and better continuity of care. (Walker et al. 2005)

An article that was based on work that looked at the methods of assessing the quality of data in EHRs and concluded that

> There is currently little consistency or potential generalizability in the methods used to assess EHR data quality. If the reuse of EHR data for clinical research is to become accepted, researchers should adopt validated, systematic methods of EHR data quality assessment. (Weiskopf and Wang 2012)

It further concluded that "there is no consistent method for doing this, so we do not have a good method of assessing the quality of data in EHRs" (Weiskopf and Wang 2012).

The Data Quality Problem

The EHR data quality challenge is widely recognized and has more than once been a topic at the Annual MIT Information Quality Industry Symposium. A panel discussion at the fifth annual symposium in 2007 (MIT 2011) is very much on-point for this. Presenters state that the presence of an EHR does not in and of itself guarantee improved quality data (MIT 2011). It is possible that, if the EHR is poorly designed, it may detract from or reduce the quality of the data. The most common source of EHR data quality issues is human error (MIT 2011). So the problem can often be incorrect data at the source. How and why does that happen? The panel presented a list of the typical reasons:

- Active error—someone entering the wrong value
- Passive error—a system default value was not reset to a correct value

- Not having data due to [it] being overlooked (clutter) or not in a logical location
- Data in multiple locations do not coincide
- Information captured does not contain all required elements—some data is present but not all components
- When data elements are not definitive, uncertainty regarding interpretation can be common
- Source data on same observation or event resides in more than one location dependent on updates—which location is the definitive source? (MIT 2011)

Active error is obvious—someone can enter the wrong data while charting. System designs can increase or decrease the likelihood of this. For example, it can be easy for a busy provider to pick the wrong choice from a poorly constructed or presented drop down list. Passive error may be not quite as obvious. EHR systems often offer a default value, and it is certainly possible that the EHR may not reset that to a correct value (which may be no value) when, for example, a new patient is charted, or even more likely, the latest episode of care is charted for a previously seen patient. This is one of the difficult issues that all EHR system designers grapple with. Specifically, is it good design to bring forward data from the previous episodes of care so that the clinician can chart the current episode by only modifying what has changed? This approach introduces the very real risk that the user will overlook default values from before that are not valid now. Alternately, does the EHR require providers to start over each time with a "blank slate" for each new patient? This is more time consuming for busy and often impatient healthcare providers. The choice of offering the prior episode as a default starting point is often touted by vendors as a time saver during the sales process. This chapter will later discuss some innovative approaches to this vexing problem. Next, the data can just be overlooked or not entered because of a very cluttered or illogical screen design. Data can be collected from multiple locations or multiple encounters with the patient, and they can be inconsistent. In summary, there are a number of reasons why data in EHRs can be incomplete, inconsistent, or wrong, and many of them involve, in whole or in part, EHR design issues. These data quality issues not only threaten proper patient care, but they substantially complicate efforts to achieve care coordination and to use digital clinical data for research and other secondary purposes.

This section will now take a deeper look at the core problem of collecting data in an EHR at the point-of-care to understand why it is such a difficult design issue by looking at how various EHR designers have approached the data collection problem. As previously noted, there are hundreds of EHRs being offered commercially. The choices as to which EHRs to discuss in this book should not be construed as indicating that the systems are the only choices, the preferred choices, or the best choices for an individual provider.

The nature of the data being collected needs to be addressed before looking at specific EHR design solutions. Will it be the same free, unstructured text that providers typically record in their paper charts, or will it be structured data essentially representing choices from the increasingly sophisticated medical ontologies, such as SNOMED CT (Systemized Nomenclature of Medicine Clinical Terms)? "Avoiding need for 'notes' or comment field entries by using discrete data fields is most common and effective solution" (MIT 2011).

However, today computing may well be on the threshold of technology that works well to provide clinical decision support based mostly on unstructured data. Tools are available that are specifically designed to extract clinical concepts from free text medical notes and other clinical documents such as pathology reports. Examples include MedLEE, which was developed at Brandeis University (Friedman 2000) and MetaMap developed at the

National Library of Medicine (NLM) to translate text into the NLM's very comprehensive Unified Medical Language System (UMLS). The most visible example of this approach is IBM's computer system (Watson), which has been deployed at Memorial Sloan-Kettering Cancer Center to help oncologists make better treatment decisions. The belief behind much of this approach is that free text information is the predominant form for both the medical literature and patient charts. IBM's Ed Nazarko makes the point that the information in the unstructured part of medical records may be richer, more detailed, and even more accurate than structured data, in part because clinicians do not like entering structured data and do it poorly and, in part, because no single existing medical ontology can be used practically to elicit the amount of clinical detail needed to describe real-world patients (Nazarko 2013). The Watson project at Memorial Sloan-Kettering Cancer Center will be discussed in more detail in chapter 10.

A key purpose of data standards is to facilitate the collection of structured clinical data. Doing this in practice is difficult with one of the root causes being complexity. Providers often complain about digital charting taking too much time. This may well be, at least in part, the result of the complexity of the data and data structures that is being navigated for charting purposes. SNOMED is the most sophisticated and complete ontology of medical terms. Keep in mind that ontologies represent not just the data items but their relationships to each other. SNOMED CT is the "simplified" version of SNOMED focused on clinical practice. However, SNOMED CT still contains 311,000 concepts connected to each other through over 1,300,000 relationships. How does one write software that allows busy clinicians to navigate through something that complex and still maintain the efficiency of care? In short, how does one collect high quality data from clinicians without slowing down their practice to the point that it is just not acceptable to them and is not economically sustainable? A similar issue arises with the increasing complexity of the International Classification of Disease (ICD) as it evolves into an ontology capable of representing clinical concepts that further define and refine the diagnoses that have traditionally been its core component. Logical Observation Identifiers Names and Codes (LOINC) is yet another commonly used but increasingly complex data standard. It relates mostly to lab tests and other clinical observations but still contains nearly 60,000 codes, and for each of those, there are six axes descriptive of the test or observation: once again, a lot of complexity. Medications are the simplest clinical element to code. The National Drug Code (NDC) system has been in use since the 1970s, long before most other data standards were widely used. It is a US specific system, consisting of ten digits that identifies the producer of the drug, the drug, and the package form. There are over 86,000 NDC codes in the version currently posted on the National Library of Medicine website. This is still more complexity for providers to navigate. Imagine having to do it *all*: identifying the correct SNOMED CT, ICD, LOINC, CPT (Current Procedural Terminology), and NDC codes for the current patient.

Historically, the goal has been to avoid as much free text, unstructured data as possible because it can be vague, difficult to use or even read, and is not a usable platform for reminders and clinical decision support and other secondary purposes. Structured data have been viewed as more precise and reliable and certainly more useful for supporting clinical decisions and for other purposes such as public health surveillance and research. But how does one collect this data? There are, of course, a number of approaches given the large number of EHR systems. The most common is called "templates," essentially the electronic version of the paper check forms that many providers have developed for use in their paper-based charts. These forms often relate to a specific clinical problem, particularly for a specialist who frequently sees the same problems. In templates, all the common issues and all the common answers are predefined and laid out so that the provider just checks whatever is appropriate for each patient. The commonly expressed criticism of this approach is that it represents "cookie cutter medicine" that does not allow providers to fully express the clinical information necessary to justify their decisions and fully communicate each patient's situation. On the other hand, computer-based versions of this approach typically allow for many (even thousands in some cases) templates that can provide a high degree of patient specificity if they are used appropriately.

Another less common approach is to take advantage of the relationships built into the ontologies so that the provider can navigate up and down a tree, by expanding to reveal more detail and contracting to reveal less as they go. This allows documentation at whatever level of detail is appropriate for each patient with minimal use of free text. Typically a note is built and displayed in another window as the provider selects whatever clinical details are appropriate. The tree structure must be complex to accommodate the rich set of clinical findings that are encountered in medical practice, so there may well be a lot of clicking (or touching with today's tablet computers) involved. Providers using a highly structured approach to documentation often complain that the resulting notes lack the nuanced details that free text notes provide.

Promising Approaches

There are approaches that can overcome at least some of these issues. A healthcare-specific voice recognition technology and three commercial EHRs as illustrations of potential solutions will now be discussed. The documentation approaches discussed so far are passive—they present the provider with a way of charting but do not further intervene to make the job easier. Virtually all the template-based systems do allow each provider to customize their templates to better fit their particular patients and clinical approach. Some allow providers to exchange templates, so a generalist faced with a difficult or unusual (at least for them) problem can use a template developed by the appropriate specialist who sees that problem frequently. However, customized or not, the template is usually static at the time it is being used. Most cannot dynamically adapt to the specific patient and clinical situation, which is the root cause of the criticism commonly used against templates. Documenting against a structured medical ontology has a similar static issue, although the provider, given enough time and effort, could navigate the tree in a way that is best suited to each individual patient.

Solutions could be more clinically intelligent—they could be aware of the specifics of each patient encounter and adapt to it to make the provider's documentation task easier and to help avoid oversights in care and its documentation. The systems discussed next are built, at least in part, on a more clinically adaptive approach.

Case Study: M*Modal

M*Modal is not an EMR or EHR but an advanced healthcare-specific voice recognition technology. We first discuss it and then discuss an EHR that uses it in an attempt to provide more convenient and effective data collection. M*Modal began in 1998 when a group of three PhD students from Carnegie Mellon University spun voice recognition technology they had been working on into a company that was renamed M*Modal in 2001 with a narrowed focus on healthcare. It was acquired by MedQuist in 2012, and the entire company took the M*Modal name. It now offers a suite of web services that support speech-enabled EHRs, radiology reporting, mobile device-based clinical documentation, and traditional clinical documentation services based on human editing and billing coding, with predictive code generation from narrative text.

The technology had for years been very widely used by medical transcription services around the globe. The benefit to the services was that most of the transcription was done automatically, so expensive human labor was only needed to correct what the computer got wrong (it tells the humans what it is not certain of) or cannot transcribe at all (it also points those cases out).

Every instance of use goes back to the company's servers, which observe the corrections humans make and use that knowledge to further train the system, so over time, the system gets better even with various speaking styles, languages, and dialects. Moreover, it can now recognize text sufficiently well to put it into the proper section of a note, so that, for example, no matter the order in which the note is dictated, the chief complaint goes into that part of the note, while the physical exam, assessment, and plan go into their respective sections of the note.

In many instances clinical concepts are automatically identified in the text and are coded into structured medical terminology, such as SNOMED CT, and into various coding systems for medications, as well as into ICD, CPT, and LOINC. Here again the system has been trained over time as humans corrected coding mistakes or manually coded those things the computer could not code. The specific accuracy is highly dependent on (a) noise levels, (b) medical specialty, (c) amount of similar data previously seen, and (d) the subset of SNOMED codes of interest (for example, allergies, diseases, symptoms, procedures). Very specific clinical concepts, such as smoking history, that are normally expressed in one of a few possible ways, can be more accurately identified than concepts that can have a large number of possible expressions, such as the patient's problems. High levels of accuracy are possible. For example, the company says it has 97 to 100 percent speech understanding accuracy for radiologists dictating on high quality microphones in a quiet image reading room.

The overall accuracy is sufficient that some clients of the company use the technology to code already digital text information. They submit it from their system over the Internet to the company's Fluency for Coding service that identifies the clinical concepts and puts them into the appropriate structured nomenclature, most typically SNOMED CT. Some software is installed locally so that this process works better when there is a loss of Internet connectivity.

Several EHRs now have M*Modal technology built-in. In all such cases, it is still a web service, so the central system continues to learn and further develop from all users. Based on M*Modal's capabilities, it would appear that voice recognition has developed to the point that it can be a practical method of collecting and structuring clinical data. Greenway Medical Technologies was the first EHR vendor to take advantage of that.

Case Study: Greenway Medical Technologies

Greenway was founded in 1998 by nearly 100 physicians, clinicians, practice administrators, hospital executives, and community leaders with the goal of developing a long-term solution to rising healthcare costs, medical errors, and decreasing patient safety. Its EHR is called PrimeSUITE®. Figure 6.1 shows the integration of M*Modal's speech recognition (the speech controls are at the top) into its documentation process. In this example, the physician first imported the past medical history from the patient's face sheet into the new note and then dictated the chief complaint and the history of present illness. M*Modal software recognized what information belongs in those two sections of the chart and placed them accordingly.

Figure 6.1   A screenshot from Greenway's PrimeSuite EHR illustrates M*Modal integration into the charting process.

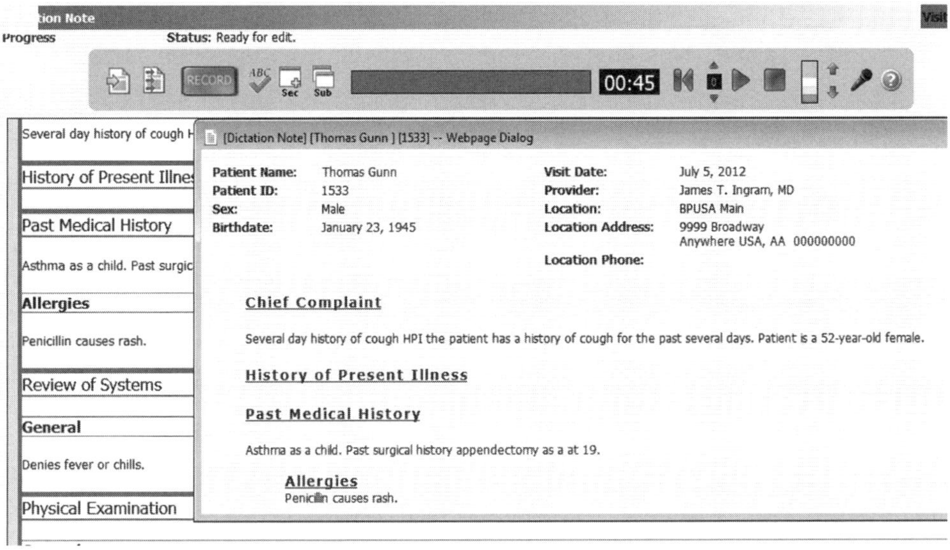

There are numerous other places where dictation can go directly into structured forms, such as the patient's cover sheet. Dictation process management is automated so that the resulting text is routed to an internal or external resource for verification and the correction of any mistakes. PrimeSUITE isn't yet converting text to structured clinical concepts, but Greenway says that this is planned for a future release.

In addition to using M*Modal's capability to convert unstructured text into SNOMED CT, the company has built an Extensible Markup Language (XML)-based document structure that conforms to Clinical Document Architecture (CDA), so key clinical documents, such as a history and physical, are standardized across most of their client sites. They take advantage of M*Modal's ability to recognize clinical concepts, so for example, if the physician says "chief complaint," the statement that follows is tagged in the underlying XML as the chief complaint (most likely the LOINC code 10154-3 or the SNOMED CT code 2476638014 for "presenting complaint"). The result is that these documents are usable for other purposes, such as extracting data for reporting or even for clinical research. To give one more example, if the physician says a patient is on 81 milligrams of aspirin that information would be tagged with an RxNorm reference code and put in the patient's medication history. RxNorm provides standardized names for clinical medications and then links them to most of the commercial medication databases used by information systems. It is part of the National Library of Medicine's Unified Medical Language System® (UMLS) effort to integrate and distribute key terminology, classification, and coding standards for healthcare.

In short, PrimeSUITE represents the use of a more clinically intelligent EHR technology. By converting free text to a structured ontology within a CDA framework, it essentially bridges the gap between what providers typically want to do—enter the same free text information they are used to noting—and making that information available for reporting, analysis, and even clinical research.

Case Study: WebChart by Medical Informatics Engineering (MIE)

MIE was founded by Doug Horner in 1995 as a HIE, including a clinical repository, mostly for lab data. This was at the very beginning of the Internet, and it is remarkable that the company was web-based from the outset and even provided the needed network connectivity to their clients' offices. Over the years their offering evolved into an EHR, starting with high-speed digital storage and management of transcribed documents. Next, they replaced paper charts using scanning integrated with bar code technology, so the system would know the type of each scanned document, technology that was previously developed for banking. They began with a group of dermatology providers who were used to dictating and transcription. Because of its image management, the service allowed MIE's clients to more compactly have their dictation and diagrams in one place. In this dermatology practice, MIE claims to have eliminated paper charts while reducing the number of transcriptionists from six to two because of productivity increases.

In 1998 MIE introduced WebChart (this was very early for a web-based EMR) and their "Minimally Invasive EMR™" around 2000. Horner feels that physicians are and should be "cognitive not clerical" (Horner 2013). The system "learns" each doctor's practice patterns and, over time, can predict what they are going to input and fills that in for them, a concept that is now widely used in the system. These learned concepts are not problem specific. Instead the system organizes answers to questions based on the patient's history and the most common questions for each chief complaint. To give a simple example, in a case typically requiring antibiotic therapy, the drug the physician has most often used in the past for similar cases would appear first on their list of choices. These preferences (for example, each physician's approach) are built into a "medical library" allowing nurses to switch libraries as they rotate among physicians. MIE provides some interesting case studies on its website.

MIE now has thousands of clients according to its website (http://www.mieweb.com/company/why-mie). The company also offers a personal health record (PHR) called NoMoreClipboard that is fully integrated with its EHR. Partially as a result of offering both capabilities, it is used extensively in occupational health clinics for major employers who typically use both an EMR and a PHR. To give one example of the integration, the EMR evaluates each patient's risk of developing particular chronic diseases, such as diabetes or hypertension, and tells the PHR what questions each patient should answer to further evaluate that risk and monitor their progression toward that disease or their success in helping to avoid it.

Case Study: Praxis by Infor-Med Corporation

Infor-Med Corporation was founded by Richard Low, a UCLA and Yale-educated physician, who first trained in surgery and did emergency medicine before shifting to internal medicine. Dr. Low recalls attending a seminar given by a physician and lawyer and first realizing how important medical documentation is. He later found out that the "average physician spends 2.5 hours per day doing paperwork, that's 8.5 years of his career" (Low 2013). He says he examined clinical records and determined that "no two doctors chart the same." His dream was to develop something that would save doctors time, while allowing them to maintain their individual approach to charting. Dr. Low says that he started the company in his native Argentina in 1989 with $15,000 of his own money, which, he says, went a great deal further there than it would have in the United States (Low 2013). The Praxis EMR was introduced in 1993, and since its second product release in 1998, the profitable company has grown with no outside financing.

The way Praxis makes documentation more efficient for physicians is itself not easy to understand. At its core is the notion of a "clinical concept." Praxis does not define concepts in a standardized way as, for example, SNOMED does. Rather they consider a concept an indivisible clinical unit in the view of an individual physician. In essence a concept is a basic element of the way a particular physician thinks about medicine.

Based on this idea, the company developed what it calls a "concept processor." The computer science term for this is an artificial neural network (ANN). An ANN is an advanced computing approach used to model complex relationships between inputs and outputs or to find patterns in data. A bank, for example, might use an ANN to find people who are more likely to be submitting fraudulent credit card charges based on patterns that might not be obvious to a person looking at the data, in part because of its massive scale. The technology is also being applied in healthcare to look for fraudulent claims.

The basic idea behind Praxis is that physicians develop a method of going from inputs—such as the history, physical exam, and lab results—to outputs, such as a diagnosis and treatment plan. Dr. Low says that its concept processor learns how each individual physician does this for the problems they see and uses that knowledge to save the physician time on subsequent visits by essentially anticipating what the physician will likely do and, therefore, document (Low 2013). The system starts as a "blank slate" in each practice but, over time, it gets better at finding the closest encounter to the current one. Dr. Low says that after around 50 iterations of a particular problem, the system is well trained and can accurately find the closest matching or even identical prior encounter (Low 2013). Based on this matching process, the EMR brings up the clinical concepts the physician has used in the past for similar patients, as illustrated in figure 6.2. The idea is that showing such similar prior patient notes will save the physician time and also serve to provide clinical reminders, reducing the chance that something will be overlooked or forgotten. Praxis has avoided the temptation to automatically document for the physician who must specifically decide

Figure 6.2   The Praxis EMR presents clinical concepts for the current patient based on the most similar previous patient(s).

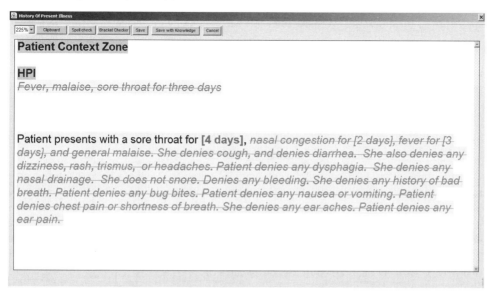

(by clicking on them) what to chart for each patient from the concepts presented from the most similar prior patient encounter. The physician can also add more or edit concepts for each case, as appropriate.

Documentation flow in Praxis is quite different than in traditional charting. Physicians are trained to begin by asking patients what brought them to the office—their chief complaint. Praxis does not begin with the chief complaint because it is typically a vague statement of the problem that usually will not provide sufficient specificity for the concept processor to find the best prior case. Physicians using Praxis are trained to first input the most clinically specific input (a "clinical finding") they can. This allows the concept processor to more accurately find the identical or best match to the patient being seen. Physicians can group subsets of an overall problem, such as acute pharyngitis (sore throat), according to whatever clinical divisions make sense to them. This further assists in getting to the best possible matching case and its associated clinical concepts. Physicians can post their own personal approach to clinical concepts so, for example, a family physician can import the approach used by an expert neurologist to evaluate headache.

Praxis is available as a hosted service or as a licensed client-server software program. Dr. Low says the company has around 3,000 clients with its largest user community being family physicians (Low 2013). Praxis scores very well in the 2012 annual survey of 3,088 family physicians done by the American Academy of Family Physicians (AAFP 2012). In that survey nearly 80 percent of the 21 Praxis users—a far higher percentage of positive ratings than for any other EMR—agreed with the statement that "This EHR helps me see more patients per day (or go home earlier) than I could with paper charts" (AAFP 2012). The survey provides some tentative confirmation (this is not a random survey so the results cannot be viewed as statistically proven) that a more clinically intelligent EMR can overcome the problem of reduced productivity with electronic versus paper charting.

The Data Visualization Challenge

Collecting high quality clinical data in a manner that is efficient for physicians is challenging but not the only major challenge facing contemporary health informatics as it is applied to medical practice. We now turn to a second challenge: visualizing that data, once collected, to optimally support high quality, efficient, and safe care.

This is a more formative area than data collection. The overall EMR visualization problem can be usefully considered against three axes, each of which presents its own more specific visualization challenges. These axes are:

- The types of patients seen in medical practice
- The medical specialties and their specific information requirements
- The clinical scenarios in which EMRs are viewed

There are, of course, many different kinds of patients. A young patient might come to the doctor with a broken arm. Such a patient usually has an acute problem that can be fully resolved in a few weeks with no long term consequences. Achieving that resolution may only require two or three clinical encounters. That patient, particularly since they are young, may have no other medical problems. The patient may not take any medications. There really is nothing else for the doctor to focus on. This patient has a very simple chart that may be entirely maintained in this physician's office.

This kind of patient is totally different than an older person with congestive heart failure who may have multiple other medical problems. The older patient might even have five or more chronic diseases. If so, the patient may well be taking 10 to 12 medication and would have been seen previously dozens of times. The patient is almost certainly receiving care from multiple providers with the inevitable differences in describing and recording clinical data, which complicates things, even if there is a functional HIE (which is often not the case) so that today's provider has access to the complete EHR. In summary, such a patient has a very complex chart. So, while this is an admittedly simple set of examples, the point should be clear. There are very different patients with very different charts.

There are also different kinds of physicians. A primary care physician seeing a hypothetical congestive heart failure patient is responsible for their total care and, at least to some level of detail, may well be interested in almost any of the data in their chart during any visit with that patient. This is very different than the specialist to whom that primary care physician might refer the patient. For example, suppose the patient has developed atrial fibrillation, a common cardiac arrhythmia (abnormal heart beat). That specialist may see the patient one time to evaluate and start the patient on what the specialist feels is the right therapy, and then send them back to their primary care system for follow up. If things go well, the specialist may never see the patient again or may just see the patient once a year to make sure the atrial fibrillation is well controlled. Such a specialist is not looking at the chart as broadly as the primary care physician is. The specialist may well investigate the patient's cardiac status more deeply but, for the most part, will ignore the rest of the chart unless it is directly relevant to the problem at hand.

Finally, there are the different reasons that a chart gets viewed. Again, let us consider a primary care physician seeing a patient for an annual checkup. Given the purpose of the visit, the physician will take a broad view of the patient and will review to some level of depth all issues, problems, medications, and so on. However, that same physician, while on call for their group, might get a telephone call from a patient in the middle of the night. Such a patient will have a clear chief complaint, which might be a fever or a cough or some other acute medical problem. In this situation, even a primary care physician is not going to go through the whole chart and review the history of all the patient's problems. The physician is going to focus on the reason for the call, and ideally would only want to look at the data that relates to that problem so the physician can make a quick decision and go back to bed. The decision most likely is whether the patient needs to go to the emergency room, can safely be seen in the office the next morning, or just needs a call in the morning to see if the problem has gotten better.

So, there are different kinds of patients, different charts, and different views of those charts depending on what kind of physician is looking at them and the reason why the physician is looking at them. The key point is that EHRs are unaware of this. For the most part, the same view of the chart is going to be available in all these situations. Of course, there is customization of views that is available in most EHRs, but really optimizing things around these different situations is probably beyond the capabilities of the customization. Moreover, were the customization features that robust, it is likely that few end users would be able to properly utilize them.

This problem falls into the domain of a relevantly new branch of computing called data visualization, and for several reasons, there is a growing interest in the field for applications including healthcare. First, there are now enormous digital data sets available in virtually all fields of endeavor—including healthcare now that electronic records are finally being widely deployed—and everywhere there is essentially the needle and hay stack problem: how to pull the useful information out of enormous amounts of data in order to optimize decision making.

Figure 6.3 is an example of a system that was developed to help with similar problems in other domains. While the tool has not yet been formally used in healthcare, this example uses data from prostate cancer patients to visualize their therapy in relationship to the staging (progression) of their disease. It is courtesy of Professor John Stasko of Georgia Tech, who is an expert in the field of data visualization. The tool, called Jigsaw, analyzes a gigantic database of text documents and visualizes them according to whatever axes a particular user finds interesting. The key is using analytics to find connections among and between data items that might otherwise not be made.

This might support the EHR visualization proposed by Dr. Jonathan Nebeker. He has a deep interest in health informatics with a particular focus on things such as clinical decision support and visualization of clinical data from EHRs. Refer back to figure 4.3 and you will see that his model groups clinical information in a chart into in four dimensions: interventions, conditions or health concerns, observations, and goals. These can and do interact, so for example, from a semantic point of view, interventions treat conditions, while conditions manifest themselves through measurable or other types of observations. Interventions may have a physiological effect that, in turn, has a manifestation. Interventions may exacerbate, improve, or have indeterminate effects on diseases. The information in a chart reflects these

Figure 6.3   Jigsaw, a data visualization and analysis tool, highlights relationships between the stage of prostate cancer (at the right), treatments (middle), and medications (left).

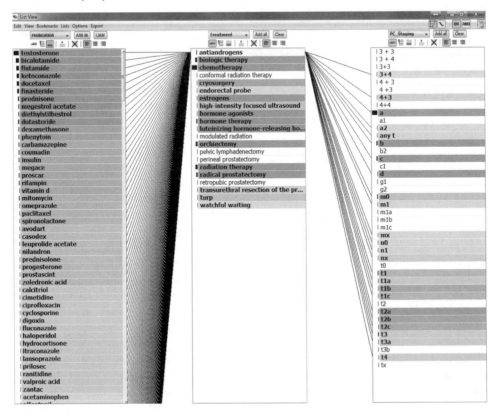

semantic relationships, so his group works on relating information across and within these four dimensions, as illustrated in figure 4.3. The highlighting shown is as if someone had clicked on hypertension in the conditions column. Based on that, the EHR, which understands clinical relationships, is highlighting the related clinically relevant information. For example, a patient might well be taking various medications only some of which are treating the hypertension. Their hypertension manifests itself through observations, such as their systolic and diastolic blood pressure.

In addition to their interest in improved visualization of clinical data, Dr. Nebeker's group emphasizes patient-centered functional goals, such as increased lifespan. These depend, of course, on the intermediate observation-based medical goals, such as maintaining blood pressure within a certain range. However, the range in figure 4.3 between the bars is not generic but is tailored to the specific patient. This hypothetical older patient with diabetes and high blood pressure gets light-headed and experiences falls when his blood pressure is within the accepted normal range for his age. The provider in this scenario can customize the patient's range to a higher intermediate medical goal. The key point is not treating the goals from the provider's perspective, but treating things that matter to patients both in terms of mortality and morbidity, with morbidity being reflected as functional status and symptom control. Dr. Nebeker contends that is the appropriate measure for quality of care.

How can this visualization relate interventions, conditions, or health concerns, observations, and goals, since for the most part, those relationships are not explicit (or even implicit) in health data standards or ontologies? Dr. Nebeker's group uses the National Drug File Reference Terminology (NDF-RT), which was developed by the VA and FDA and relates medications to the interventions they treat and their physiological effects. They have extended the terminology to map manifestations and goals. At present, the terminology is incomplete, but they are working on extending it by various means, including what is essentially "crowd sourcing" by letting providers make these associations ad hoc, just by dragging and dropping information objects among the four axes in the semantic model.

The problem of medication reconciliation is another use case for improved visualization. When patients move from one care venue to another—from home to a hospital or from the hospital to a skilled nursing facility—their medication program is often disrupted. They are either not kept on the medicines they should be on or they are put on the wrong dosage of these medicines or other issues arise. Medication reconciliation is the process of spotting these problems during, in particular, these transitions of care. An innovation visualization approach for medication reconciliation was developed by Dr. Ben Shneiderman's highly-regarded data visualization group at the University of Maryland (Plaisant 2012). The video (Plaisant 2012) provides an example of the potential for innovation in the visualization of health data. Shneiderman's group has also published *Interactive Information Visualization to Explore and Query Electronic Health Records* (Rind et al. 2013), a comprehensive overview of the whole topic of information visualization with respect to EHRs.

Another important publication that is relevant to the visualization challenge, as well as other challenges of contemporary health informatics, is entitled *Computational Technology for Effective Health Care: Immediate Steps and Strategic Directions* (Stead and Lin 2009). The group that published the report was headed by Vanderbilt's Dr. Bill Stead, one of the contemporary academic thought leaders in health informatics. The report looks broadly at the effectiveness of health information technology with respect to improving clinical care. It attempts to identify the gaps between the best of this day's technology and what is ultimately needed to improve healthcare. It concludes that computer-based tools and systems that offer clinicians and their patients assistance for thinking about and solving health problems related to specific instances of care is an imperative:

> These multiple sources of evidence—viewed from the committee's perspective—suggest that current efforts aimed at the nationwide deployment of health care IT will not be sufficient to achieve the vision of 21st century health care, and may even set back the cause if these efforts continue wholly without change from their present course. Specifically, success in this regard will require greater emphasis on providing cognitive support for health care providers and for patients and family caregivers on the part of computer science and health/biomedical informatics researchers. Vendors, health care organizations, and government will also have to pay attention to cognitive support, which refers to computer based tools and systems that offer clinicians and patients assistance for thinking about and solving problems related to specific instances of health care. This point is the central conclusion of this report. (Stead and Lin 2009)

The report goes on to describe cognitive support as systems that relate more specifically to the mental models that physicians have as they care for patients and that caregivers have as they deal with disease. This view aligns with the axes discussed at the beginning of this section and the approaches taken by some of the commercial systems and research projects that have been discussed.

The report further suggests the need for providing more evidence-based clinical decision support as an integral component of EMRs used in daily practice. This is made more explicit by a list of "seven information-intensive aspects of the IOM's vision for 21st century health care":

- Comprehensive data on patients' conditions, treatments, and outcomes;
- Cognitive support for health care professionals and patients to help integrate patient-specific data where possible and account for any uncertainties that remain;
- Cognitive support for health care professionals to help integrate evidence-based practice guidelines and research results into daily practice;
- Instruments and tools that allow clinicians to manage a portfolio of patients and to highlight problems as they arise both for an individual patient and within populations;
- Rapid integration of new instrumentation, biological knowledge, treatment modalities, and so on into a "learning" health care system that encourages early adoption of promising methods but also analyzes all patient experience as experimental data;
- Accommodation of growing heterogeneity of locales for provision of care, including home instrumentation for monitoring and treatment, lifestyle integration, and remote assistance; and
- Empowerment of patients and their families in effective management of health care decisions and their implementation, including personal health records, education about the individual's conditions and options, and support of timely and focused communication with professional health care providers. (Stead and Lin 2009)

While these recommendations go far beyond the data visualization challenge, they are intimately intertwined with it and further demonstrate the importance of having good data visualization tools built into EHR systems and of collecting quality data to drive those tools.

REFERENCES

AAFP. 2012. The 2012 EHR User Satisfaction Survey: Responses from 3,088 Family Physicians. http://www.nebrafp.org/media_area/2012EHRUserSatisfactionSurvey.pdf

American Medical Association. 2012. Exam Room Computing & Patient-Physician Interactions. http://www.ama-assn.org/assets/meeting/2013a/a13-bot-21.pdf

Brailer, D. 2005. Interoperability: The key to the future health care system. *Health Affairs* (web only). http://content.healthaffairs.org/content/suppl/2005/01/18/hlthaff.w5.19.DC1

Commonwealth Fund. 2008. 2008 Commonwealth Fund International Health Policy Survey of Sicker Adults. http://www.commonwealthfund.org/Surveys/2008/2008-Commonwealth-Fund-International-Health-Policy-Survey-of-Sicker-Adults.aspx

Commonwealth Fund. 2011. International Survey of Sicker Adults. http://www.commonwealthfund.org/Publications/In-the-Literature/2011/Nov/2011-International-Survey-Of-Patients.aspx

Deloitte. 2013. Physician Adoption of Health Information Technology. http://www.deloitte.com/view/en_US/us/Industries/health-care-providers/46fb8ec4d1a8e310VgnVCM2000003356f70aRCRD.htm

Friedman, C. 2000. A broad-coverage natural language processing system. Proceedings of the AMIA Symposium. 270–274 http://www.ncbi.nlm.nih.gov/pmc/articles/PMC2243979/

Horner, D. 2013. Interview by M. Braunstein. Skype, Spring 2013.

Low, R. 2013. Interview by M. Braunstein. Skype, Spring 2013.

MIT. 2011. Electronic health records (EHR): Benefits and challenges for data quality. *The Fifth MIT Information Quality Industry Symposium.* http://mitiq.mit.edu/IQIS/Documents/CDOIQS_201177/Papers/02_08_2B_Panel_Disc.pdf

Nazarko, E. 2013 (July 25). Personal communication with author.

Nightingale, Florence. 1863. *Notes on Hospitals. London*: Longmans, Green and Company.

Plaisant, C. 2012. "Twinlist demo (March 2012)." Video clip. YouTube. http://www.youtube.com/watch?v=YXkq9hQppOw

Rind, A., T. Wang, W. Aigner, S. Miksch, K. Wongsuphasawat, C. Plaisant, and B. Shneiderman. 2013. Interactive information visualization to explore and query electronic health records. *Foundations and Trends® in Human–Computer Interaction.* 5:3 207–298.

Stead, W.W. and H.S. Lin. 2009. *Computational Technology for Effective Health Care: Immediate Steps and Strategic Directions.* The National Academies Press. http://www.ncbi.nlm.nih.gov/books/NBK20640/

University of Washington School of Medicine. 1998. Ethics in Medicine. http://depts.washington.edu/bioethx/topics/mistks.html

Walker, J., E. Pan, D. Johnston, J. Adler-Milstein, D.W. Bates, and B. Middleton. 2005. The Value Of Health Care Information Exchange And Interoperability. http://content.healthaffairs.org/content/suppl/2005/02/07/hlthaff.w5.10.DC1

Weed, L. 1969. Medical Records, Medical Education, and Patient Care: The Problem-Oriented Medical Record as a Basic Tool. Cleveland, OH: Press of Case Western Reserve University.

Weiskopf, N.G. and C. Wang. 2012. Methods and dimensions of electronic health record data quality assessment: Enabling reuse for clinical research. http://jamia.bmj.com/content/early/2012/06/24/amiajnl-2011-000681.long

Wilcox, A., S.S. Jones, D.A. Dorr, W. Cannon, L. Burns, K. Radican, K. Christensen, C. Brunker, A. Larsen, S.P. Narus, S.N. Thornton, and P.D. Clayton. 2005. Use and Impact of a Computer-Generated Patient Summary Worksheet for Primary Care. *AMIA Annual Symposium Proceedings.* 824–828. http://www.ncbi.nlm.nih.gov/pmc/articles/PMC1560720/#!po=70.0000

RECOMMENDED READING AND RESOURCES

A recent and up-to-date primer on the problems of using electronic health record data for research: http://online.liebertpub.com/doi/full/10.1089/big.2013.0023.

A discussion of the interoperability issue by the first director of ONC is found in this reference: Brailer, D. 2005. Interoperability: The key to the future health care system. *Health Affairs* (web only). http://content.healthaffairs.org/content/suppl/2005/01/18/hlthaff.w5.19.DC1.

MIE WebChart Case Studies: http://www.mieweb.com/solutions/webchart-ehr-case-studies/.

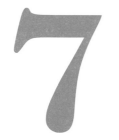

Chapter

7

Empowering the Patient

Chronic diseases can be caused by lifestyle and behavior decisions. Success in treating chronic disease involves patients making different choices and changing the behaviors that can lead to development of the diseases. The management of these diseases is ideally on a continuous basis (the usual term for this is *continuity of care*), which necessarily requires patient involvement from home. From an informatics point of view this all implies that healthcare data exchange take place not only among providers but between providers and their patients. Patient-facing tools are required to do this, and this chapter will deal with specific technologies for use by patients. These technologies must address several important issues: where can the data come from to manage patients on a more continuous basis; how can this data be turned into useful and actionable information for busy providers; and how can informatics engage patients to help them better manage and even prevent chronic disease?

Overview

For many years, chronic disease patients have been encouraged by their provider to keep logs of information, such as their blood pressure or their compliance with the use of certain important medications. Interestingly, the term "personal health record" apparently first appeared in 1978 in *Health Visitor*, the official journal of the Health Visitors Association (the term home healthcare is used in the United States) in the United Kingdom (Anonymous 1978). The ability to take this idea entirely into the digital age necessitated the common availability of the Internet and of patient-facing tools such as modern browsers, smartphones and mobile apps. Even with those technologic advances, the concept has not yet gained wide traction for reasons that will be discussed after a more detailed view of what a personal health record (PHR) is and can do.

The Markle Foundation's Personal Health Working Group's final report on PHRs released in 2003 defined a PHR as an:

> Internet-based set of tools that allow people to access and coordinate their life-long health information and make appropriate parts of it available to those who need it. PHRs offer an integrated and comprehensive view of health information, including information people generate themselves such as symptoms and medication use, information from doctors such as diagnoses and test results, and information from their pharmacies and insurance companies. (Markle Foundation 2003)

The report listed these key attributes of a PHR:

- Gives each person control of his or her own PHR
- Allows individuals to decide which parts of their PHR can be accessed, by whom, and for how long
- Contains information from the patient's entire lifetime
- Contains information from all healthcare providers
- Is accessible from any place at any time
- Is private and secure
- Is "transparent," individuals can see who entered each piece of data, where it was transferred from, and who has viewed it
- Permits easy exchange of information with other health information systems and health professionals (Markle Foundation 2003)

The report presents data that shows that substantial majorities of patients would use a PHR for key health functions with the interest higher among chronic disease patients and their caregivers. Functions that patients found particularly interesting were:

- E-mail my doctor (75 percent)
- Track immunizations (69 percent)
- Note mistakes in my record (69 percent)
- Transfer information to new doctors (65 percent)
- Get and track my test results (63 percent) (Markle Foundation 2003)

These same patients saw the following list of potential benefits from using a PHR:

- Help me understand my doctor's instructions (71 percent)
- Prevent medical mistakes (65 percent)
- Give me more control over my care (64 percent)
- Help me ask better questions (62 percent)
- Change how I take care of myself (60 percent) (Markle Foundation 2003)

Finally, virtually all patients (91 percent) expressed concerns about the privacy and security of their health data, but only 25 percent felt that these concerns were sufficient to prevent them from using a PHR because of their view that sufficient protective technologies exist (Markle Foundation 2003).

PHRs can provide services that patients value because they can see the potential benefits and, despite real concerns about privacy and security, are willing to embrace the technology. Yet, according to the IDC Health Insights' survey in 2011, only 7 percent of respondents reported ever having used a PHR, and less than half of these respondents (47.6 percent) are still using one to manage their family's health (Dunbrack 2011). Further, the majority of respondents (50.6 percent) said that the reason why they had not used the online technology was that they were not familiar with the concept of a PHR (Dunbrack 2011). This suggests that providers have a key role to play in introducing patients to information technology for their use and in encouraging patients to use it, a concept that is supported by two studies (Fotsch 2006; Jimison et al. 2008). Indeed, both Kaiser Permanente and the Veteran's Administration, organizations that are known to encourage patient use of technology, report much higher utilization (Kaiser Permanente 2012; Tsai and Rosenheck 2012). As discussed, one of the key objectives of Meaningful Use Stage 2 is to encourage providers to help patients with adoption of technologies that will enable and encourage patient participation in their own care.

Given the wide interest and the perception of benefits, why have PHRs not already gained more widespread adoption? This is a question with a complex set of answers. The need for more providers to help patients understand and adopt the technologies has already been discussed. However, there have been issues with the technologies themselves. Among them are issues that are similar, in many respects, to the barriers that have impeded the adoption and effective use of electronic medical records (EMRs) and health information exchange (HIE). First is the data entry issue. Until recently patients wanting to use a PHR had to enter their own medical information. Convincing people to spend the time to do that has been an issue. Perhaps an even larger problem is the collection of structured data. In one way this is similar to what has been discussed with respect to providers and EMRs. It can take too much time. In addition medical terminology can be complex and foreign for patients. Despite this, to get structured information that could support providing feedback and other services to the PHR users, developers have generally asked patients to enter information by selecting among terms that might be unfamiliar to them. Google left the PHR field in 2012, but when students in a Georgia Tech graduate seminar were asked to create their own PHR using Google Health, they were often intimidated by the quantity of data they had to input and the complex and unfamiliar medical terminology they had to use to enter their data. Given this, it is not hard to imagine how difficult this would be for less technically sophisticated patients. At least one recent study determined that the "key variable explaining patient willingness to adopt a PHR was the patient's health literacy" (Noblin et al. 2012).

More recently, as discussed, standards have emerged for the sharing of basic health records using the Consolidated Continuity of Care Document (CCCD) and the Blue Button + format, both files that can contain a reasonably comprehensive and structured patient record. These have been embraced by the PHR developers who are aware of the barrier to adoption that the data collection problem creates and most PHRs will now upload patient data from the provider's EHR if it is in these formats.

For a patient to be able to import their health data via a CCCD or the Blue Button +, their physician(s) must have adopted EHRs that can export data in these formats. Here the requirements of electronic health record (EHR) certification and Meaningful Use come into play. Stage 2 of Meaningful Use requires that a minimum percentage of a provider's practice seen within each reporting period must actually access their records electronically. An export of a CCCD or Blue Button + file from the provider's EHR and import of that data into the patient's PHR is an attractive and relatively easy solution to this requirement.

The Blue Button + pull initiative is setting the stage for patients to be able to "register" their Direct e-mail address with their provider and get automated updates sent to their PHR whenever new information becomes available. This might include sending automated reminders to patients with specific health conditions or the need for age and gender-specific check-ups. It might also include secure delivery of visit summaries and patient instructions after a healthcare visit. The approach is based upon HTTP RESTful (Hypertext Transfer Protocol Representational State Transfer) transport protocols, which allow an automated interaction between a server (in this case the EHR) and a client (in this case the PHR). Measures are included to assure trust, a potential problem whenever patients are interacting with their providers electronically, particularly if the patients registered independently of their provider for their PHR. The PHR goes through a patient registration process that establishes what it is called, where to find it, what permissions it might ask patients for, and how to display an authorization screen to patients. It is not difficult to envision how important widespread use of this approach might be for the multiple chronic disease patients for whom requesting data from their multiple providers might itself be a difficult task. A Markle Foundation report goes beyond the one provider scenario and calls for "PHRs [to] contain information from all health care providers" (Markle Foundation 2003). Ideally the multiple chronic disease patients can use one PHR to bring together all of their basic health data from all of their providers. That puts the patient in the position to provide an overview of their care when and where it is needed, fulfilling a very old idea: the patient should be the ultimate repository of their own health record. Should this happen, PHRs would be increasingly able to provide valuable information and services to those patients and their providers.

PHR Case Study: HealthVault

HealthVault was funded and incubated within Microsoft, starting in 2005, by Peter Neupert and Sean Nolan. Mr. Nolan, now a distinguished engineer at Microsoft, says he learned over the ensuing years that interoperability and innovation in healthcare were harder and took longer than he had expected (Nolan 2013). Today, based on the many factors we've been discussing, he feels they are finally in the right place at the right time, something he expressed by saying that "patients as a hub of information sharing are going to be a key part of our healthcare system" (Nolan 2013).

So far HealthVault has been most successfully introduced to people when they are having a life event, such as a baby, getting a new medical diagnosis, having a medical emergency, or having a parent getting older and needing help. At that point, a key advisor, such as a physician, can best introduce people to PHR technology. HealthVault agrees with others that employers also make sense as a point to introduce PHRs, but has not focused on them yet.

Over the next few years, Mr. Nolan feels that there will be sufficient saturation of interoperability that PHR adoption will increase (Nolan 2013). HealthVault has very successfully implemented an app platform, and today there are some 140 apps, which, along with around 220 medical devices, can interact with a patient's PHR, often to provide personalized support based on the data stored there or to serve as the data warehouse for information patients collect (Nolan 2013). The HealthVault API is platform agnostic (it even works with iPhones) (Nolan 2013). Through the API, a developer could ask HealthVault for "all this patient's blood pressures" or "all of those blood pressures with a systolic component over 120." Consent for use of their data, along with all other stored information, is entirely managed by the patient.

Both the American Heart Association (AHA) and the American Diabetes Association (ADA) have used the HealthVault API as part of tools they have created for patient management of diseases within their respective domains. AHA's Heart360 app allows patients to track and manage their heart-related health data, access additional information and resources on how to be heart healthy, and share their results with their provider. A separate app for providers allows them to see how their patients with a heart condition are doing. Again, the HealthVault system manages consent to assure that patients are always in full control of access to their data. The ADA provides similar capabilities to diabetics through its Diabetes 24/7 HealthVault app.

Example of a HealthVault App

PHR apps can be used for very serious purposes and can have both patient- and provider-facing components. The Interoperability & Integration Innovation Lab (I3L) at Georgia Tech has developed a HealthVault app in support of an Office of the National Coordinator for Health Information Technology (ONC) HIE Challenge Grant funded project in Rome, Georgia. Breast cancer patients use an Android tablet to access credible education content specific to their clinical situation. They use a HealthVault app (MyJourney Compass) that tracks five symptoms common to cancer and provides bidirectional capability between patients and their ambulatory providers. Symptoms are captured in the tablet, stored in patients' HealthVault PHR and transmitted using GA Direct, Georgia's Health Information Network's Direct HISP (Health Information Service Provider). Also using GA Direct, the provider organizations push clinical summaries to patients for inclusion in their PHRs. In the case of one provider, a Consolidated Clinical Document Architecture (CCDA) Extensible Markup Language (XML) formatted clinical summary meeting the stage 2 Meaningful Use requirement is provided via a patient portal using a Blue Button format. The other two provider organizations are providing patients with PDF versions of their clinical summaries until the providers' EHR systems are upgraded to meet the stage 2 requirements at which time they will convert to sending a CCDA summary. In figure 7.1, one of the clinical symptoms the patient is tracking is pain, a very common problem in cancer and one where input from the patient to the provider is a key to good management. Also note the use of a special Direct e-mail address, which would be given out after the established trust process has been completed to verify the identity of the provider or patient using that address.

Figure 7.1   Cancer patients can use the MyJourney Compass HealthVault app to record their pain level and four other measures and can send the results for the past two weeks, along with a comment, to their provider using GeorgiaDirect (Direct messaging) via the GA Health Information Network (GAHIN)—the statewide HIE in Georgia.

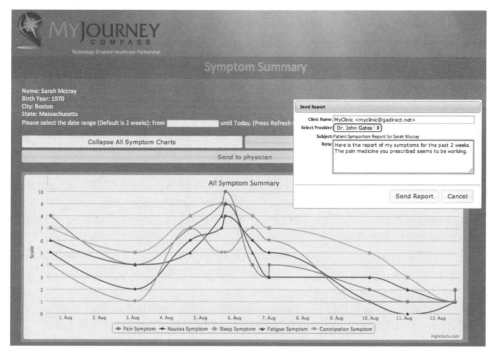

Other PHRs

There are, of course, other providers of PHRs. The Dossia Consortium, a not-for-profit association of major employers, was formed in 2006 and provides an open-source, secure, PHR platform supporting apps for consumer, patients, and providers. An example in public health was developed with the New York City Department of Health and Mental Hygiene and consists of two components: (1) a dashboard (external to the PHR) that provides volunteer workers with graphical population and individual level tracking and reporting, intervention, communication, and contextual education materials; and (2) a Dossia PHR app that tracks a hypertension initiative. Other PHR apps provide health risk assessment, medication management, and other capabilities, along with an integrated health record that includes data from medical devices (wireless blood pressure cuff and scale).

PHRs may be morphing into app platforms, but they are hardly the only, or even the major, home for these new and convenient patient-facing tools. The predominant base for healthcare apps is the smartphone.

Health Apps

In January 2007, Apple introduced the iPhone and the idea that virtually anyone could create relatively simple programs (apps) and efficiently sell them through an online store without having to deal with the details of software distribution and online e-commerce. Today the iPhone and Google's Android are the two most popular smartphones, and there are hundreds of thousands of apps in their respective stores. A site that tracks mobile technology publishes *Consumer Health Apps for Apple's iPhone*, and its August 2012 version claims to list over 13,000 apps (mobihealthnews 2011).

As would be expected, the patient health apps vary enormously in sophistication, functionality, and the degree to which they are directly involved in patient care rather than in other important areas, such as maintaining health and wellness. A search of the Apple app store for "blood pressure" finds 539 iPhone apps and 236 iPad apps. Most of these that record data have patients manually enter their blood pressure readings so they can graph and track them and even send them by e-mail to their physicians. Patients are not covered by HIPAA, so they can even do this using regular e-mail, if they wish. More sophisticated apps, such as the iHealth™ Blood Pressure Dock, automatically collect the data, in this case by connecting to the company's US Food and Drug Administration (FDA)-cleared wrist blood pressure measurement device. This company also offers a digital scale that communicates wirelessly with an iPhone via Bluetooth®. Data collection by smartphones may potentially even include an ECG. AliveCor has announced a technology in which the ECG leads are embedded in a special smartphone case. This approach has been FDA cleared and is available for sale to licensed providers and patients via a prescription. Given the sophistication of these apps, it is not surprising that the FDA announced, just before the end of the 2013 federal fiscal year, that it would begin regulating health apps that:

- [Were developed] to be used as accessories to regulated medical devices, such as apps that allow health care providers to make diagnoses by viewing medical images on smartphones or tablets
- [Can] transform mobile devices into regulated medical devices, such as apps that allow a smartphone to be used as an electrocardiography machine (FDA 2013)

Legislation has been introduced in the US Congress to "provide regulatory clarity regarding mobile medical applications, clinical decision support, electronic health records and other healthcare related software" (Slabodkin 2013).

There are other examples of a smartphone being used as a health measurement device. A group at Georgia Tech Research Institute is developing iTrem, an app that measures patient's tremors using the accelerometers built into smartphones. SkinScan™ uses the smartphone's camera to take pictures of lesions of concern to the patient and even analyzes them to advise the patient if they need to see a dermatologist.

Other apps are offered for use by clinicians for functions such as assistance in interpreting ECGs. Apps are being offered as devices for use in hospitals and even in critical care. AirStrip™ is marketing an FDA-cleared platform that allows waveforms and other clinical information from sophisticated hospital patient monitoring systems to be accessed by their clinician via a smartphone or tablet computer.

This technology will become more embedded in healthcare delivery over time, particularly as the apps implement the data representation and transport standards that are increasingly in use by EHR systems. At the same time they introduce new problems in securing and insuring the privacy of protected health information (PHI) and in verifying the trust necessary to know that health data is being sent where it is intended to go.

Before leaving health apps, it is worth noting that there is some evidence that mobile phones, and specifically their SMS text messaging capability, can be used to change patient behavior, a critical issue in prevention and management of chronic disease. A 2009 literature review of 14 studies that met the inclusion criteria found that behavior change interventions delivered by SMS can have positive short-term outcome but suggested that more and better research was needed (Fjeldsoe, Marshall, and Miller 2009). A literature review found 21 studies published in 27 papers looking at the use of SMS to improve diabetes management and found "some positive trends were noted, such as improved self-efficacy, hemoglobin A1c, and self-management behaviors," but that "many of these studies lacked sufficient sample sizes or intervention lengths to determine whether the results might be clinically or statistically significant" (Holtz and Lauckner 2012). One recent and widely publicized study suggests that SMS text messaging can be cost effectively used to achieve at least short-term reductions in smoking (Wells et al. 2012). Similar results were found by a group of Georgia Tech researchers for management of pediatric asthma patients (Tae-Jung et al. 2012).

The author is not aware of any studies in peer reviewed journals on the impact of actual mobile apps on patient behavior or clinical outcomes. A significant challenge for the app model is gaining an understanding of what aspects of the design of an application makes it effective, particularly in terms of patient engagement. Health communication research and psychology research, such as social cognitive theory, have long sought to understand what influences human behavior, and more to the point, what influences a person to change their behavior. Health apps offer the possibility to answer long standing questions by making it possible to monitor what information a person pays attention to and how they communicate with care providers and people in their social network. Health apps also suggest new questions, such as how an online game can catalyze learning about a health condition and motivate healthy behavior. For example the MAHI app for diabetes management increased patients' internal locus of control (an individual's belief that they can influence future health outcomes) and their willingness to experiment with healthy eating alternatives (Mamykina et al. 2008). However, currently there are wide gulfs between the design of new health apps and understanding what makes them effective. This is clearly an area in need of more study.

Health Websites

Health websites are an area of health informatics with a large potential but with many unresolved issues. According to the Centers for Disease Control and Prevention (CDC):

> research has shown that 74% of all U.S. adults use the Internet, and 61% have used it to look for health or medical information. Additionally, 49% have accessed a website that provides information about a specific medical condition or problem. (Cohen and Adams 2009)

"Patients are increasingly using the internet for health-related information and may bring this to a GP consultation" (Bowes et al. 2012). The issue of how providers incorporate these new patient tools into their practice is far from resolved (Forkner-Dunn 2003; Gerber and Eiser 2001).

Health websites can be usefully divided into several groups based on their level of sophistication: patient education, patient search, patient communities, and PatientsLikeMe®.

Patient Education: The Mayo Clinic's site is probably the best known example of a patient-facing health education site. It is a rich site providing well written monographs, describing a huge list of diseases and conditions. Some monographs include a video. There is also information on how conditions are diagnosed and treated at Mayo, available clinical trials, Mayo research into the condition, as well as profiles of the researchers in that area, and actual patient stories. Not all of these are available for every condition. There are many other well-known general patient education sites and numerous sites focused on a specific diagnosis or disease class.

Patient Search: As mentioned earlier, best practices have yet to be developed for incorporating web tools into clinical practice. The physician concerns in this regard are clearer. They include the lack of reimbursement of e-mail interaction with patients and time wasted with patients who bring in concerns, suggested treatments, or diagnoses based on unreliable or inappropriate information.

Personalized search could substantially remedy this. The basic idea is to equip a specialized health search tool with clinical knowledge about the individual patient or health consumer using it. This idea is already commonplace—perhaps too commonplace. Use any of the major search engines and you will be presented with ads that somehow relate to your interests. What is happening is that the search engines are paying attention to what you look for and learning even more detail about you based on what you show interest in by clicking on it. Simply put, if you search for information about cars, then it is far more likely you are in the market to buy one.

Health is a more complex challenge for personalization. People may not know the right terms to use to describe their problem or interest. In addition, many unapproved "cures" and "treatments" are offered and the sites promoting them can be a wealth of misinformation. The Internet in general provides a great deal of misinformation and biased or inexpert opinions. However, it can be particularly problematic if people decide they have some rare, life threatening disease based on an Internet search, or if they do have a serious illness, they become enamored of a bogus remedy that will not cure it and may even do them harm.

A solution may be linking some form of search to trusted and reliable information about the patient. This might come from a PHR that is populated with data from the patient, from health claims, or from the patient's EHR. This is yet another area where the semantic web might be of great value. The data from a patient's PHR could theoretically inform an intelligent search engine that could use the semantic web to find the best results, even considering the sort of data relationships we discussed earlier with respect to health ontologies, since it is likely that these ontologies will be encompassed by the web's Resource Description Framework (RDF) framework.

Patient Communities: In the past few years the Internet has morphed from a place where people primarily consume information to one where they are actively involved in contributing it. This "social networking" is arguably the primary use of the Internet today. There are several advantages of social networking, particularly for patients with rare or unusual conditions or patients with no local support system. Virtual communities provide a way to engage with people with similar problems, identify medical resources, share experiences, prepare for what is ahead or even explore the success others have had with specific treatments. They can also be a source of practical advice on coping with the personal and family issues associated with disease.

PatientsLikeMe®: PatientsLikeMe may be the most sophisticated health social networking site. The company was cofounded in 2004 by three MIT-trained engineers: Benjamin and James Heywood (brothers) and longtime friend Jeff Cole. Five years earlier, the Heywoods' brother, Stephen Heywood, had been diagnosed with amyotrophic lateral sclerosis (ALS, also known as Lou Gehrig's disease) at the age of 29. The Heywood family soon began searching the world for ideas that would extend and improve Stephen's life. They envisioned an environment for sharing and collecting data, typically on innovative treatments for incurable disease. To accomplish this, social networking was built on a research platform. Getting patients engaged in aggregated clinical research was their primary mission.

The site is free to patients and accepts no advertising, but it is not a non-profit business. The objective is to gather data from patients about the illness experience and make that available in aggregated form to organizations that are interested in particular populations of patients. Examples would be pharmaceutical companies or companies with early stage products that want to learn from patients that have the condition they seek to treat. For example, a pharmaceutical company might partner with the site to create a portal for engaging organ transplant recipients, a site within the site, where it can talk to patients and learn from them, while at the same time considering the aggregated data. The site now has well over 1,000 conditions, but prior to April 2011 there were 20 (Okun 2013).

To create a clinically relevant research platform, PatientsLikeMe uses structured surveys to collect patient-reported data. Novel treatment, symptom, and condition data enter the "User Voice dashboard," where it is reviewed and curated to assure data integrity. The company receives around 75 "user voice" entries per day (Okun 2013). Some may already be in the system. For example, there could be a spelling difference, or the patient could have entered two concepts together, such as "pain and depression." These are split so the patient can monitor each separately and each can be aggregated for research purposes.

All clinical data is coded in the background using standardized terminologies. Symptoms and side effects are coded into Systemized Nomenclature of Medicine Clinical Terms (SNOMED CT) and Medical Dictionary for Regulatory Activities (MedDRA), a medical terminology used to classify adverse events associated with the use of biopharmaceuticals and other medical products. Diagnoses are coded into ICD-10, the next generation of this coding system that, as you should know, is not yet widely used in the United States. Despite this high degree of coding, as much as possible the "patient voice" is maintained.

PatientsLikeMe points out that the patient self-manages around 90 percent of their care (Okun 2013). As shown in figure 7.2, the site helps patients put their conditions in context; organize the status of symptoms, treatments, and side effects; and prepare themselves for a clinician encounter through the use of a clinician visit sheet. They try to help patients

Figure 7.2   A multiple sclerosis member of PatientsLikeMe has an integrated view of their care.

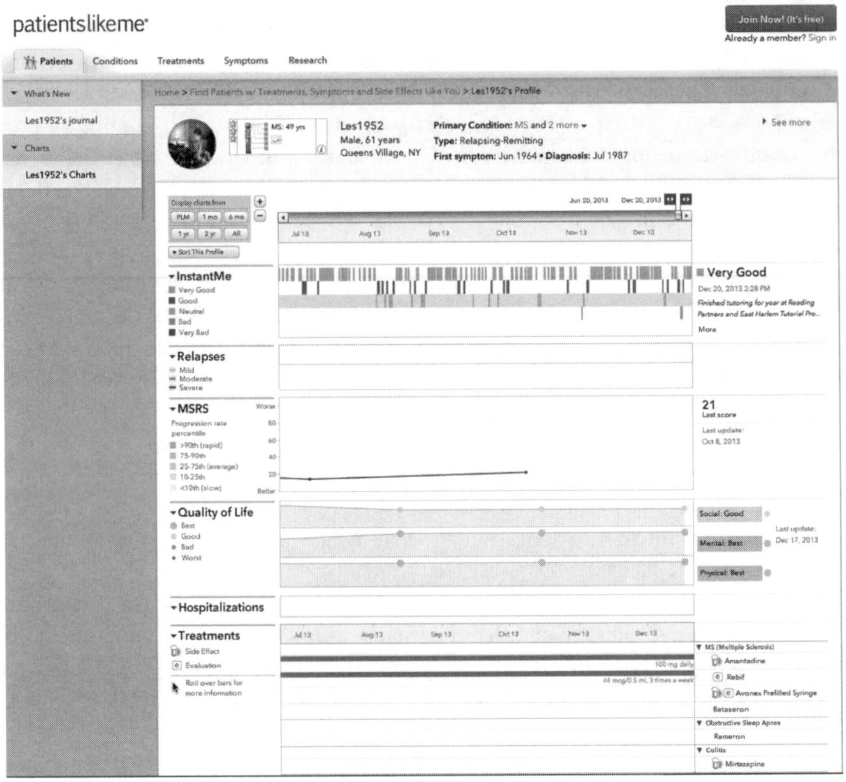

answer the question "given my status, what is the best outcome I can hope to achieve and how do I get there"? They offer patients connections to other similar patients and patient communities.

PatientsLikeMe is perhaps best known for a dramatic research study initiated by the patients themselves. After a report from Italy suggested that Lithium might slow the progression of their disease, a group of patients with ALS decided to experiment on their own with lithium carbonate treatment. Patients using lithium asked for support to find the effects, if any (Okun 2013). In 12 months using the tools on the site, patients showed that Lithium had no effect on their disease progression (Wick et al. 2011). A traditional clinical trial would almost certainly have taken several years. This study dramatically illustrates the potential for patient participation in their own health and in clinical research through making data more accessible and easier to share, aggregate, and analyze.

Patient Portals

The concept of a web-based patient portal preceded the PHR and is still in wide use today. McKesson Technology Solutions, whose RelayHealth division is a leader in this space, has a patent for an electronic method of communication between healthcare providers and patients involving personalized webpages for doctors and their patients.

Figure 7.3   Patients can export or download their health data using RelayHealth. Note that the Blue Button is available to patients to upload EMR data into their RelayHealth record.

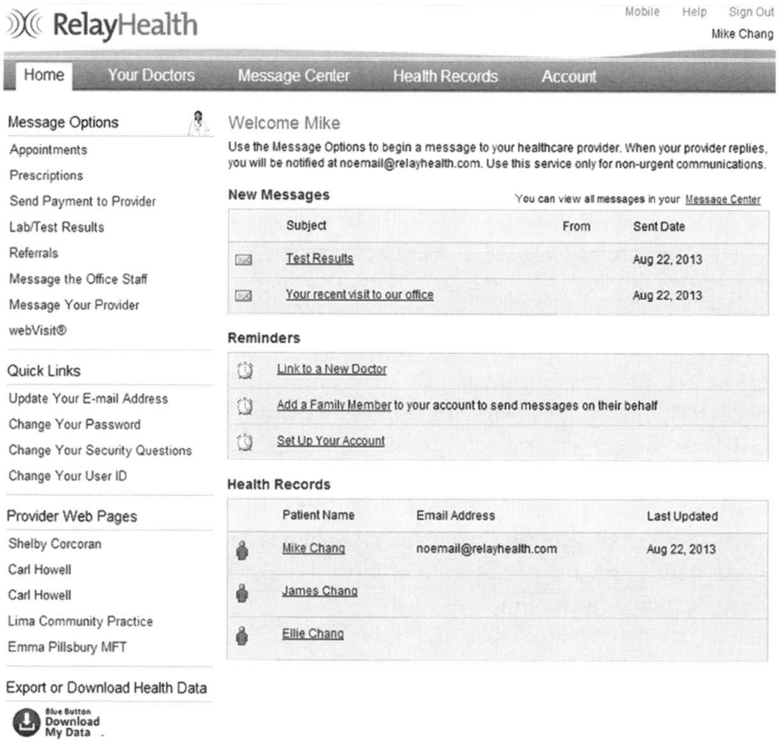

A patient portal is a webpage that facilitates communication between patients and their health providers. Potential functions include secure e-mail, making appointments, and viewing test results. In general patients do not input their own clinical data into a portal. Some portals now include the capability for a patient to upload their clinical data in the Continuity of Care Document (CCD) or Blue Button format (or the newer CCDA and Blue Button + formats) from their provider's EHR into their PHR.

RelayHealth

RelayHealth was originally founded in 1999 as Healinx by Assaf Morag. Today their patient portal serves over 2,000,000 activated patients and is interfaced to all of the major health enterprise systems (Kahlon 2013). A health system typically provides RelayHealth's health information exchange capabilities for use by its employed providers or those that commonly refer patients to the health system. RelayHealth's platform facilitates clinical integration of data (using HL7, CCD, Blue Button, and other standards) among EHR systems (figure 7.3), and also includes a frontend portal for those users who do not have an EHR. In 2011 RelayHealth won the Blue Button for All Americans Challenge by being the first vendor to support the Blue Button for more than 25,000 physicians and other clinical providers (Kahlon 2013).

The platform is optimized to build a longitudinal patient record by integrating with clinical inpatient systems, such as the billing system, the emergency department system, the inpatient EHR, the laboratory system, the radiology system, and the transcription system via Health Level 7 (HL7) and CCD standards. Ambulatory EHRs can use either the CCD format or HL7, as well integrate with RelayHealth. They also provide support for Direct and the new Transitions of Care (ToC) Consolidated CDA (CCDA) format. An example of ToC would be discharge from a hospital to a rehabilitation facility after surgery. RelayHealth was one of the first six companies in the CommonWell Health Alliance to promote and facilitate health data interchange (CommonWell Health Alliance 2013).

The end goal is that patients get an integrated inpatient/outpatient longitudinal patient record, as well as tools to manage their care. They can also get a total family record—parents' and children's health records—in one place. Patients can contribute most of their data, and RelayHealth also supports a connection to Microsoft HealthVault to access information from some connected devices.

Patients can request appointments using the portal. These requests are routed to the staff members within a practice who are trained to interface with the portal. Patients can also request prescription renewals and refills through the system. The majority of these transactions are routed to pharmacies through SureScripts.

The system provides patient-to-provider and provider-to-provider secure messaging, as well as management of sending orders and receiving their results. The patient's primary care physician gets automatic notification of any emergency department visits, an important feature to help assure continuity of care.

To support all this functionality, RelayHealth provides a cross-organizational master patient index (XMPI) and does extensive terminology mapping to and from its base nomenclature of SNOMED for clinical problems, International Classification of Disease (ICD) for diagnoses, and Medi-Span (a commercial provider of medication databases) for medications.

Home Telehealth

Patients with chronic diseases can face a daunting challenge. They must manage chronic disease in their homes every day for the rest of their lives. This can involve medications, diet, exercise, and tracking physiologic or other biologic parameters. Changes in reimbursement are fostering a growing interest on the part of providers in knowing how their chronic disease patients are doing on a more continuous basis. As a result technology for patient use at home is an active area for research and development as well as commercial activity and has been so for many years. These technologies divide into several sub areas that are listed in order of increasing sophistication and potential value:

- Subjective data about symptoms or status that patients enter into a portal or PHR can be of value to their care providers.
- Significantly more value can be obtained from objective data, such as weight, blood pressure, or blood glucose. It is becoming more common for patients at home to obtain their own physiologic measurements.
- Technology could provide ongoing advice and assistance to patients in managing their diet, exercise, and medications.
- With relatively inexpensive equipment and a high speed Internet connection, a care coordinator could make virtual home visits when the data from the patient indicates one might be appropriate.

Research suggests that, in time, it might be possible that technology in the home could monitor patient behavior to help detect issues like a decline in clinical status for a patient with congestive heart failure, based on changes in their movement patterns or even a failure to take prescribed medications (Georgia Institute of Technology 2010). This field is called "behavior imaging," essentially sensing and understanding patient behavior remotely through various technologies. The technology is already being provided commercially by companies, such as Behavior Imaging Solutions, for use in the assessment and treatment of disorders such as autism.

These functions, taken as a whole, comprise the still developing field of home telemedicine. One of the first people to think deeply about the field was Steve Kaufman, who founded HealthTech Services in 1988, where he developed a device called HANC (Home Assisted Nursing Care), a physically large and quite expensive home care nursing robot and assistant to aid a broad range of home care patients in achieving what is called "supported independence." Today, with the huge reductions in their size and cost, the use of robots as assistive devices in the home is now an area of active research and may even reach commercialization in the coming years (Broekens et al. 2009).

However, financial incentives in healthcare do not yet generally facilitate the use of robotic or most other far less expensive technologies for patient care in the home. In many ways, the reimbursement problem is similar to provider use of EMRs or even e-mail, in that the adoption of technology may not happen unless providers have an incentive to use it. Using e-mail to communicate with patients makes perfect sense and is probably preferred by many patients, but it will not happen as often as it could if providers only get paid for physical visits. The advent of outcome-based payment could change this dynamic. If providers are interested in achieving the best and most economical outcomes, and if technology in the home is shown to more than pay for itself by helping achieve these outcomes, then it would be logical for providers to see that technology in the home is provided, even if they have to pay for it.

Despite the reimbursement issue, there are numerous commercial home telehealth products on the market. The simplest and least expensive deliver a single physiologic measurement, such as blood pressure. They may be Bluetooth® enabled, so that the data can go to a cell phone, and from there, to a website. Often this data flow is a service provided for a monthly fee by the device maker. While this business model is attractive to companies, since recurring revenue is far more lucrative, and hence more valuable, than one time device purchases, it risks creating a series of proprietary databases (often termed "walled gardens"), each of which has its own narrow view of the patient.

There are initiatives and offerings designed to avoid this happening. The Continua™ Health Alliance was created in 2006 by a group of technology, medical device, and healthcare delivery organizations, and it now has more than 200 members (Continua Health Alliance 2013). The goal is to create standards for interoperable home telehealth devices and services in three major categories: chronic disease management, aging independently, and health and physical fitness.

Even without such standards, exporting telehealth data from the home to a PHR can integrate it with data from other devices and with the rest of the patient's clinical record. Qualcomm's Health Management division offers their own approach to this integration. Their 2net™ Hub Platform includes two components. The first is a small hub device that plugs into an electrical outlet and provides single point collection of wireless health data in the home. It supports the Bluetooth®, Bluetooth Low Energy, Wi-Fi, and ANT+ local area radio protocols. It is also Continua™ certified. The second component is a cloud-based service for aggregation and analysis of the data. The data can be sent from there to EHRs and other systems operated by providers or other organizations interested in the patient's status. It can also be sent to the patient's PHR. According to the company the system was designed and engineered to meet all HIPAA requirements (Qualcomm Life 2013). A new company, humanAPI, also proposes to collect patient data from many sources and unify access to it into a single pipeline. However, access to the data (similarly to FHIR and Health eDecisions) is via a RESTful API. This company also claims to meet all HIPAA requirements.

The Future

Much progress has been made in home telehealth. Scales, blood pressure, and other measurement devices now typically incorporate Bluetooth®, and that technology now works well enough that the need for managing wires has been largely eliminated, so devices can be placed more conveniently for the patient. The scale, for example, can more likely be placed in its traditional bathroom location. The user interface is facilitated because touch technology is far better and less expensive because touch panels are now so widely used in cars, new tablet computers, and other devices. However, for the most part, today's in-home telehealth products are surprisingly similar, both functionally and technologically, to what was offered a decade or more ago.

What might change this? Certainly outcome-based contracting may have a large impact on deployment, but what will improve the usability and acceptability of the technology itself? What will lead to greater success in changing patient behaviors?

All current telehealth technologies represent, to one degree or another, an intrusion of "foreign" devices into the home. To some this can be threatening or intimidating. Suppose the patient's interface to this new technology was through something far more familiar, such as a TV. Largely homebound patients often watch TV on a regular, daily basis. The screens are large enough that even people with poor eyesight can easily read them. Digital TVs are really a specialized computer. Most are now capable of being connected to the Internet. Some even provide an "app platform," but the user interfaces tend to be very poor and getting to the apps involves leaving the "TV world" and going into a quite different space that is unfamiliar to the user. What if these limitations were overcome and the app and TV worlds were seamlessly integrated? If, as is widely rumored, Apple or Microsoft introduce TVs, would they go much further? Microsoft has developed a new app layer for Windows 8 that is claimed to work seamlessly across smartphones, tablet computers, and regular PCs. Might the TV be next?

Apple and Microsoft already offer devices to turn an existing TV into an app platform. Apple's device is called Apple TV and is currently used mostly for streaming media from the Internet to a local television. Microsoft may be further down that road for health, since they have HealthVault, which is available as a Windows 8 app. The Windows 8 app platform will apparently soon work with Microsoft's Xbox, a device most people think of as a game console but one that is Internet-enabled and supports apps, including some for health and fitness. They also produce a device called Kinect that could potentially allow people to control their TV with gestures. At least one company, 5Plus, is using Kinect to image patient movements as part of physical therapy at home (Five Plus. 2013). Kinect might also be a future part of in-home behavior imaging. Samsung's Smart Interaction technology, built right into its high-end TVs, uses a camera and microphone to enable watchers to control TV functions via voice and gestures. Google's Chromecast is a device that plugs into any TV's High-Definition Multimedia Interface (HDMI) slot and turns that TV into a high definition Internet-enabled device. Through it hundreds of apps in the "Health and Fitness" category in the Google play store can now be displayed on any HDMI equipped TV. Apple

AirPlay-enabled Apps can be used on a TV via the Apple TV device but currently only a few are listed in the health and fitness section and none are listed in the medical section of the Apple TV guide (Apple 2013). For patients at home, could the TV be the long-sought gateway to a more active role in their own care?

Conclusion

Technology for patients, particularly as it finds its way into the home, has the potential to help make healthcare a more complete and effective system with respect to prevention and wellness and the management of chronic disease. Many challenges remain. They begin with proving the value of these technologies sufficiently for reimbursement for them to become more widely available. Doing that may well require adapting technologies, such as the TV, from the consumer electronics domain to take advantage of their lower cost, ease of use, and consumer familiarity.

Many feel the next stage of the evolution of technology will include the "Internet of Things" described by McKinsey in a way that closely mirrors the long held goals of health technology in the home:

> the physical world itself is becoming a type of information system. In what's called the Internet of Things, sensors and actuators embedded in physical objects—from roadways to pacemakers—are linked through wired and wireless networks, often using the same Internet Protocol (IP) that connects the Internet. These networks churn out huge volumes of data that flow to computers for analysis. When objects can both sense the environment and communicate, they become tools for understanding complexity and responding to it swiftly. (Chui et al 2010)

REFERENCES

Anonymous. 1978. Computerisation of personal health records. *Health Visitor* 51(6): 227.

Apple. 2013. AirPlay Apps List. http://theapple.tv/apps/list-of-airplay-enabled-apps/

Bowes, P., F. Stevenson, S. Ahluwalia, and E. Murray. 2012 (Nov.). "I need her to be a doctor": Patients' experiences of presenting health information from the internet in GP consultations. *Br J Gen Pract* 62(604). http://www.ncbi.nlm.nih.gov/pubmed/23211176

Broekens, J., M. Heerink, and H. Rosendal. 2009. Assistive social robots in elderly care: A review. *Gerontechnology* 8(2):94–103. http://mmi.tudelft.nl/~joostb/files/Broekens%20et%20al%20 2009.pdf

Chui, M, M. Löffler, and R. Roberts. 2010. The Internet of Things. McKinsey Quarterly. March. http://www.mckinsey.com/insights/high_tech_telecoms_internet/the_internet_of_things

Cohen, R.A. and P.F. Adams. 2009. Use of the Internet for health information: United States, *NCHS Data Brief no. 66.*

CommonWell Health Alliance. 2013. CommonWell Members. http://www.commonwellalliance .org/members

Continua Health Alliance. 2013. About the Alliance. http://www.continuaalliance.org/about-the-alliance

Dunbrack, L.A. 2011. Vendor Assessment: When Will PHR Platforms Gain Consumer Acceptance? http://www.idc-hi.com/getdoc.jsp?containerId=HI227550

Five Plus. 2013. http://www.5plustherapy.com/

Fjeldsoe, B.S., A.L. Marshall, and Y.D. Miller. 2009. Behavior change interventions delivered by mobile telephone short-message service. *Am J Prev Med* 36(2):65–173.

Forkner-Dunn, J. 2003. Internet-based patient self-care: The next generation of healthcare delivery. *J Med Internet Res.* 5(2):e8.

Fotsch, E. 2006. AHIC Chronic Care Workgroup Testimony. Secure messaging and online services to enhance care and health. http://www.webcitation.org/6C9ZNgdMjGeorgia Institute of Technology. 2010. Overview of Expedition in Computational Behavioral Science. http://www.cbs.gatech.edu/

Gerber, B.S. and A.R. Eiser. 2001. The patient–physician relationship in the Internet age: Future prospects and the research agenda. *J Med Internet Res* 3(2):e15.

Greenway. 2013. http://www.greenwaymedical.com/solutions/primesuite/

Holtz, B. and C. Lauckner. 2012 (Apr.). Diabetes management via mobile phones: A systematic review. *Telemed J E Health*18(3):175–84.

Jimison, H., P. Gorman, S. Woods, P. Nygren, M. Walker, S. Norris, and W. Hersh. 2008. Barriers and drivers of health information technology use for the elderly, chronically ill, and underserved. *Evid Rep Technol Assess* 175:1–1422. http://www.ahrq.gov/research/findings/evidence-based-reports/hitbar-evidence-report.pdf

Kahlon, S. 2013. Interview by M. Braunstein. Skype, Spring 2013.

Kaiser Permanente. 2012. News Center: Kaiser Permanente HealthConnect Electronic Health Record. http://xnet.kp.org/newscenter/aboutkp/healthconnect/faqs.html

Mamykina, L., E.D. Mynatt, P.R. Davidson, and D. Greenblatt. 2008. MAHI: Investigation of social scaffolding for reflective thinking in diabetes management. *Proceeding of the twenty-sixth annual SIGCHI conference on Human factors in computing systems ACM,* 477–486.

Markle Foundation. 2003. The Personal Health Working Group Final Report. http://www.policyarchive.org/handle/10207/bitstreams/15473.pdf

mobihealthnews. 2011. Consumer Health Apps for Apple's iPhone. Chester Street Publishing, Inc. http://mobihealthnews.com/research/consumer-health-apps-for-apples-iphone/)

Noblin, A.M., T.T.H. Wan, and M. Fottler. 2012. The impact of health literacy on a patient's decision to adopt a personal health. *Perspect Health Inf Manag* 9:1–13. http://www.ncbi.nlm.nih.gov/pmc/articles/PMC3510648/

Nolan, S. 2013. Interview by M. Braunstein. Skype, Spring 2013.

Okun, S. 2013. Interview by M. Braunstein. Skype, Spring 2013.

PatientsLikeMe. 2013. http://www.patientslikeme.com/

Praxis. 2013. http://www.praxisemr.com/

Qualcomm Life. 2013. Introducing the Award-Winning 2net Platform. http://www.qualcommlife.com/wireless-health

RelayHealth. 2013. http://www.relayhealth.com/

Slabodkin, G. 2013. Bill Provides Guidance on FDA Mobile Medical Apps Regulation. http://www.fiercemobilehealthcare.com/story/bill-provides-guidance-fda-mobile-medical-apps-regulation/2013-10-22.

Stasko, J., C. Görg, Z. Liu, A. Sainath, and C. Stolper. 2013. Jigsaw. http://www.cc.gatech.edu/gvu/ii/jigsaw/

Tae-Jung, Y., H. Young Jeong, T.D. Hill, B. Lesnick, R. Brown, G.D. Abowd, and R.I. Arriaga. 2012. Using SMS to provide continuous assessment and improve health outcomes for children with asthma. *Proceedings of the 2nd ACM SIGHIT International Health Informatics Symposium (IHI '12).* ACM. 621–630.

Tsai, J. and R.A. Rosenheck. 2012. Use of the internet and an online personal health record system by US veterans: Comparison of Veterans Affairs mental health service users and other veterans nationally. *J Am Med Inform Assoc* 19(6):1089–1094.

US Food and Drug Administration. 2013. FDA Issues Final Guidance on Mobile Medical Apps. http://www.fda.gov/NewsEvents/Newsroom/PressAnnouncements/ucm369431.htm

Wells, J., A. Srinath, C. Free, G. Forde, and C. Forde. 2012. Cost-effectiveness analysis of a mobile phone SMS text-based smoking cessation intervention. *UTMJ* 89(3):160–165.

Wick, P., T.E. Vaughan, M.P. Massagli, and J. Heywood. 2011. Accelerated clinical discovery using self-reported patient data collected online and a patient-matching algorithm. *Nat Biotechnol* 29(5):411–414.

RECOMMENDED READING AND RESOURCES

The Blue Button + Pull API can be found here: http://blue-button.github.io/blue-button-plus-pull/.

To see how far HealthVault apps have come, take the American Heart Association's Heart360 Guided Tour at http://www.youtube.com/watch?v=aWI7ziYz7Hg.

A later day embodiment of HANC is here: http://www.youtube.com/watch?v=EU4pTB6JeEY.

Georgia Tech's Healthcare Robotics Lab works on assisting patients at home: http://www.hsi.gatech.edu/hrl/.

A sample Blue Button ASCII file posted by the VA: http://www.va.gov/BLUEBUTTON/docs/sample_file.txt.

Examples of the use of the Blue Button: http://www.va.gov/BLUEBUTTON/Resources.asp.

The Blue Button + Implementation Guide site provides a wealth of information: http://bluebuttonplus.org/.

Chapter 8

Population Health Management

Population health is a relatively new term that has been defined as "the health outcomes of a group of individuals, including the distribution of such outcomes within the group" (Kindig and Stoddart 2003). One of the earliest publications in the field was *Why Are Some People Healthy and Others Not? The Determinants of Health of Populations* (Evans et al. 1994), a book which grew out of the work of the Population Health Program of the Canadian Institute for Advanced Research. Its authors state the concept's "linking thread [is] the common focus on trying to understand the determinants of health of populations" (Evans et al. 1994).

More recently, with the more widespread adoption of electronic health records (EHRs) and the development and deployment of cloud-based tools for aggregating and analyzing data derived from them across an entire population of patients, the term has come into use as a component of clinical practice. Throughout this book there has been a focus on patients with chronic disease and multiple chronic diseases in particular. Chronic disease accounts for the majority of healthcare spending, and most patients over 65 have one or more chronic diseases, so these patients are common in medical practices, particularly those of primary care physicians. Chronic disease is a lifelong condition requiring care over years or even decades. Each chronic disease patient should ideally be managed according to well-defined care processes. Certain tests should be done periodically to ascertain their degree of control or to screen for impending complications of their chronic disease. The usual design of electronic medical records (EMRs) is based on traditional medical practice in which patients are seen one at a time. A medical record, particularly if it provides clinical reminders and decision support, can help assure that each patient receives the proper care when in their provider's office and that other needed care is not overlooked. However, a primary care provider may have hundreds of chronic disease patients in their practice, not all of whom will be seen on a timely basis. Some patients may be brought in at a predetermined interval for a visit that was not required. Others may not be brought in soon enough to detect an exacerbation of their condition in time to avoid an emergency department visit or hospitalization. Digital tools have been developed to manage the population of patients in a provider's practice or even in a group of practices that are typically affiliated in some way, and these tools are the focus of this chapter.

As with many things in health informatics, the impetus for the use of these tools is in large part financial. In the past decade or so there has been growing interest in alternative payment approaches, starting with pay-for-performance (P4P) and the more advanced version of P4P called outcomes-based contracting.

According to a group at the Research Triangle Park Institute:

> A common criticism of [fee-for-service] FFS, which P4P is intended to address, is that FFS rewards providers for producing higher volumes of health care services without direct assessment of the effect on quality of care or overall costs of the healthcare system. By providing direct financial incentives tied to quality of care performance measures and cost of care performance measures, P4P should provide countervailing incentives that directly promote improved quality and reduced costs. (Cromwell et al. 2011)

In some cases (such as outcomes-based contracting) there can be a formal sharing of efficiency gains and cost savings, and there can even be penalties (so called loss sharing) if costs increase, stay the same, or even do not decrease by some agreed upon minimum amount.

Individual providers do not typically contract under P4P or outcomes-based payment systems. Instead, groups of providers, who are often aligned with or even employed by a hospital, do the contracting. For obvious reasons these groups want to monitor the care being delivered by their members against the quality and cost metrics that will determine what they are paid, identify individual providers who are not meeting objectives, and possibly even identify individual patients whose care does not meet standards or whose clinical status seems to be deteriorating in a way that could lead to expensive hospital care.

The informatics challenges that these new payment approaches raise have to do with capturing the data to measure quality and cost of care in aggregate across providers and visualizing the results at the individual-provider and even individual-patient level. This can be easier to do if all those providers have the same electronic health record (EHR) system, although even that does not necessarily assure consistency in the way data is collected or represented. The clinical data that will be specifically reported to the payer to assess the quality of care being delivered will be collected as structured data (International Classification of Disease [ICD], Current Procedural Terminology [CPT], and specified quality metrics, such as those discussed in chapter 2), and this data is collected using a consistent list of choices to avoid as much inaccuracy as possible. Even this, of course, does not eliminate the possibility of inaccurate reporting by individual providers and the same data quality issues discussed in the chapter 6. However, under the new payment models, there can be actual revenue implications for poor data quality, something that is virtually guaranteed to place a greater emphasis on the issue.

Moreover, in many situations, the individual providers do not have the same EHR system, substantially complicating the task of assembling a uniform dataset that can be usefully analyzed and reported. It is even possible that some providers are using paper records, a problem that is diminishing as EHR adoption grows. Some open source solutions have been developed and entrepreneurs have spotted an opportunity and have created a new class of commercial health informatics systems focused on population health management. This is a very important new class of technologies that can best be covered by looking at some specific case studies. As with the case studies in the prior two chapters, some of these are commercial systems, but their inclusion should not be interpreted to mean they are the best available systems or best suited for the particular purposes of any reader of this book.

Case Study: popHealth

popHealth is an open-source quality-measurement system funded by Office of the National Coordinator for Health Information Technology (ONC) and developed by the Mitre Corporation. It runs over Laika, an open-source EHR-testing framework intended to analyze

Figure 8.1   popHealth queries are run within the provider's firewall so protected health information (PHI) never leaves provider control.

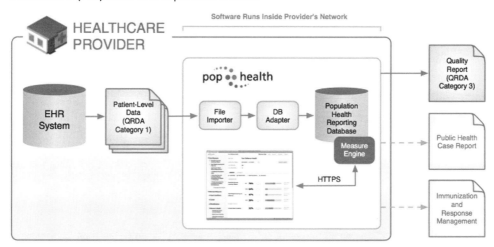

Source: ONC 2013

and report on the interoperability capabilities of EHR systems as a part of the EHR certification process. The technology approach is similar to hQuery, another ONC funded open source effort that automates a more generalized set of distributed queries across diverse EHRs for purposes such as clinical research. hQuery will be discussed in more detail in chapter 9. popHealth captures summary clinical data from healthcare providers' EHRs in one of the standard formats that will be discussed.

Figure 8.1 illustrates the data aggregation process. In it certified EHRs produce patient-level aggregated data formatted according to the Quality Reporting Document Architecture (QRDA), which is a Clinical Document Architecture (CDA) compliant standard that is discussed in more detail in chapter 9. These reports are in response to a query typically sent in Health Quality Measure Format (HQMF), a standard for representing health quality measures as an electronic document that is also discussed in more detail in chapter 9.

The QRDA files can provide data at a patient level (Category I), as a list of patients (Category II), or as aggregated data (Category III). In this example Category I data is being collected. A QRDA Category I report contains quality data for one patient for one or more quality metrics, and the data elements in the report are defined by the particular measure(s) being reported.

> A QRDA Category I report contains raw applicable patient data (e.g., the specific dates of an encounter, the clinical condition) using standardized coded data (e.g., ICD-9-CM, SNOMED CT). When pooled and analyzed, each report contributes the quality data necessary to calculate population measure metrics. (HL7 2012)

Software at the provider's site extracts the needed data from an EMR, packages it in the QRDA format, and sends it to the popHealth system, which then aggregates it and generates summary quality measure reports on the providers' patient population, as shown in Figure 8.2. Here data from 500 patients has been aggregated from a hypothetical practice consisting of 10 providers who could be using different EHRs. This is a key point. The use of query standards facilitates data collection, aggregation, and reporting, no matter what

Figure 8.2   popHealth aggregates and summarizes quality metrics for 500 patients from a 10-provider practice (providers could be using different EMRs).

Source: ONC 2013

the underlying EMRs. Of course, the EMRs or some other software in each provider's practice must be capable of interpreting the HQMF queries and packaging the data according to the QRDA format, but these are both relatively simple Extensible Markup Language (XML) documents formatted according to CDA, as shown in chapter 9. The underlying data structures, data representations, and database technologies in the multiple EMRs involved will typically be different, but this cloud-based process bridges those differences, at least for certain well-defined quality metrics.

The measures shown in Figure 8.2 should be familiar from our discussion of Meaningful Use in chapter 2. For each measure there is a goal (screening for the use of tobacco in the case of Preventive Care and Screening: Tobacco), a denominator (the number of patients for whom the measure is applicable), and a numerator (the number of patients who met the goal). This leads to the calculation of a percentage that is often compared against a contractually specified minimum for each quality metric. Adult weight screening illustrates the use of patient-specific information—in this case age—to stratify patients into two groups: those adults under 65 years of age and those aged 65 or above.

While reporting for Meaningful Use may be the most widespread use case for population health technologies, it is certainly not the only one. Another typical use case would be a physician network that has contracted with an insurance company, or even an employer, to provide care under a P4P approach. Under such a contract, common quality metrics, such as those illustrated in Figure 8.2, may have to be collected, aggregated, and reported. Managers in the physician network will be interested not only in the overall performance of

Figure 8.3 Several individual providers are compared with respect to a National Quality Forum (NQF) quality metric for screening for tobacco use.

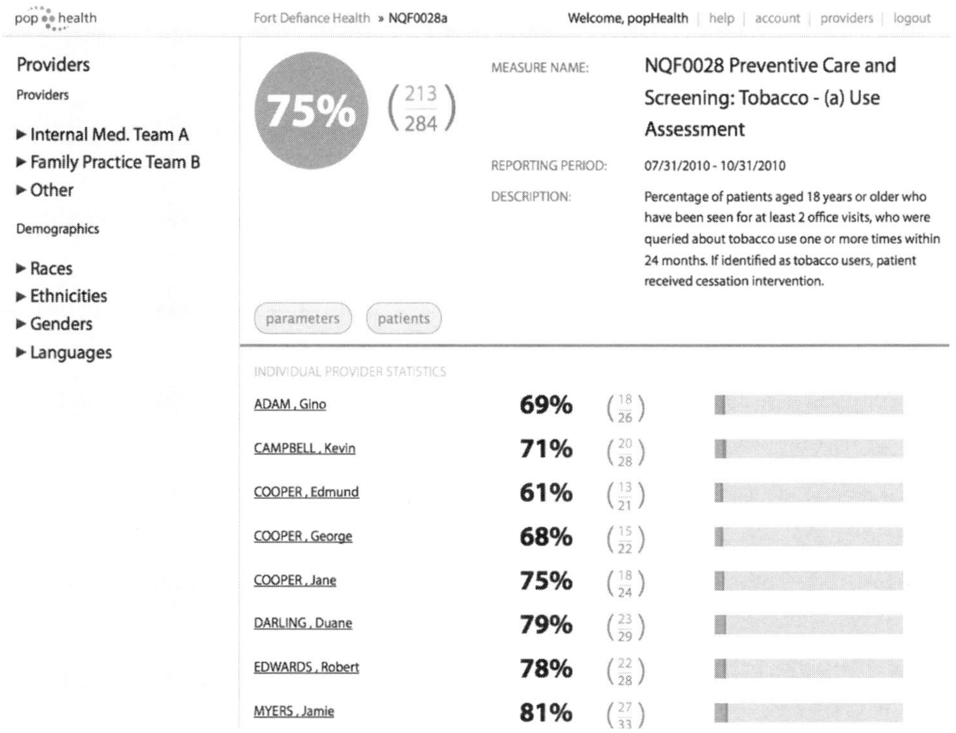

| pop ●● health | Fort Defiance Health » NQF0028a | Welcome, popHealth | help | account | providers | logout |

Providers

Providers

► Internal Med. Team A
► Family Practice Team B
► Other

Demographics

► Races
► Ethnicities
► Genders
► Languages

75% $\left(\frac{213}{284}\right)$

MEASURE NAME: **NQF0028 Preventive Care and Screening: Tobacco - (a) Use Assessment**

REPORTING PERIOD: 07/31/2010 - 10/31/2010

DESCRIPTION: Percentage of patients aged 18 years or older who have been seen for at least 2 office visits, who were queried about tobacco use one or more times within 24 months. If identified as tobacco users, patient received cessation intervention.

(parameters) (patients)

INDIVIDUAL PROVIDER STATISTICS

ADAM , Gino	69%	$\left(\frac{18}{26}\right)$
CAMPBELL , Kevin	71%	$\left(\frac{20}{28}\right)$
COOPER , Edmund	61%	$\left(\frac{13}{21}\right)$
COOPER , George	68%	$\left(\frac{15}{22}\right)$
COOPER , Jane	75%	$\left(\frac{18}{24}\right)$
DARLING , Duane	79%	$\left(\frac{23}{29}\right)$
EDWARDS , Robert	78%	$\left(\frac{22}{28}\right)$
MYERS , Jamie	81%	$\left(\frac{27}{33}\right)$

Source: ONC 2013

the network but with comparing the performance of individual providers against a chosen quality metric, as shown in figure 8.3. Figure 8.2 showed overall practice performance for several quality metrics. Figure 8.3 focuses on one metric but reports performance against it for several providers. Note as well, the menu on the left side of the figure, which provides a number of ways to sub-aggregate and report the data for this metric.

Finally, metrics for a specific patient can be summarized, as shown in figure 8.4. Note in the left side of the screen that outstanding quality metrics for this patient are flagged with dots (in red on the actual screens). Other clinical data for this patient is presented in the main part of the screen, giving the provider-focused dashboard from which the overall care of the patient can be considered.

This illustration of population health management brings together many of the key technologies and concepts from the earlier chapters in the book. Standards are critical to being able to collect and meaningfully aggregate the needed clinical data. Standards are also critical to having a single, machine-readable definition of the data that is required (the query) and of the results that are sent back. Such a distributed query framework greatly facilitates the exchange of data across the diverse EMRs that will typically be found in the United States. While it is not specifically illustrated in the figures, since both the query and the response are CDA-formatted XML documents, they could be attached to a Direct e-mail, further facilitating the needed information exchange, even from practices in a remote area not served by a formal health information exchange (HIE). The next section will turn to population health in a situation where such a formal exchange exists.

Figure 8.4   Quality metrics are summarized for an individual patient, and those that fail to meet a goal are highlighted on the left.

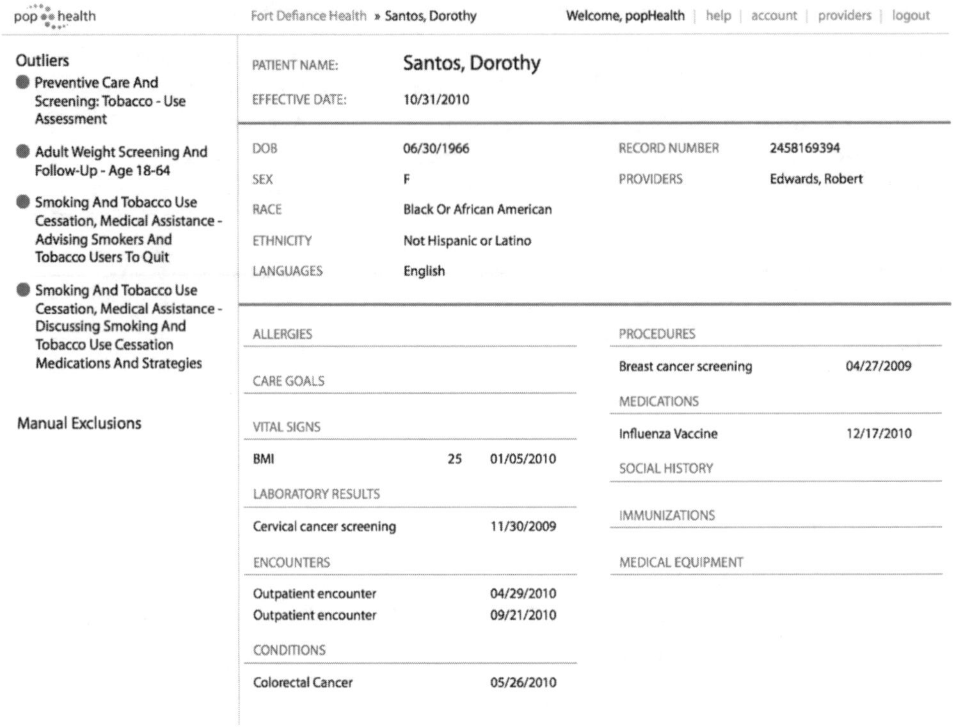

Source: ONC 2013

Case Study: Quality Health First

The Indiana Health Information Exchange's Quality Health First initiative provides a number of important services including:

- Tracking patients who are due for preventive screenings
- Reminders to providers of needed health screening interventions
- Disease-specific summaries based on each provider's patient population
- Comparisons of each provider to the provider community as a whole

These tools align well with the information necessary to manage care under a P4P or outcomes-based reimbursement system. Figure 8.5 shows a query capability to find specified subsets of patients based on a richer set of demographic, clinical, and financial factors than were illustrated by popHealth, a tool with a simpler data model to facilitate aggregating data from multiple EMRs. Indiana Health Information Exchange (IHIE) is, of course, a centralized HIE. IHIE normalizes a rich data set from the contributing EMRs and other sources and stores it in a central database. This facilitates more robust queries including those for population management against quality metrics. As a result, the data available are not limited to elements that are relatively standardized across EHRs because they are included in required reporting for Meaningful Use or are commonly required by P4P contracts.

Figure 8.5   The Quality Health First service from IHIE provides more detailed searching and query capabilities than would normally be available via a distributed query framework that uses a simpler data model to facilitate data aggregation from many different EMRs.

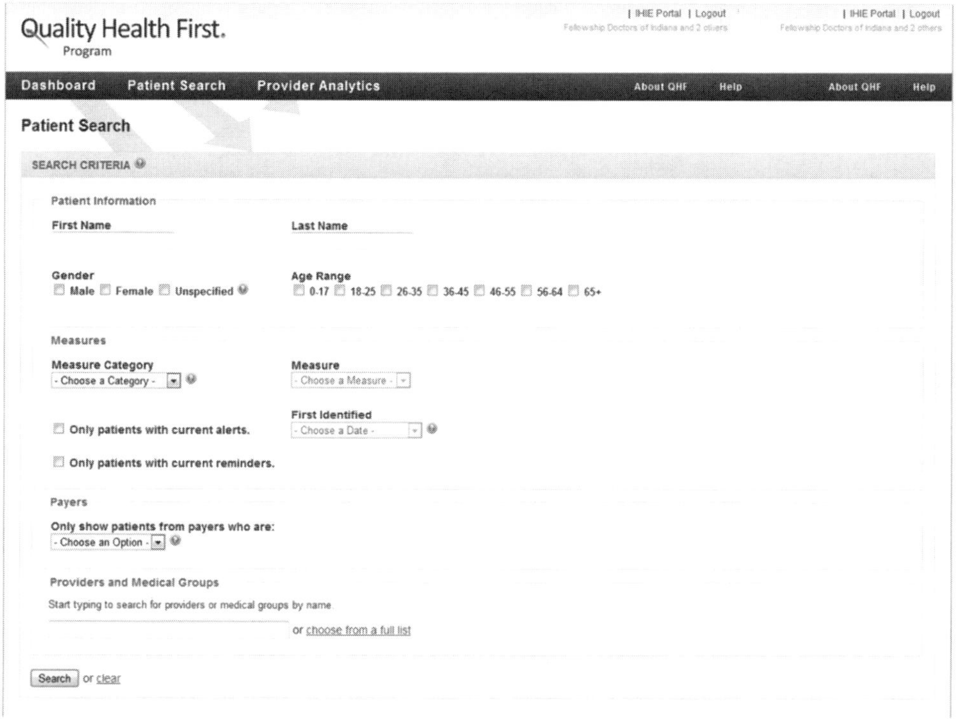

An aspect of Quality Health First is the public reporting of practice quality scores. Reporting practices must have a minimum of 30 patients in any measure and may comprise several physicians, including internists, family practitioners, and pediatricians, as well as nurse practitioners and physician assistants (IHIE 2013). Figures 8.6 and 8.7 are examples of this and show the wide variation among some of the reporting practices (this is not individual physician-level data) in their success in managing diabetes as indicated by the practice-to-practice variations in the process metric of obtaining an annual HbA1c (figure 8.6) and the percentage of diabetic patients that are under control as indicated by the outcome metric of a HbA1c equal to or less than 9 percent (figure 8.7). This data is publicly posted, introducing a level of transparency into the health system in Indiana, something many people believe is essential to increasing quality (IHIE 2013).

Transparency is a vehicle to achieve what the federal government calls "value-driven care." The motivation is that "consumers deserve to know the quality and cost of their health care. Health care transparency provides consumers with the information necessary, and the incentive, to choose health care providers based on value" (HHS 2013). To promote transparency, the federal government's Medicare program is also publicly posting its own quality metrics for participating hospitals. At the Hospital Compare website (http://www.medicare.gov/hospitalcompare/search.html), patients who are at risk might be concerned about the care given by their local hospitals for heart attacks (acute myocardial infarction or AMI). This site allows them to compare the performance of nearby hospitals on various metrics,

Figure 8.6   A Quality Health First report of the *process* metric for obtaining regular HbA1C levels for diabetic patients. The data is across many practices (only a partial list is shown here) and shows that three of the practices are below the state average (the yellow line) and two are below their regional average (the light gray line).

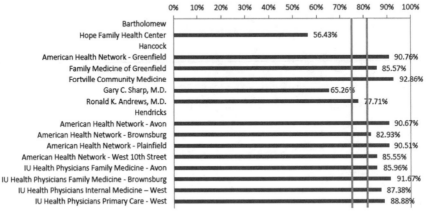

Figure 8.7   A Quality Health First report of the *outcome* metric for HbA1C levels for diabetic patients. The data is across many practices (only a partial list is shown here) and shows that seven of the practices are below the state average (the yellow line) and five are below their regional average (the light gray line).

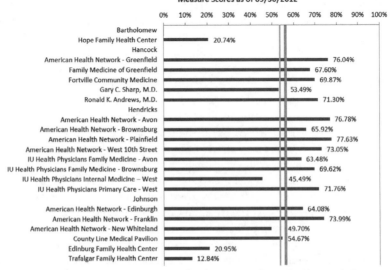

such as the percentage of the time that AMI patients being seen in the emergency department have an intervention done to open blocked vessels in their heart within the 90-minute window the best available current medical evidence says is appropriate for this care (Keeley et al. 2003). Medicare also offers a Physician Compare website (http://www.medicare.gov/physiciancompare/). Although currently no specific quality metrics are reported, physician participation in the Physician Quality Reporting System (PQRS), Electronic Prescribing (eRx) Incentive Program, and Electronic Health Record (EHR) Incentive Program is noted. The site says that "Beginning in 2014, Physician Compare will also include quality of care ratings for Group Practices. Ratings for individual physicians and other healthcare professionals will be added in the future." (Medicare.gov 2013)

Hospitals and physicians can't choose whether or not to participate in the federal quality comparison programs, but they do have to opt-in to the public reporting on Quality Health First. Molly Hale, IHIE's director of marketing and communications says:

> Developing the public reporting site the way it is now took a fair amount of community discussion among provider stakeholders as well as employers and payers. The practice site level reporting was the preferred approach, rather than individual physician level reporting, because some physicians don't have enough patients with particular conditions to make measures related to those conditions statistically significant. Also, only primary care practices are included in public reporting because specialists don't participate in QHF. The data is risk-adjusted for each practice's payer mix, broken down into commercial, Medicare, and Medicaid patients. In the case of solo practitioners, scores would be reflective of one physician; however the majority of the reports are for group practices. (Hale 2013)

Risk adjusted data is a particularly important issue for comparative quality reporting, as is illustrated by these comments. To give but one example, a physician working in a low income neighborhood may well be seeing sicker patients with more advanced disease and with more limited resources than a similar physician working in a middle class or wealthy neighborhood. In general it would be unreasonable to expect these two physicians to have comparable results. Risk adjustment compensates for these differences, so quality data can be more meaningfully compared across physicians and practices.

Case Study: Wellcentive

Wellcentive was founded in 2005 by Mason Beard in Georgia and Paul Taylor, a practicing physician in Michigan. Dr. Taylor's organization, a physician hospital organization (PHO) was under a P4P contract with Blue Cross. As discussed, a P4P contract places demands on the physician group to produce superior clinical outcomes. By law, a PHO must be clinically integrated to provide coordinated care, but Dr. Taylor's organization was attempting to achieve this essentially using spreadsheets. There were a variety of EHRs in use, but many practices were documenting on paper.

The two company founders felt that their payers, who were only able to look at retrospective claims data, had an inferior view of care to the more timely view that could be assembled from the practices in the PHO if clinical data were aggregated in "real time." Providers also had more detail. For example, the payer might know that a hemoglobin A1c (HbA1c), the important test discussed in chapter 2 to follow the clinical status of diabetics, was done, but they would not know the value, so it was very hard for them to see if the test was being followed up appropriately. Also, each payer saw their claims but not the claims paid by other payers, while the patient's physician could, in theory, have a much more comprehensive view of the care, particularly if data was aggregated from all the practices caring for a patient.

They decided to develop a solution. The needed data were in the systems that supported each practice. The key challenge was gathering it and putting it into a useable, more standardized and structured form. The original proof of concept was web based and was integrated with a few systems, mainly in clinical laboratories. It also had a generic tool for loading data from other systems. Despite the fact that the system was primitive by today's standards, the PHO rose significantly in the Blue Cross Blue Shield of Michigan's Physician Group Incentive Program (PGIP) quality rankings.

Today, Wellcentive's data collection and aggregation is most commonly from ANSI 837 claims data—the same data that is sent to the payer (we saw part of the 837 electronic claim format in chapter 5) via a direct feed from the practice management system that does billing for the provider office; transfer of Logical Observation Identifiers Names and Codes (LOINC) from the major lab companies; and Health Level 7 (HL7) feeds from the local health systems for information about hospitalizations and discharges. Where an HIE is present, it is possible to get much of the needed data via an interface to it. The company can accept data in a CCD format via a Direct connection but says this is just now starting to happen in any volume.

The Wellcentive Advance™ suite of products includes the Data Manager, Analytics Manager, Outcomes Manager, and Community Quality Manager and is used by providers in all 50 states. The company says their customers include some of the nation's best-known health systems (Beard 2013). Data Manager helps these customers map data from their systems to Wellcentive, in order to bridge any differences in terminology. The tool takes advantage of the web, so customers can collaborate with their business partners to build these maps. For example, a provider network might allow a lab technician in the local hospital to help build a map between the terms used in that laboratory and those used in Wellcentive. The tool also logs and tracks data errors. A common example is a patient not found in one of the systems in the network because of a naming or other difference in key demographic data. These tools are designed to help clients identify and fix data quality issues. Interestingly, this function is increasingly becoming the responsibility of office managers because the tool simplifies what was once thought of as a highly technical function. In most practices, office managers are the people who have historically dealt with coding issues. Analytics Manager allows larger provider networks to incorporate data from loosely affiliated practices, even though those practices are not formally using Wellcentive.

Outcomes Manager uses the data, once collected and aggregated, to provide proactive management of wellness and chronic disease in the patient population being cared for by the provider network. The user might be a care coordinator in a patient-centered medical home (PCMH)-model clinic, but many smaller clinics are now outsourcing this function to a new class of independent professionals often referred to as a Care Manager. This allows providers to have access to this needed service without having a full-time employee devoted to the task.

Figure 8.8 from Outcomes Manager shows a list of alerts defined by a practice. For each, the number of qualifying patients (the denominator in the percentage calculation) is shown along with the percentage of patients who do not meet this quality metric. Adjacent to that is a graphical representation of the practice's current quality performance versus their goal for each metric. Red flags indicate metrics below the corresponding goal set by the practice. Practices can define the provider cohort against which these metrics are calculated, so for example, cardiologists could be compared only to other cardiologists. The View Patients link brings up the individual patients who do not meet the goal. The practice then has a number of options, including an automated system the company provides to contact each patient to provide reminders, patient education, or to request the patients make an appointment. These calls can be customized based on known clinical data so that, for example, a patient with an elevated low-density lipoprotein (LDL) could be asked to come in to be evaluated for statin therapy (statins are widely used drugs that can lower LDL).

Figure 8.8   A report of overall performance for a list of practice-defined alerts illustrates the need to consider metrics by health plan (such as United Healthcare, a major health insurance company).

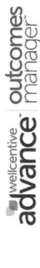
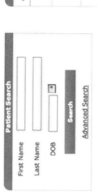

advance wellcentive | **outcomes** manager

Patient Search

First Name

Last Name

DOB

Search

Advanced Search

Favorite Alerts

Alert Name	Patient Count	%	Show [My Performance ‡]	Patient List
☆ Care Gap - Order HbA1c re-test (> 7 and > 90 days)	63	24%	20%	View
☆ Concert Health Plan - Women, Age 40 - 75, Last Mammogram > 1 Yr, Excludes Bilateral Mastectomy	157	65%	15%	View
☆ United Healthcare - Women, Age 40 - 75, Last Mammogram < 365 days, Excludes Bilateral Mastectomy	4	0%	20%	View
☆ United Healthcare: Asthma Action Plan > 1 year old	10	16%	15%	View

Inbox

From	Date
☒ Sue Caremanager	Jun 24, 2013
☒ WellCentive Administrator	Jun 17, 2013
☒ Jim Clifford	May 13, 2013
☒ WellCentive Administrator	Dec 7, 2012
☒ LANIE HESTER	Aug 13, 2012

Favorite Reports

Report Name	Report Type	PCP	Both	SCP	Generate
☆ Annual Mammo	Administrative (Provider)	○	◉	○	pdf html csv xls
☆ Coronary Artery Disease	Administrative (Provider)	○	◉	○	pdf html csv xls
☆ Diabetes LDL < 100 < 1 year	Administrative (Provider)	○	◉	○	pdf html csv xls
☆ Hypertension BP < 140 90 within 1 year	Administrative (Provider)	○	◉	○	pdf html csv xls
☆ Patients on Statin Medications	Personal (Provider)	○	◉		pdf html csv xls

Figure 8.9   An analysis of the use of lipid-lowering drugs (LLDs) for patients at risk for coronary heart disease helps providers find patients whose treatments may fall outside of accepted standards of care.

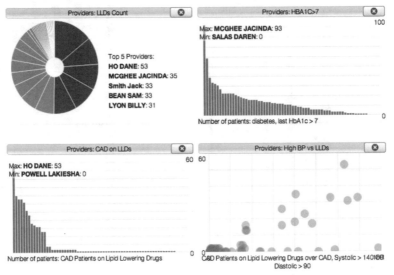

Figure 8.9 is a visualization of patient use of lipid-lowering drugs (LLDs) such as statins with the providers with highest and lowest percentages of LLD use shown. Separate analyses are given for patients with known coronary artery disease (CAD) and those at increased risk of CAD because of an elevated HbA1c or blood pressure. These tools were developed specifically with outcomes-based contracting in mind.

The company's Community Care Plan (CCP) allows a provider or care manager to track specific interventions and outreach dates for patients in order to close preventative care gaps and/or failures to use best practices for chronic disease management. It also offers a PHR. Any patient-entered data is considered unverified. The provider is alerted when it is input and, if they verify the data, it can then be used by the quality management system. Thus, for example, if the patient reports an increased blood pressure that data, once verified, might trigger a "blood pressure not under control" alert for the patient.

Population Management for Public Health

This chapter has focused on population health management within the context of care delivery. Before concluding it is important to recognize that there is another broad area of application for similar tools and technologies in the public health domain. Here, as shown in figure 8.10, data are collected from populations of patients in order to understand the impact of factors and determinants of health, such as genetics, the environment, and individual behavior on health and health outcomes, including health disparities. Data such as this can be used to consider or even model the potential impact of policies and programs on any problems or disparities that are revealed by the analysis.

Surveillance for disease outbreaks or incidents of bioterrorism is another key public health issue. The Centers for Disease Control and Prevention (CDC) has developed Biosense 2.0 specifically for these purposes. It will be a topic for discussion in chapter 9.

Figure 8.10   Public health includes using data collected from populations of patients in order to understand the impact of factors and determinants of health such as genetics, the environment, and individual behavior on health and health outcomes, including health disparities. It also looks at the potential impact of policies and programs on any problems or disparities that are revealed by the analyses (SES is socio-economic status).

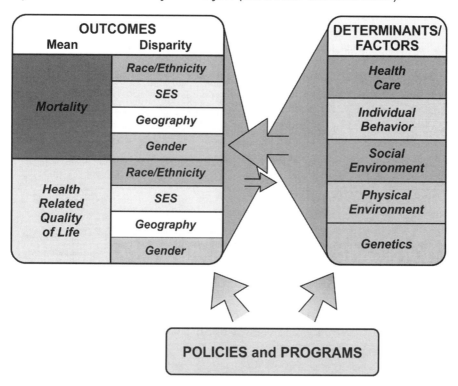

Conclusion

Managing populations has many aspects and applications, from improved delivery of care, to understanding disease patterns, and their causes in the population to protecting the public against outbreaks of infectious diseases. All of these require the coordinated application of all of the core technologies of health informatics on a wide geographic basis. As a result, these applications of health informatics are among the best illustrations of these technologies in use and are also (along with the research applications discussed in chapter 10) among the most compelling arguments for full adoption of EMRs.

REFERENCES

Beard, M and K. Elder. 2013. Interview by M. Braunstein. Skype, Spring 2013.

Cromwell, J., M.G. Trisolini, G.C. Pope, J.B. Mitchell, and L.M. Greenwald. 2011. *Pay for Performance in Health Care: Methods and Approaches.* RTI Press http://www.rti.org/pubs/bk-0002-1103-mitchell.pdf

Department of Health and Human Services. 2013. Value-Driven Health Care Home. http://www .hhs.gov/valuedriven

Evans, R., M.L Barer, and T.R. Marmor. 1994. *Why Are Some People Healthy and Others Not? The Determinants of Health of Populations.* New York, NY: Aldine de Gruyter.

Hale, M. 2013. Interview by M. Braunstein. Skype, Spring 2013.

HL7. 2012. Category I (QRDA) DSTU Release 2. http://www.hl7.org/implement/standards/ product_brief.cfm?product_id=35

Indiana Health Information Exchange. 2013. Public Reporting. http://www.ihie.org/public-reporting.

Keeley, E.C., J.A. Boura, and C.L. Grines. 2003 (Jan 4). Primary angioplasty versus intravenous thrombolytic therapy for acute myocardial infarction: A quantitative review of 23 randomised trials. *Lancet* 361(9351):13–20.

Kindig, D. and G. Stoddart G. 2003. What is population health? *American Journal of Public Health* 93:(3)380–383.

Medicare.gov. 2013. About the Data. http://www.medicare.gov/physiciancompare/staticpages/ data/aboutthedata.html

ONC. 2013. popHealth. http://projectpophealth.org/

RESOURCES AND RECOMMENDED READINGS

A journal for those with a particular interest in population health management: http://www .liebertpub.com/POP.

A thought piece on population health management for health system executives: http://www .advisory.com/~/media/Advisory-com/Research/HCAB/Research-Study/2013/ Three-Elements-for-Successful-Population-Health-Management/Three-Key-Elements-for-Successful-Population-Health-Management.pdf.

A recent report on population health management by the Patient-Centered Primary Care Collaborative (PCPCC): http://www.pcpcc.org/resource/managing-populations-maximizing-technology.

Health Data
and Analytics

Chapter 9

Data Query in a Federated Environment

The primary use of clinical data is caring for patients. Secondary use refers to the other purposes for which that data can be utilized. Population health management to improve the quality of outcomes for chronic diseases is a common example of secondary use that was discussed in chapter 8. Quality reporting is yet another important secondary use of clinical data, but one where data collection currently derives entirely from providers and their electronic health records (EHRs). If the patient's goals are to be manifest in quality reporting, the data collection process may need to be extended to include such sources as personal health records (PHRs) and even mobile apps.

Public health surveillance is another secondary use that involves mining data from these same sources in order to improve the understanding of the health of an entire population, and the ability to spot disease outbreaks or detect and track changes in aggregate health, such as the obesity epidemic in the United States and in many countries around the world. A fourth example of secondary use is clinical effectiveness: determining if the treatments that are prescribed for patients actually work as intended and are safe and cost-effective ways to manage their conditions. Finally, there are countless opportunities for secondary use of clinical data for research. Examples include mining data to understand how problems are related or interrelated, what the symptoms and manifestations for disease are in a natural population of patients, and to enhance our ability to properly diagnose and treat diseases.

To understand the opportunities more clearly, consider a specific use case—mining clinical data derived from clinical practice for adverse drug reactions. Before medications are approved by the US Food and Drug Administration (FDA) for marketing and widespread use in the United States, there are three phases of human testing, each with increasing numbers of subjects for different purposes. The earlier phases involve testing in very limited and carefully controlled patient groups. The third phase gathers information about safety and effectiveness by studying different populations and different dosages and using the drug in combination with other drugs. The number of subjects usually ranges from several hundred to around 3,000 people (FDA 2012). The three stages of testing typically take place over many years.

Many people are not aware that there is a fourth phase called post-marketing *surveillance*. This takes place in the real world, after the medication is released for use by patients. So, if these drugs have already been tested in three phases, why is this necessary? The poster child for the fourth phase of clinical testing is thalidomide, a drug that was marketed in Europe as a mild sleeping pill but not in the United States because of the FDA's more cautious procedures. The drug was thought to be safe, even for pregnant women, a group in which the use of medications is done with particular care for fear of damaging the fetus. However, it caused thousands of babies worldwide to be born with deformed limbs. People began to understand that testing could not stop when drugs were brought to market. As a result, the concept of post-marketing surveillance was introduced, based on the understanding that even the most well-designed controlled trials may not uncover every problem that can become apparent once a medication is widely used. The rationale for this surveillance leads directly to the potential role of health informatics as a source for the needed data:

> Even the most well-designed phase 3 studies might not uncover every problem that could become apparent once a product is widely used. Furthermore, the new product might be more widely used by groups that might not have been well studied in the clinical trials, such as elderly patients. A crucial element in this process is that physicians report any untoward complications. (Lipsky and Sharp 2001)

Clearly mining electronic records for the surveillance data is appealing because it eliminates potentially costly, time-consuming and error-prone extra manual collection processes and is therefore more likely to be accepted by physicians who are generally not required to report the results of drug therapy after market approval. The FDA's Sentinel Initiative is designed to facilitate this automated reporting, beginning with a mini-Sentinel pilot project that, among other things, looks at mining multiple existing electronic healthcare data systems for side effects and problems with medication therapy. There are currently around 25 collaborators that include many of the leading and largest health organizations, so this is already a substantial effort (Mini-Sentinel 2013). The architecture of the system leads to the concept of distributed query. In Mini-Sentinel queries for specific data are sent to the participating organizations and are responded to while the protected health information (PHI) stays at the source. This has a number of advantages that will be discussed in the next section. While mining electronic health records (EHRs) is a key part of the project, there are other potentially interesting data sources, such as databases created for other purposes and even the Internet.

For example, one study mined the FDA's own adverse drug and reporting system and discovered some previously unrecognized adverse drug reactions (Tatonetti et al. 2011). The Stanford-based study group went on to confirm that 47 of these drug interactions were substantiated when they analyzed electronic records of actual patients. Another example of using nontraditional data sources was done by a study group from Microsoft, Stanford, and Columbia University that mined logs of millions of web search queries to find evidence of unreported drug side effects before they were found by the FDA's warning system (White et al. 2013). Taken together, these two studies suggest the near certainty of a future in which many traditional and nontraditional data sources contribute to the advancement of medical knowledge through data mining and analysis.

Two challenges should be familiar by now: the multiplicity of EHRs and the inconsistent data representation among those records. The EHR certification process and meaningful use require that EHRs can produce a Continuity of Care Document (CCD), but these are not comprehensive and they can contain inconsistent data representations across sources. Beyond these two challenges, dealing with privacy concerns and regulations can be particularly complex for secondary use of clinical data. In routine patient care, consent is generally received to share the entire patient record with anyone involved in that patient's treatment. However, this data cannot be used for purposes other than treatment, payment, and healthcare operations (TPO). This is the TPO exclusion that permits providers, insurance companies, and other healthcare entities to exchange data for these specific purposes. This allows, for example, quality reporting to be done without obtaining each patient's explicit approval. Research is not covered under TPO, so patient consent must be obtained for the use of medical record data for research. It is complex, as discussed in chapter 4, to provide patients with a usable mechanism for designating those parts of their record they are willing to share for a particular research purpose. Finally, there are institutional concerns. Health systems and other providers worry about how their data will be used. A common concern is that it might cast the performance of their institutions in a negative way in comparison with other institutions. Distributed query is a process for mining data from diverse electronic records in ways that can address at least some of these problems, concerns, and issues.

Distributed Query

Distributed query is a technology solution to mining health data from diverse federated EHRs. There are several reasons why it may not be wise to put data into a central database, beginning with public acceptance. Patients generally do not want their data to be widely shared and many patients express concerns about the protection of their data once it is shared. Moreover, patients typically do not want their data shared without their explicit permission (which is a violation of HIPAA for anything but the TPO exceptions mentioned earlier).

With respect to cloud-based medical data sharing, a 2010 international consumer survey commissioned by Fujitsu and conducted by ORC International Limited found that patient attitudes may be shifting but that the majority of patients still have concerns:

> Giving access to centralized medical data, ensuring that patients get the correct treatment quickly and potentially saving lives, was more contentious [than five other potentially sensitive applications of personal data in the cloud], but still approved of on balance. "I've been in hospital many times," commented a consumer in Chicago, "but none of it is connected. If I get a new doctor, they won't know what operation I had or when I had it, so it would be good to have that information available instantly. Some of my previous doctors are dead: I don't even know what has happened to their records." This person was not alone: although there were concerns about the loss and misuse of such data, 40% of people surveyed thought that the benefits of centralized medical records were more important than the issues, compared to 21% who thought the opposite. (Fujitsu 2010, 8)

There were significant differences from country-to-country with respect to medical data sharing, with German consumers being the most opposed (28 percent felt the potential benefits outweigh their concerns) and consumers in the United States, Singapore, and Australia being the least opposed (over 40 percent in each country felt the potential benefits outweigh their concerns). In no case, however, did the majority of patients feel the benefits of sharing outweigh the risks (Fujitsu 2010, 10).

Patients might feel more secure if they know that their data stays in their provider's EHR, located in their office (of course, with the increasing use of cloud computing, the records—even hospital records—may well be located in a remote data center, but this is largely invisible to patients).

Another interesting reason for distributed query is the usefulness of the data itself. If the data partners—the organizations that are providing the data—are active participants and the data are under their control, they can contribute their own knowledge of the data and the issues surrounding the data to studies. This is particularly important in an environment, such as in the United States, where there are still not comprehensive and widely used standards for data representation. A third reason for distributed query is willingness to participate. It should be self-evident that data partners, organizations, or entities that are asked to contribute their data, are probably more likely to participate if they feel they are still in control of their data. In many of the distributed query architectures they will know precisely what is being asked for and how it is going to be used. They may even be asked to approve each query before it is executed and may be able to review their results before they are released. Governance is also easier since there is no need for a comprehensive set of rules for accessing the data. Each data partner manages their own decisions about what data should be accessed and how they are going to obtain patient participation. Finally, an argument can be made that this approach is technically simpler, since there is no need for a high-security central data repository.

The basic concepts of distributed query can be simply stated. Since the data are federated, queries must be done where the data are stored. If there are multiple EHRs involved, as will commonly be the case, the technical solution is to have a standard query framework. If there is inconsistent data representation across the multiple EHRs, there must be some intermediate, higher-level ontology in which the needed data are represented. To deal with privacy concerns, each data source must manage their patient permissions.

The query itself is formulated by the organization, group, or person that has a question they want answered. The means of stating it is ideally a high-level terminology that is easily understood by a non-computer technical researcher. The query is then distributed to each of these multiple EHRs through a standard query framework. On arrival, the query is interpreted in each of the recipient's sites into a form that will be understood by their particular EHR (this is similar in many respects to the curly braces problem with the Arden Syntax). The query will express the data that is required and any data related issues in a standard ontology that is received in the same form by all the EHRs. These standardized queries will have to be interpreted into terminology that is understood by each EHR. There are a number of query frameworks designed to provide all of these technical capabilities.

Examples of Distributed Query

This section will discuss three distributed query frameworks that, taken together, represent the varying approaches being used currently. As with health information exchange (HIE), there is a trade-off between complexity and functionality. As a result, each framework is typically applied against a specific use case or set of use cases where its functionality is sufficient and its technology is appropriate for the task at hand. The three frameworks are:

- **hQuery** was designed to keep things as simple as possible. popHealth, the population health management system discussed in chapter 8, has a very similar architecture. hQuery has largely been supplanted by the ONC Query Health initiative but because of its simplicity, is very useful for illustrating the concept of distributed query.

- **i2b2** is designed for use in more complex research environments.

- **PopMedNet** is an interesting model of data collaboration with a data warehouse, somewhat similar in concept to a hybrid HIE.

hQuery

hQuery is a modern, open-source, cloud-based system, with an attractive web interface (figure 9.1) and a simplified standard information model. The goal is that nontechnical users, including healthcare providers, can specify queries using a simple point-and-click user interface. Generic queries can be made against and summarized responses received from various clinical data sources. All PHI stays behind the provider firewall. It integrates with

Figure 9.1 hQuery provides an attractive, modern point-and-click interface to the query builder, who could even be a nontechnical healthcare provider.

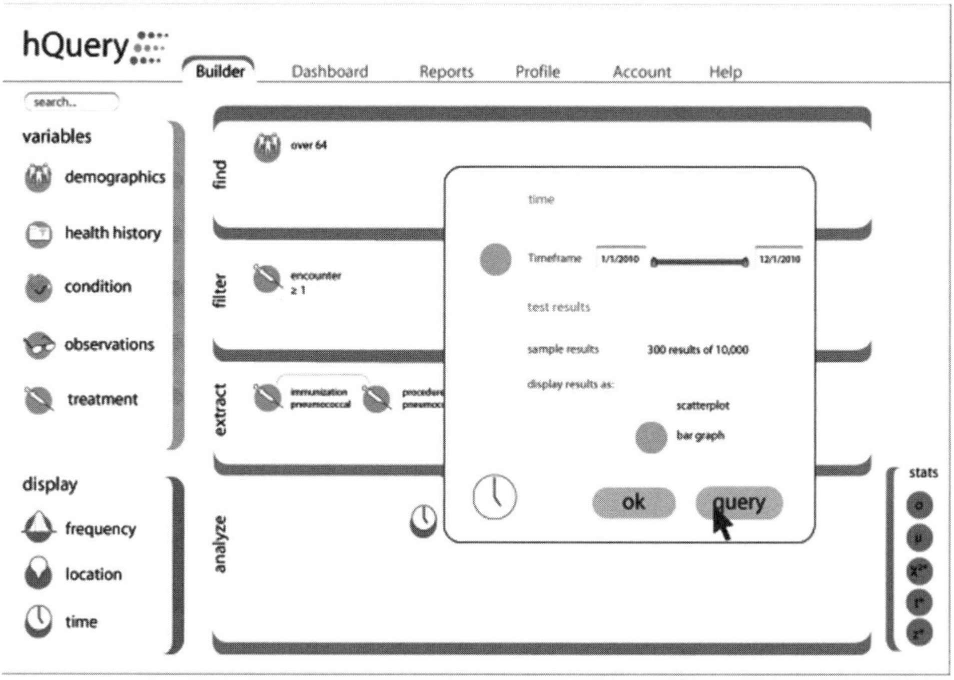

Source: Gregorowicz and Hadley 2011. © Query Health. http://wiki.siframework.org/Query+Health

certified EHRs mainly by leveraging their ability to product a CCD or CCR, further contributing to a simplified standard information model because these two Extensible Markup Language (XML) documents have a well-defined but limited data domain. This is essentially a trade off in which the data that are available are limited but are much more readily available. A similar trade off was identified as part of quality reporting discussion in chapter 8. It is possible that the amount of standard information in these documents will increase over time. In the hQuery architecture, the query is sent out to participating systems that can be healthcare providers, hospitals, or even a HIE. The patient information model (PIM) is simple, standardized and subdivided into various domains (medications, encounters, conditions) and, critically, is independent of the source of the data (see figure 9.2). The PIM supports the queries, which are probably made by someone who is not a physician and who does not know the information models of the individual systems that are being queried. This enables generic queries, regardless of how the data sources are organized or how clinical data are represented in the target systems. hQuery provides the visualization capabilities we expect of modern, web-based tools. As shown in figure 9.3, data can be attractively presented in a variety of ways, including geographically against maps, which of course, is very useful for purposes such as public health surveillance.

Informatics for Integrating Biology and the Bedside (i2b2)

Integrating Biology and the Bedside (i2b2) is a substantial research tool with a primary goal of supporting the joint exploration of genomic and clinical data for research purposes. The

Figure 9.2   hQuery provides a simple patient information model to facilitate query building by nontechnical users and interoperability with various EMRs.

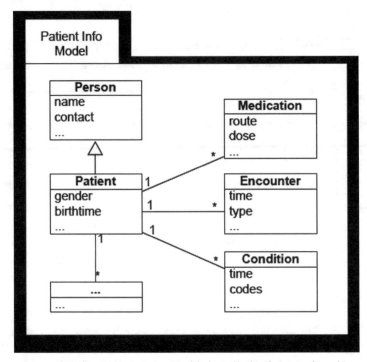

Source: Gregorowicz and Hadley 2011. © Query Health. http://wiki.siframework.org/Query+Health

Figure 9.3   hQuery presents query results in an attractive way that, in this example, includes frequency, time, and geographic distributions.

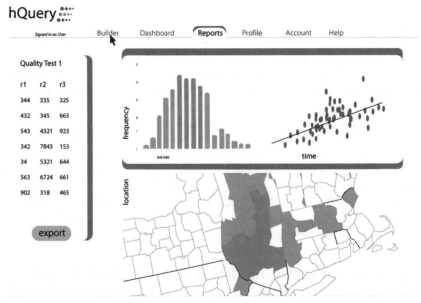

Source: Gregorowicz and Hadley 2011. © Query Health. http://wiki.siframework.org/Query+Health

genome is the DNA in most of our cells. It is the storehouse of the inherited properties that, in large part, govern how we work. Clinical data includes the problems and the symptoms that manifest themselves with disease, the lab and other tests and procedures, and of course, any treatments the patient may have had. There is now enormous interest in bringing these two data sets together to understand how differences in the human genome express themselves in clinical problems, their manifestations as symptoms, and individual variations in response to treatments. Cancer is a particular focus because cancers to which have historically been assigned a single label are actually a whole family of diseases, based in part on the genomic sequence of each individual patient and of their cancer. In fact, it is now clear that most cancers consist of multiple cell types with different genomic properties. If this can be understood in more detail, it is hoped that treatments can be tailored to specific patients—an example of a new field of medicine called personalized health. This will be discussed further in chapter 10.

To give a noncancer example of this, in a research project using i2b2, the researcher has a hypothesis that mutations in a particular gene contribute to the risk of a particular clinical heart problem. The researcher wants to know if there are associations in any animal models between that gene and heart disease and needs to search a database. She finds such an association because i2b2 is a robust platform that can support this kind of sophisticated clinical research.

i2b2 is much more complex than hQuery and is not a true distributed query technology but rather a hybrid query model, where some data is centrally stored. An i2b2 implementation includes a data mart, where deidentified clinical, research, and administrative data (data that, at least in theory, cannot be traced back to an individual patient) are stored, and an interface to construct and manage queries and data sets. Researchers can use i2b2 to perform as hoc queries to find patients who might be a fit for their proposed research study or to check the hypothesis underlying the study. If they wish to proceed, they must obtain Institutional Review Board (IRB) approval before i2b2 can be used to retrieve protected health information for research using queries stored from their earlier exploratory work. Plug-ins and extensions to i2b2 are available to add additional data capture, extraction, and analysis functionalities to the platform's core capabilities. I2b2 enjoys broad support in academic centers, research networks devoted to clinical and translational research and in industry. The i2b2 website presents interesting, actual use cases, such as this one from a group of collaborating medical centers in the Boston, Massachusetts, area:

> Can we identify genes that influence risk of rheumatoid arthritis (RA), multiple sclerosis (MS) and inflammatory bowel disease (IBD)? Moreover, can we query electronic medical records for patient characteristics that predict preclinical manifestations (e.g., demyelinating disease on MRI for pre-MS), severe disease (e.g., fistulas for IBD), and treatment response (e.g., anti-TNF therapy for RA)? In particular, we will focus on coronary artery disease (CAD) in all three autoimmune diseases to search for immune-mediated mechanisms that underlie CAD. (i2b2 2013)

PopMedNet

In the PopMedNet the partners contribute data to what are effectively data lockers that they individually control. Before any query can be run against their data, they can review and approve it, and they can review all results before sending them back to the portal. This makes a query simpler because all the data is in one place, but the data partners are always in control of which queries they respond to and whether they want to contribute their results, once they see them. This hybrid approach is an interesting middle ground between a purely federated approach and a pure centralized approach, and one that offers many of the advantages of each while minimizing their disadvantages. The FDA's Mini-Sentinel system uses the PopMedNet framework in large part because of the advantages of the data locker approach in assuring the various state health departments that they will maintain control of their data and how it is used thereby encouraging participation in the program.

Biosense 2.0

The Centers for Disease Control and Prevention's (CDC) BioSense 2.0 is another example of the success of the data locker approach where collaboration is essential. In an earlier model, the CDC proposed to house the data, an approach that reportedly exacerbated some of the issues and concerns we discussed earlier. In the new model, hospitals, health exchanges, and other entities get permission from state authorities and then send data to GovCloud that is operated for the US government by Amazon Web Services. The data is stored in a locker controlled by each state. Individual states also have the option of collecting data locally and then transmitting the data to their state locker. The data is then made available through the BioSense front end, allowing public health professionals to study trends or make other analyses involving single or multiple jurisdictions. Some data comes to BioSense with ICD-9 codes, allowing it to be normalized into syndrome and sub-syndrome levels. Data are stored in both raw and normalized formats for access through the BioSense front end.

BioSense is open architecture, to facilitate open data sharing through application programming interfaces (APIs), but always after state authorities grant permission. An early example was the use of BioSense by the Tarrant County Public Health Department in Texas to visualize health data collected by BioSense using Google Fusion Table technology, and making that visualization publicly available. The data include aggregated figures of emergency room illnesses, including gastrointestinal illness, rashes, heat-related illness, and upper respiratory issues in a six-county area of northeastern Texas. Some of the data are public and the link is in the resources at the end of this chapter.

Access to the secure data is currently limited to authorized state and local health administrators, as well as CDC users. Since the value of this massive data aggregation lies in its widespread availability, future plans for BioSense include providing data to universities and other public users.

Distributed Query Standards

The ONC is very interested in distributed query and their Query Health Initiative has posted a scenario in which an information requester sends a query to an intermediary, which could be a HIE that distributes that query to the sources of the data (S&I Framework 2013). The query will be in a standardized form that will then be interpreted and implemented. The necessary software to do that is located on the data source side where the query is then executed, the results are formatted and returned to the initiating agency.

To accomplish this, the Query Health Initiative has identified the need for four kinds of standards:

- The **query envelope** is the package in which queries are sent and results are received.
- The **query format** expresses the queries in a declarative format.
- The **results format** specifies how the data, found in each responding system based on the query, should be formatted and packaged for return to the query source.
- The **data model** promotes common data element definitions across organizations.

To understand queries it is important to understand the difference between declarative and procedural expressions. For example, below is an illustration based on the preparation of a cake:

Declarative	"Make me a cake."
Procedural	Mix 3 cups of flour, 2 ¼ cups of sugar, 2 tsp. of baking powder, 1 tsp. salt, 3 sticks of butter, ½ tsp. of vanilla extract, 1 cup milk, and 8 large egg whites. Bake at 350 for 40 minutes.

The declarative statement says *what* is desired, but it does not say *how* to achieve the desired result. Below it is the procedural statement, that is, the recipe for making the cake. A similar issue would exist in sending queries to diverse EHR or other systems. The declarative statement might be "how many diabetic patients do you have between the ages of 35 and 50 who are on this drug and are having fainting spells." That is the logical query, but it is not something that can be interpreted and executed by most computers yet, so it has to be turned into terms that the computer system understands and use some sort of explicit data query procedure that the system can then implement to obtain the desired results against its data model and database architecture (yet another example of something similar to the "curly braces problem" encountered in discussing the Arden Syntax in chapter 5).

To facilitate doing this across multiple EHRs the Query Health Initiative has selected standards for each of the four requirements listed earlier.

Query Envelope

The query envelope is a set of requirements and data elements that are necessary to securely exchange queries and result between organizations. It is agnostic as to formats and results and the repositories that house the data. In other words, it is a universal format that can be used by any system. It contains the following metadata:

- **Query Identification**: A Query Id that is a unique identifier within the Query Network
- **Information Requestor Identification**: e-mail, name, organization name
- **Query Purpose and Priority**: Purpose codes are TREAT, HPAYMT, HOPERAT, HRESCH, HMARKT, PATRQT, PUBHLTH; Priority is 1 to 5, with 1 being the highest
- **Query Type**: Format of 1–20 characters; Level of PHI Disclosure codes are Aggregated, Limited, Deidentified, PHI
- **Query Timing**: Submission date and time; optional date and time for execution

Query Format

The query format is in a standard called the Health Quality Measure Format (HQMF). HQMF is designed to represent health quality measures as an electronic document. Similarly to CDA, it uses the Health Level 7 (HL7) standard XML document format for documenting the content and structure of a quality measure based on the HL7 Reference Information Model (RIM), but instead of describing what happens in a patient encounter, the HQMF standard describes how to compute a quality measure.

HQMF is a different standard from any that have been discussed, since it is a procedural description of how to calculate a quality measure. However, for generality it is not at the level of detail that it can actually be executed by the system receiving the query request, but at a level of detail such that it can be interpreted into something that the system can compute.

Like any good CDA document it has a header and a body that is divided into sections with the section names specifying their purpose.

For example:

```
<patientPopulationCriteria classCode="OBS" moodCode="EVN">
<id root="c75181d0-73eb-11de-8a39-0800200c9a66"/>
<code code="IPP" codeSystem="2.16.840.1.113883.5.1063"
   codeSystemName="HL7 Observation Value">
<displayName value="Included in Initial Patient Population"/>
</code>
<isCriterionInd value="true"/>
<precondition typeCode="PRCN">
<!-- Weight measured -->
<observationReference classCode="OBS" moodCode="EVN">
<id root="f92aa450-73c0-11de-8a39-0800200c9a66"/>
</observationReference>
</precondition>
</patientPopulationCriteria>
```

(HL7 2012)

This XML specifies the patients who qualify for the query are those who have had their weight measured. The example is taken from a HL7 draft document that describes HQMF in great detail (HL7 2012).

Note that it takes quite a bit of XML to say in a computer-readable form something that can be said in English as "include only patients who have had their weight measured." Moreover, this is only the part that is describing the need for patients who have had at least one weight measurement and says nothing about the desired range of weights, if that is an issue for the research. The XML for HQMF can get very complex. There are critics who say that HQMF is far too complex and verbose, and that there are much simpler ways of describing queries (Beller 2013). Others defend HQMF as

> a powerful language for developing and computing measures of population health. Despite complexity concerns, we believe this format can be supported, which will be important in stage two of meaningful use and possibly required in stage three. HQMF is also a key component in Query Health and will likely play important roles in other health informatics initiatives. (Klann et al. 2012)

Query Results

The query results are formatted using the Quality Reporting Document Architecture (QRDA), which is a CDA compliant standard that encompasses the aggregate quality report containing all the calculated summary data for one or more measures for a population of patients within a particular system over a particular time period. Like HQMF, QRDA makes use of CDA templates, the rules for representing clinical data consistently, as discussed in chapter 5. Many QRDA templates are reused from the HL7 Consolidated CDA (CCDA) library of commonly used templates that, as also discussed in chapter 5, have been harmonized for Meaningful Use Stage 2.

There are three major categories within QRDA:

- **Category I (Patient-level) Report**: This contains quality data for *one patient* for one or more clinical quality measures, where the data elements in the report are defined by the particular measure(s) being reported. A QRDA Category I report contains raw applicable patient data (for example, the specific dates of an encounter, the clinical condition) using standardized coded data (for example, ICD-9-CM, SNOMED CT®). When pooled and analyzed, each report contributes the quality data necessary to calculate population measure metrics.

- **Category II (Patient-list) Report**: This is a multipatient-level report. Each report contains quality data for a *set of patients* for one or more clinical quality measures, where the data elements in the report are defined by the particular measure(s) being reported on.

  Whereas a QRDA Category I report contains only raw applicable patient data, a QRDA Category II report includes flags for each patient, indicating whether the patient qualifies for a measure's numerator, denominator, exclusion, or other aggregate data element. These qualifications can be pooled and counted to create the QRDA Category III report.

- **Category III (Aggregate-level) Report**: This contains aggregate quality data for *one provider* for one or more clinical quality measures. These reports provide organizations with the statistical information needed to track diseases, monitor quality of healthcare delivery, track the results of particular measures over time, and determine results from specific populations for those measures. Using quality query systems, researchers can ask questions of the data residing in health information systems and receive relevant data that are stripped of all patient identifiers, protecting patients and healthcare providers from the risks of inadvertent privacy loss (HL7 2013).

Below is an example of part of a result in QRDA XML:

```
<templateId root="2.16.840.1.113883.3.117.1.2.4.3" displayable="Use of
relievers for Inpatient Asthma (CAC-1)"/>
<templateId root="2.16.840.1.113883.3.117.1.2.4.4" displayable="Use of
Systemic Corticosteroids for Inpatient Asthma (CAC-2)"/>
```

(HL7 2013)

These again point to the use of templates, a technique we discussed earlier as a key component of CDA documents and HQMF.

In this example, the function of each of the two QRDA templates and the XML that they consist of is explained in the display name that is part of each line. While the CDA format is familiar, the content is obviously different, given the purpose of this document. For example, CAC-1 and CAC-2 (colored in the example) refer to National Quality Forum (NQF) defined quality measures for inpatient asthma care, each of which has its own complex definition developed by NQF.

Query Data Dictionary

The final technical standard is the Clinical Element Data Dictionary (CEDD), the intermediate data ontology that is neutral with respect to all of the systems that might receive these requests. Keep in mind that the query request is based on clinical concepts. This issue is similar in many respects to the idea of declarative requests that we discussed earlier. These are standardized conceptual representations of the desired data that can be mapped by the receiving system into the particular clinical concepts that are represented in that system—a similar process conceptually to what has to be done to interpret and execute the procedural statement discussed earlier. There are nearly 50 sub-domains within the CEDD. See the Recommended Reading and Resources for an online CEDD dictionary.

Conclusion

Distributed query frameworks are a specialized technology for HIE. Unlike traditional exchange, their goal is to support secondary use of patient data for purposes other than direct patient care. These technologies serve both the needs of population health, as discussed in chapter 8, and the requirements for data to drive the sophisticated models and simulations, to be discussed in chapter 10. From the earliest days of the EMR, pioneers (such as Dr. Larry Weed) saw this as an opportunity. Even dating back to Florence Nightingale, it has been the hope that health data would serve beyond its primary purpose to help improve care processes and increase medical knowledge. Now that the background and understanding of the underlying informatics technologies has been given, chapter 10 will focus on these final goals, at the top of the spectrum of contemporary health informatics systems shown in figure 2.9, and the tools and methods that are being used to achieve them.

REFERENCES

Beller, S. 2013. Dealing with EHR Dissatisfaction (Part 5). Curing Healthcare. http://curinghealthcare.blogspot.com/

Fujitsu. 2010. Personal data in the cloud: A global survey of consumer attitudes. Tokyo, Japan: Fujitsu Limited. http://www.fujitsu.com/downloads/SOL/fai/reports/fujitsu_personal-data-in-the-cloud.pdf

Gregorowicz, A., and M. Hadley. 2011. "hQuery." Presentation at the hQuery Summer Concert Presentation, August 11, 2011. http://wiki.siframework.org/Query+Health

HL7 Clinical Decision Support Workgroup and HL7 Structured Documents Workgroup. 2012. Health Quality Measures Format: eMeasures. http://www.hl7.org/implement/standards/product_brief.cfm?product_id=97

HL7 International. 2013. HL7 Implementation Guide for CDA® R2: Quality Reporting. Document Architecture—Category I (QRDA) DSTU Release 2 (US Realm). http://www.hl7.org/implement/standards/product_brief.cfm?product_id=35.

i2b2. 2013. Autoimmune/CV Diseases. Partners Healthcare. https://www.i2b2.org/disease/autoimmune_cv.html.

Klann, J.G., and S.N. Murphy. 2012. Computing health quality measures using informatics for integrating biology and the bedside. *Journal of Medical Internet Research* 15:4. http://www.jmir.org/2013/4/e75/?utm_source=feedburner&utm_medium=feed&utm_campaign=Feed%3A+JMedInternetRes+%28Journal+of+Medical+Internet+Research+%28atom%29%29#table1

Lipsky, M.S. and L.K. Sharp. 2001 (Sep.–Oct.). From idea to market: The drug approval process. *J Am Board Fam Pract* 14(5):362–367. http://www.ncbi.nlm.nih.gov/pubmed/11572541

Mini-Sentinel. 2013. Collaborators. http://mini-sentinel.org/about_us/collaborators.aspx

S&I Framework. 2013. Query Health—Project Charter. http://wiki.siframework.org/Query+Health+-+Project+Charter

Tatonetti, N.P., J.C. Denny, S.N. Murphy, G.H. Fernald, G. Krishnan, V. Castro, P. Yue, P.S. Tsau, I. Kohane, D.M. Roden, and R.B. Altman. 2011. Detecting drug interactions from adverse-event reports: Interaction between paroxetine and pravastatin increases blood glucose levels. *Clin Pharmacol Ther* 90:133–142. http://www.nature.com/clpt/journal/v90/n1/full/clpt201183a.html

US Food and Drug Administration. 2012. The FDA's Drug Review Process: Ensuring Drugs Are Safe and Effective. http://www.fda.gov/drugs/resourcesforyou/consumers/ucm143534.htm.

White, R.W., N.P. Tatonetti, N.H. Shah, R.B. Altman, and E. Horvitz. 2013. Web-scale pharmacovigilance: listening to signals from the crowd. *J Am Med Inform Assoc* amiajnl-2012-001482.

RECOMMENDED READING AND RESOURCES

More technically inclined students with an interest in distributed query should review this document: http://wiki.siframework.org/file/detail/ONC%20Summer%20Series-%20Query%20 health_Brown%20PlattV1.pdf.

An interactive i2b2 demonstration system: http://webservices.i2b2.org/webclient/.

More technically inclined readers or readers with a specific interest in i2be may wish to read this paper, which explains an actual use case for i2b2 in predicting asthma exacerbations: http://www.ncbi.nlm.nih.gov/pmc/articles/PMC2815458/.

The i2b2 website at https://www.i2b2.org/index.html provides information on a number of use cases, as well as extensive technical information on i2b2.

A list of academic institutions (and a few large healthcare providers and health related companies) are listed on the i2b2 website at https://www.i2b2.org/work/i2b2_installations.html.

Interactive Google Fusion presentation of Tarrant County Public Health data: http://www.google. com/publicdata/explore?ds=z46e2n1b69u8mu_&ctype=l&met_y=cds_rate.

The ONC is interested in distributed query and has created a query health group that has a Wiki at http://wiki.siframework.org/Query+Health. The schema posted on it is helpful for understanding distributed query in more depth, so the author suggests you review their presentation on this. If you are technically inclined and want more detail, view http://wiki.siframework.org/file/view/ OWG%20Technical%20Approach%20Primer%2002012012%20v2.2.pptx/311808624/OWG%20 Technical%20Approach%20Primer%2002012012%20v2.2.pptx.

A detailed description of HQMF is here: http://wiki.siframework.org/file/view/ Critique+of+HQMF-XML.pdf.

A presentation on QRDA is here: http://www.cms.gov/Regulations-and-Guidance/Legislation/ EHRIncentivePrograms/Downloads/VendorWorkgroupCall_April16.pdf.

An online dictionary of CEDD objects is available here: http://ushik.org/lists/FunctionalGroups? system=si&objectClass=CEDD%20Object.

The detailed NQF quality criteria can be explored using the search function on this page: http:// www.qualityforum.org/QPS/.

Chapter

10

Big Data Meets Healthcare

Many of the immediate opportunities to help address the problems of healthcare delivery require the widespread adoption of health informatics: adoption of electronic records, managing chronic disease at the population level, deployment of in-home monitoring and care management systems, and increased patient engagement through technologies from websites to smartphone apps. As a byproduct of their primary, shorter-term objectives these technologies are creating a plethora of digital data that many feel can be used to help define and refine longer-term, more effective solutions. Some observers are brimming with confidence about the potential:

> The application of big data to health care is inevitable. The first information technology revolution in medicine was the digitization of the medical record. The second is surely to leverage the information contained therein and combine it with other sources. Big data has the potential to transform medical practice by using information generated every day to improve the quality and efficiency of care. (Murdoch et al. 2013)

The ability of health informatics to help optimize both clinical and financial results is limited by our current knowledge, which is based on best evidence. The future ability to more fundamentally transform healthcare will rest on the ability to mine, analyze, and visualize this data in ways that can inform better clinical decisions, the development of new policies, and the ability to construct novel systems of care delivery that are responsive to the problems that have been outlined in this book. This is the classic problem of converting data into information, an often-overlooked distinction. Having vast storehouses of data does not, in itself, lead to insights or progress. Data only leads to change when processed, organized, structured, and presented in a context that provides actionable information that is relevant to a particular question or problem.

The nature and quality of the data also matters in limiting the scope of what can be done with it. An assistant professor at MIT's Media Lab, argues that, to be potentially transformative, data must be big in size, resolution, and scope (Hidalgo 2012). To reframe this idea in a way that is directly relevant to the main topic, to transform healthcare delivery systems, data must represent many patients and providers, must do so in detail, and must be combined with other data to give the context within which care is delivered and the external rules and policies within which that delivery system must operate. The data must, in summary, be sufficient to represent the behavior of a complex adaptive system.

From Statistics to Simulation

How can data be turned into useful information? The answer has substantially changed with the advent of modern computers with enormous power available at low cost that facilitates tackling problems in ways that would have previously been intractable or unaffordable. The gold standard for classic medical research is the randomized controlled trial. A common use case is determining if a new medication or treatment is, in fact, superior to the currently accepted approach. Does it prolong survival in a cohort of cancer patients? Does it produce fewer or less severe side effects? Increasingly policy makers and payers are questioning proposed new treatments, asking not only if they work and are safe but wondering if they are also "clinically effective"—is the cost more than justified by the clinical benefits?

In a randomized controlled trial, a cohort of similar patients is assigned by lot to one of two groups—a study group that gets the new treatment and a control group that gets the current treatment (or, in some cases, gets a placebo, that is, no treatment at all). Data are carefully and systematically collected by researchers who are ideally blind to which group each patient has been assigned. Data are then analyzed statistically to answer the questions that were posed at the outset of the research. The data are also analyzed to see if any unexpected, but statistically significant, differences occurred between the study and control patient groups.

Suppose that a different kind of question is being asked. Given a specific set of clinical facts what is the optimal treatment strategy? If a particular chronic care model were changed in a specific way, what would the outcomes be on clinical quality and cost? As opposed to these classic research questions, here, in the first case, determining optimal treatment would require many alternative experiments, that is, trying every possible treatment strategy on groups of similar patients. To answer the second question (How might a change in care process affect outcomes and cost?) an experiment could be conducted by changing the clinical process in half of the clinic and comparing it to the other half that is operated as before. However, this would often be too costly and complex to do. These are the types of questions best answered through modeling and simulation—questions that "can help inform and possibly persuade decision makers to make the best decisions possible" (Stahl 2008).

Stahl goes on to say:

> We create models and simulations (i) when direct experimentation is impossible; (ii) in order to better understand and predict the world or system (real or strategy or structure of the system being studied, the hypothetical) that we are examining in terms we can comprehend; and (iii) to aid in decision making. (Stahl 2008)

Many, if not most, of the strategic challenges facing healthcare will only be resolved by making better decisions, such as:

- Earlier and more accurate diagnosis of chronic diseases so they can be more easily and inexpensively managed;
- Better, more clinically effective treatment choices;

- More effective and efficient designs for care delivery systems, for the IT systems that support them, and for the spaces in which they operate; and

- Policies and financial incentives that cause the healthcare system to operate optimally rather than according to the unpredictable results of decisions made within a complex adaptive system.

The remainder of this chapter will look at some real world examples of modeling and simulation as they are being used to tackle these types of problems. Understanding the research will require first discussing the common approaches used to modeling and simulation, so the terminology and experimental design will be more clear. First, the terms modeling and simulation need to be defined. Modeling is "a simplified representation of reality that captures some of that reality's essential properties and relationships (e.g. logical, quantitative, cause/effect)." (Stahl 2008) Simulation is "a model in which an actual or proposed system is replaced by a functioning or interactive representation of the system under study as opposed purely conceptual models such as mathematical formulae." (Stahl 2008)

Stahl lists several methods for computer-based simulation and these are most often applied in healthcare: decision trees, Markov models, discrete-event simulation (DES), and agent-based simulations.

Decision trees

These are directed graphs without recursion (one-way, no cycling back) that consist of decision nodes (the moment in time when a decision is made), some representation of the strategy by which the decision is made, and outcome nodes that represent the value of the outcomes of the strategy. In a healthcare scenario, this might be life expectancy, cost, or some representation of clinical effectiveness. Importantly, while a specific time frame is assumed over which the scenario plays out, time is not explicitly represented.

Markov models

Unlike decision trees, Markov models do explicitly use recursion (events can repeat) and represent time. In fact, the entities being modeled change from state-to-state from cycle-to-cycle, as the model is run, based on the knowledge and relationships embedded in the structure of the model. Markov models are ideally suited to many of the questions posed for healthcare where, for example, patient risks can change over time. They require that the entities being modeled exist in only one state at a particular moment in time, and these states may not overlap. For example, if patients with a specific medical condition are being modeled, a list of the possible clinical states of that condition must be developed and must clearly delineate these possible clinical states into discrete, nonoverlapping groups. Moreover, Markov models have no memory, so each transition to the next state is based solely on the status of things at the current state (although there are variations to the classic Markov approach that introduce memory). There are several sub-types of Markov models, with the Markov Decision Process (MDP) being of particular interest in what follows. MDPs are a series of probability-driven decision trees, where the output of each is the input to the next. The goal is to define the strategy that optimizes the cumulative value (called "utility") of the results gained along the way. The decision rules can be preprogrammed to change over time or based on a reward at the end of each cycle, so for example, treatment strategies might change over time based on results obtained so far. It should be clear that the Markov approach has many attractive characteristics for modeling the behavior of healthcare.

Discrete-event simulation (DES)

The key concepts of discrete-event simulation (DES) are entities, attributes, queues, and resources. Entities can be physical objects, people, or even information, such as emails. Attributes define the specific characteristics of an entity (for example, demographic factors and medical problems). Queues are where entities wait for resources if they are otherwise occupied. Queues have logic so that, for example, an emergency room will see the sickest entities in the queue first. Unlike Markov models, DES models can have a memory, such that the attributes of an entity can change over time to represent changes in their state. This is in contrast to a Markov model where this information must be embedded in the structure of the model itself. The net result is that entities are more fluid and in many respects more realistic with respect to moving about in the system represented by a DES model.

Agent-based simulations

Agent-based simulations are similar to DESs but agents have a richer set of attributes that allow them to make decisions about how to communicate or interact with each other and their environment. Agents can also be grouped hierarchically to create, for example, a cohort of patients or even social groups or entire institutions. The key use of agent-based modeling is exploring "the influence of agents on each other and the influence of the environment on agents" (Stahl 2008).

Case Study: Center for Health Discovery and Well Being™ (CHDWB)

Within the Emory-Georgia Tech Predictive Health Institute (PHI), the Center for Health Discovery and Well Being™ (CHDWB) was a demonstration project (it has subsequently been closed) focusing on health in its broadest context, exploring novel biomarkers that predict health or its loss, and affecting lifestyles in ways that favorably affect health risks. The model was an experiment to determine if CHDWB could be expanded to the entire Emory employee base in an economically attractive manner (essentially demonstrating that the discounted value of the future reduction in Emory's healthcare expenditures could, under the right model, exceed the cost that would be incurred in the near term) (Park et al. 2012).

The approach was to combine modeling and simulation technologies to gain a better understanding of existing clinical processes and to provide policy makers at Emory with a "what if" tool to explore possible new designs for PHI under which the existing demonstration model could be substantially expanded.

The computational model contained four levels in order to represent the specific "complex adaptive system" that included and surrounded CHDWB: the ecosystem level, the organization level, the process level, and the people level. Each level introduces a corresponding conceptual set of issues and decisions for both the payer and the provider. In this case, the ecosystem level was defined by the Human Resources Department, the payer responsible for healthcare costs for university employees. PHI constitutes the organization level that conducts the business. CHDWB is the provider focused on prevention and maintenance of employee health, and which defines and operates the process level. The people level represents the Emory employees that participate in the experiment.

As with any complex adaptive system, goals of the different stakeholders can conflict. Emory's Human Resource Department was interested in paying as little as possible in the near term, while getting the greatest return through reduced future health costs (Park et al. 2012). PHI was interested in reducing the future risk of disease, while obtaining sufficient revenue to be sustainable. The question was: is there a set of assumptions and policies under which both can achieve their goals?

Since CHDWB's goal was maintaining health, each person's risk for developing diabetes or coronary heart disease was calculated based on the comprehensive initial individual assessments of each participant. This included variables, such as blood pressure, fasting glucose level, and so on. Subsequent assessment data were used to estimate annual risk changes as a function of initial risks for each disease. Decreased risks imply increased average times until disease onset. This results in cost savings in terms of more years without the cost of treating the disease and a reduction in lost productivity due to absenteeism or appearing at work but performing sub-optimally (presenteeism).

The model helped to show that, under the right set of policies, the future return on investment due to reduced health costs could more than justify current investment in a program to accomplish those future reductions and PHI could be economically sustainable—a conclusion that was far from obvious at the outset (Park et al. 2012).

The heart of the model is shown in figure 10.1, a simulation of the operation of CHDWB. It represents all of the steps through which people are registered into CHDWB, are assessed, have a personalized plan developed, and receive coaching tailored to their plan.

The simulated volunteer participants go through these processes, and the economic results are based on the ability of CHDWB to mitigate their entering risk factors for diabetes and coronary heart disease. Each person's entering risk factors and their individual

Figure 10.1   The model provides this visualization of the simulation of the operational processes of CHDWB.

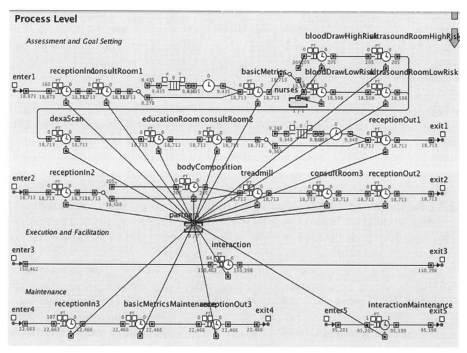

Reprinted by permission, Park et al. 2012, Multilevel Simulations of Health Delivery Systems: A Prospective Tool for Policy, Strategy, Planning and Management. *Service Science*. 4(3):253–268. © 2012, the Institute for Operations Research and the Management Sciences, 5521 Research Park Drive, Suite 200, Catonsville, MD 21228 USA.

risk factor reductions are based on probabilities (are stochastic) which, in turn, are driven by data on CHDWB's results in risk factor reduction collected during the two-year demonstration phase. Professor Peter Wilson's risk models (derived from the famous Framingham Study of the effect of risk factors on the long-term development of heart disease) were used to drive the probabilities of disease progression (Wilson et al. 1998).

This model lacked the first of Dr. Hidalgo's characteristics in that it was not "big" (there were only 700 people), but PHI was only a demonstration project and the sample was representative of Emory's 40,000 employees (Park et al. 2012). It did have resolution—some 2,000 data points were assessed for each individual participant—and it did have scope, since the model encompasses the entire "complex adaptive system" within which CHDWB operated (Park et al. 2012).

Case Study: Modeling Clinical Processes

This research focused on improving the quality and effectiveness of care for behavioral health disorders (Bennett and Hauser 2013). The clinical collaborator was Centerstone Research Institute (CRI), an affiliate of Centerstone, the nation's largest not-for-profit provider of community-based behavioral healthcare for mental health and addiction.

The goal of the research was to create a general purpose (not disease-specific) Markov Decision Process simulation for exploring policies, including payment methods, and for improved clinical decision making. The simulation is capable of sequential decision making, mimicking the treatment of chronic diseases over a period of time. According to the authors, their approach can "learn from clinical data and develop complex plans via simulation of alternative sequential decision paths while capturing the sometimes conflicting, sometimes synergistic interactions of various components in the healthcare system" (Bennett and Hauser 2013). They evaluated their simulation using real patient data from electronic health records (EHRs). Their simulation was both able to improve clinical effectiveness (as measured by a cost per unit of outcome change) and improve outcomes (as compared to the current treatment approach). In addition, the researchers were able to use the simulation to compare the results under different financial incentive scenarios that resemble the approaches used in current, real-world healthcare.

The simulation uses partially observable Markov decision processes (POMDP), one of the variations on the classic approach that introduces memory. As a result, the simulation can maintain what the researchers call "belief states"—the cognitive model clinicians bring to patient care—and this allows the simulation to deal with noisy and missing data, common characteristics of real-world healthcare and something actual clinicians do almost without thinking about it. It also allows the entities in the model to determine the optimal policy at each time point based on new information or the observed effects of prior actions, thereby becoming what the authors term "online AI agents" that more closely mimic the behavior of practicing clinicians (Bennett and Hauser 2013).

Based on these belief states, the POMDP simulates a sort of "game of chess against nature" by exploring how candidate treatment actions and potential observations affect future beliefs. In this game, the clinician takes the role of the player choosing treatment and diagnostic actions, while nature takes the role of the "opponent," choosing which information the clinician might receive after an action. Nature's "choices" are assumed to be taken according to a probability distribution matching historical data from an EHR or controlled studies. Given this model, the POMDP explores all possible future evolutions of belief states, until it reaches some maximum prediction horizon (the time interval over which the simulation operates). Then, thinking backwards, it computes a plan that consists of the optimal clinician's action for every possible observation—including contingencies for rare outcomes. Regardless of whether the clinician follows the system's advice or not, at the next stage of treatment the POMDP is given the new information and the process begins again.

The experiment was performed using comprehensive electronic records for 5,807 Centerstone patients, primarily with depression as their major diagnosis. The majority of patients had co-morbidities, such as hypertension, diabetes, chronic pain, or cardiovascular disease. For each simulation 500 patients were randomly selected from this cohort and were treated by a single physician agent (Bennett and Hauser 2013). The physician makes a treatment decision for each patient over the course of seven sessions. The clinical results are evaluated using the Outcome Rating Scale (ORS), an ultra-brief, validated functional and symptom measure for both chronic and acute mental disorders that produces a score from 0 to 40 (Miller et al. 2003). The utility metric is the cost per unit improvement in the ORS (CPUC in the results table shown here).

The authors also modeled several simpler decision-making approaches to provide context for the MDP results. The first they termed a Raw Effect model, in which the clinician considers only the effect of the currently proposed treatment, with no consideration of the long-term outcome. They argue that this mimics the currently dominant pay-for-procedure model in US healthcare (Bennett and Hauser 2013). They also modeled what they term a Hard Stop approach that ends treatment after some arbitrary time point. While this may seem strange, it is often the case that health insurance plans limit the number of outpatient mental health visits that they will reimburse, so this is not an unrealistic scenario. Max Improve assumes the most likely treatment effect always occurs. The final Probabilistic model selects an action at random but is biased based on the prediction that a treatment will improve the ORS score. With the exception of Hard Stop, where care is rigidly limited, the other models differ from MDP in that they only consider the immediate probability of a treatment effect. Their purpose was to see if the MDP model creates sufficient value to justify the complexity it adds to decision making.

Finally, three approaches were used for modeling each patient's history to predict the probability distribution of the health state at the next time point. The 0th Order uses the overall probability distribution and does not consider patient history. The 1st Order uses only the change in clinical status since the prior time point. The Global approach considers each patient's entire history.

The results are shown in table 10.1. Keep in mind that CPUC—the cost per unit improvement in the clinical outcome as measured by the ORS—is the key metric for clinical effectiveness while Final Delta is the change in the ORS score from the inception to the end of treatment. The final column shows the percentage of patients receiving the maximum number of treatment sessions.

Overall, the MDP decision-making models were the most clinically effective (smallest CPUC) using both the 1st Order and Global approaches to prediction. The Global approach performed significantly better, arguably validating the importance of having a complete view of each patient. However, MDP improved Final Delta (outcome improvement not considering cost) slightly less than a more aggressive strategy, such as Max Improve. This mimics the dilemma often faced by healthcare policy makers—is it worth paying for a major incremental expenditure that will produce only marginal improvements?

It is also worth noting that the MDP CPUC was even lower than Hard Stop (in both cases with no missing observations), presumably because it produced the lowest Final Delta. However, selecting the best CPUC performance for each model and multiplying the CPUC and the Final Delta, yields an $844 estimate for the total cost of Hard Stop, which is substantially less than the equivalent $1,103 cost estimate for MDP. This mimics yet

Table 10.1   The results of the model demonstrate that it produced nearly the best outcomes at a very attractive cost.

Decision Model	Transition Model	Missing Observations	CPUC	Avg. Final Delta	Std. Dev Final Delta	Avg. Sessions	% Max Sessions
Hard Stop	N/A	No	262.30	3.22	7.80	3.00	0%
Hard Stop	N/A	Yes	305.53	2.56	8.07	3.00	0%
Raw Effect	0th Order	No	470.33	4.69	8.66	8.00	100%
Raw Effect	0th Order	Yes	497.00	4.73	8.45	8.00	100%
Max Improve	1st Order	No	297.47	6.24	7.87	5.35	30%
Max Improve	1st Order	Yes	303.85	5.77	8.25	5.32	29%
MDP	1st Order	No	228.91	5.85	7.12	4.11	4%
MDP	1st Order	Yes	237.21	5.11	7.37	4.03	3%
Max Improve	Global	No	256.44	6.41	6.92	4.79	24%
Max Improve	Global	Yes	251.83	6.07	6.90	4.76	20%
MDP	Global	No	181.72	6.07	6.42	4.23	11%
MDP	Global	Yes	189.93	5.59	6.44	4.11	9%

Reprinted from *Artificial Intelligence in Medicine*, 57(1), C.C. Bennett and K. Hauser, Artificial intelligence framework for simulating clinical decisionmaking: A Markov decision process approach., Pages 9–19, Copyright 2013, with permission from Elsevier.

another common healthcare policy dilemma: is the optimal objective spending as little as possible in the short term or getting the most cost-effective long-term clinical result?

These same metrics were calculated for the broader patient population served by Centerstone under a fee-for-service model and CPUC was approximately $540 with a Final Delta of around 4.4. This yields an approximate cost of care of $2,376 which, once again, mimics the real world where the cost of care often substantially exceeds what is believed to be the best that could be done under an optimal model of care.

Case Study: Earlier Diagnosis of Congestive Heart Failure

Congestive Heart failure (CHF) is already the most expensive International Classification of Disease (ICD) code for Medicare, with an annual direct cost of $33 billion, and both its prevalence and cost is rising. These trends will continue unless novel and cost-effective strategies are developed to better manage this disease. While hospital admissions and readmissions are being reduced in large part because of strong financial disincentives (Medicare no longer pays for readmissions for CHF within 30 days of discharge from a CHF admission), the cost benefit is modest, self-limiting, and too infrequently does little to improve patient quality of life.

One potential strategy is earlier detection because, if CHF could be detected early enough, there would be more time to implement lifestyle and pharmacologic interventions that can delay and possibly even prevent disease progression. Early CHF detection is challenging because it is a clinically complex and heterogeneous diagnosis that encompasses a number of disease states. The 17 heart failure risk factors, developed from the Framingham study (Wilson et al. 1998), are shown in table 10.2 (along with their Extracted Criteria Code Names used in the project) and are well validated. They are also clinically useful, since most are already routinely documented in primary care and require no specialized testing.

Table 10.2   The 17 heart failure risk factors.

Framingham Major Criteria	
Criteria	**Extracted Criteria Code Names**
Paroxysmal nocturnal dyspnea or orthopnea	PNDyspnea (PND)
Neck vein distention	JVDistension (JVD)
Rales	Rales (RALE)
Radiographic cardiomegaly	RCardiomegaly (RC)
Acute pulmonary edema	APEdema (APED)
S3 gallop	S3Gallop (S3G)
Central venous pressure > 16 cm of H2O	ICVPressure (ICV)
Circulation time of 25 seconds	(not extracted)
Hepatojugular reflux	HJReflux (HJR)
Weight loss of 4.5 kg in 5 days, in response to HF treatment	WeightLoss (WTL)
Framingham Minor Criteria	
Bilateral ankle edema	AnkleEdema (ANKED)
Nocturnal cough	NightCough (NC)
Dyspnea on ordinary exertion	DOExertion (DOE)
Hepatomegaly	Hepatomegaly (HEP)
Pleural effusion	PleuralEffusion (PLE)
A decrease in vital capacity by 1/3 of max	(not extracted)
Tachycardia (rate of ≥ 120/min)	Tachycardia (TACH)

Source: Courtesy Dr. Jimeng Sun of IBM Research, Dr. Steve Steinhubl of Geisinger Health System, and Dr. Walter Stewart of Sutter Health.

However, other disease processes common in older patients can obscure the interpretation of these signs and symptoms. Moreover, CHF can be the result of a number of physiologic changes and can affect virtually all organ systems, leading to substantial overlap with the clinical manifestations of other common health problems.

This research was undertaken by Dr. Jimeng Sun of IBM Research, in collaboration with Dr. Steve Steinhubl of Geisinger Health System and Dr. Walter Stewart of Sutter Health, organizations that have the means to translate the tools that are developed into use in clinical practice to determine their impact on patient outcomes and costs.

The purpose of the project was to develop robust, valid predictive models and practical means of early CHF detection that can be widely applied in primary care practices using EHRs. The research team was motivated in part by recent work suggesting that the signs and symptoms of CHF are often documented years before the diagnosis is made, and that the pattern of documentation is likely to offer clinically useful signals for early detection. However, a clinician's often hurried manual review of patient data is typically inadequate to detect, analyze, and act upon these imbedded signs and symptoms. Another key factor in the project timing was the rapid growth in EHR adoption, which the research team viewed as an opportunity to develop novel, cost-effective strategies to detect CHF in its earliest stage, as a means to monitor patient status, motivate engagement, initiate proven disease-modifying interventions, and test preventive treatments.

The current goals of the project are to develop:

1. More sensitive and specific criteria for use of the already recognized signs and symptoms in the early detection of CHF in primary care.

2. An accurate predictive model for the diagnosis of CHF based on EHR data.

Longer-term goals are to:

3. Determine how digital ECG related measures can be used alone and in combination with other data to improve early detection of CHF.

4. Develop preliminary operational protocols for early detection of CHF in primary care.

As shown in figure 10.2, structured clinical data (such as diagnoses, medications, and lab tests) are extracted from EHR records, and unstructured text data are annotated using natural language processing (NLP) to extract symptoms (physical signs and patient reported symptoms) that may be related to CHF. These results are stored as features in a relational database. The features are variables that correspond to clinical events about the patients. In particular, each ICD-9 diagnosis code becomes a feature that counts the number of occurrences of that code. For example, a hypertension diagnosis of ICD-9 401.X becomes a separate feature recording the number of occurrences of 401.X in the patients' EHRs. The researchers also constructed features for medications, lab results, and NLP extracted symptoms. The number of all possible features can be very large, on the order of 10 to 100 thousand. To find the relevant features for predicting CHF, all features are then ranked using a selection module that is described under Goal 2 in what follows. Classification or predictive model construction is then trained using logistic regression and random forest algorithms (these are two statistical techniques for classifying objects into groups). After evaluation, the resulting models were deployed to score patients' future encounters.

Figure 10.2   Structured data (for example, diagnosis, medication, labs) are processed through the feature extraction module. Unstructured data (for example, physician notes) are annotated by a set of customized Unstructured Information Management Architecture (UIMA) pipelines (a technology developed by IBM) to extract CHF related symptoms. All results from structured and unstructured information are stored as features and subsequently ranked by the feature selection module. Classification is done using logistic regression (a statistical technique commonly used to predict whether a patient has a condition based on characteristics of the patient) and random forest (a method that uses multiple methods to classify objects).

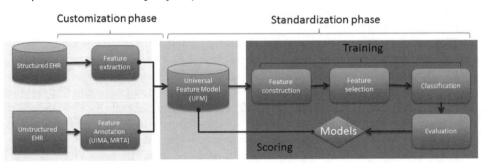

Source: Courtesy Dr. Jimeng Sun of IBM Research, Dr. Steve Steinhubl of Geisinger Health System, and Dr. Walter Stewart of Sutter Health.

Goal 1: Earlier recognition of CHF based on known risk factors. The resulting system of feature annotation analyzed the unstructured clinical notes at two levels: (1) at the sentence level (within clinical notes), a rule-based NLP system annotates all affirmative and negative mentions of CHF risk factors (table 10.2) in patient records; and (2) each encounter is also scored based on the status (asserted, denied, or unknown) of known CHF risk factors.

The criteria mention extractions achieved a precision (the fraction of retrieved instances that are relevant) of 0.925, a recall (the fraction of relevant instances that are retrieved) of 0.896, and an F-score (a statistical measure that combines precision and recall) of 0.910. Encounter scoring achieved an F-score of 0.932. With this degree of accuracy, the NLP extraction program can now efficiently process a large collection of clinical notes for Framingham CHF risk factors. When it did, the team observed that, as expected, there are many patients with CHF risk factors in their EHRs years before the clinical diagnosis. A practical benefit of this is to provide evidence-based treatment earlier based on those early signals.

Goal 2: A predictive model for CHF based on EHR data. Existing approaches for risk factor identification are either knowledge driven (from guidelines or the medical literature) or data driven (from observational data). No existing method provides a model to effectively combine expert knowledge with data-driven insight for the identification of previously unrecognized risk factors.

There are standard feature selection algorithms, such as information gain and Fisher score. The researchers designed a customized algorithm using sparse learning to combine existing knowledge about CHF risk factors with other predictive data-driven features. The main idea was to start with known risk factors (as shown earlier) and then to programmatically enhance those risk factors with additional predictive and complementary features derived from EHRs. For example, many antihypertensive medication orders become risk

Figure 10.3   The area under the curve (AUC) (a measure of how well the model discriminates between patients with CHF and those who do not have the condition) significantly improves as complementary data-driven features are added to existing knowledge-based risk factors. A significant AUC increase occurred with the addition of as few as 50 data-driven features.

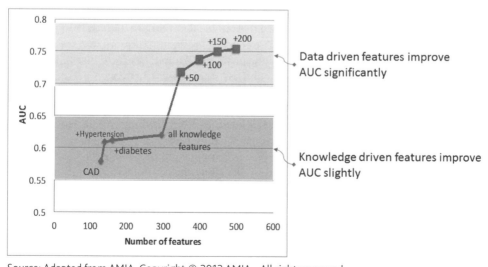

factors, since use of those medications further enforces the hypertension risk factor, which is itself a known major CHF risk factor. More specifically, the research developed a sparse regression model with regularization terms (a statistical process for estimating the relationships among variables) that correspond to both knowledge and data-driven risk factors and validated it using a large data set containing 4,644 CHF cases and 45,981 controls. The proposed method identified previously unrecognized risk factors and can better predict the onset of CHF. To demonstrate this, the researchers tested the ability of different sets of risk factors to predict the onset of CHF using the area under the curve (AUC) as the metric (figure 10.3). AUC shows how well the technique in question separates the group being analyzed into those with and without the disease. The combined risk factors significantly outperform knowledge-based risk factors alone. Furthermore, the additional risk factors were confirmed to be clinically meaningful by a cardiologist.

Case Study: Personalized Cancer Care

Over the past few decades, we have moved into an era of high technology medicine. However, "unlike in many other areas, the cost of medical technology is not declining and its increasing use contributes to the spiraling healthcare costs" (Kumar 2011). A reason for personalized medicine is to lower costs and improve results by selecting treatments that are most likely to work in a specific patient, based on their individual genomic and clinical situation:

> Personalized medicine promises to offer the right treatment for the right patient at the right time. Although that promise might seem far off, there is clear evidence that the traditional trial-and-error practice of medicine is eroding in favor of more precise marker assisted diagnosis and treatment. For the patient, the benefits are clear: safer and more effective treatment of disease. For industry there appears an equally desirable outcome of this approach: increased efficiency, productivity and better product lines. Society as a whole will also realize a benefit: more focused application of precious healthcare resources to those in need of them most. (Ginsburg and McCarthy 2001)

Personalizing medicine requires tools to more precisely identify subgroups of patients that are likely to respond to a proposed therapy.

Cancer is arguably the best target disease for personalizing medicine. Biology tells us most of our cells contain 23 pairs of DNA molecules that are divided into functionally specific regions we call genes (the genome). Some 20,000 or more (no one is sure of the exact number) of these genes code for proteins (Sanger Institute 2012). However, this constitutes a small percentage of our DNA (perhaps as little as 5 percent, this is not yet known for certain), and until a few years ago, the other regions were thought to be unimportant (and were often even labeled as "junk"). We now know that much of the DNA in these regions codes for special forms of RNA (a slightly different molecule than DNA) that are intimately involved in what is now called the "gene expression control network." Even though the genome is complicated, the gene expression control network is even more complex. This network can be thought of as a biologic computer program that takes as its input molecules that may be in or around the cell, the environment around the cell and other factors that may not yet even be fully understood and uses those inputs to make decisions as to whether specific genes should be active or inactive at any point in time.

Science has long known that each patient has a unique genome (DNA sequence), but it is also now known that cancer is, at least in part, a disorder of the gene expression control network; that the DNA of cancer cells is different from the DNA of the host (patient) cells and that there is variation in the DNA of different cancer cells within a single patient (Singer 2013). Cancer is most often treated with drugs, radiation, or surgery. The drugs can be divided into two groups: chemotherapy and mechanistic. Chemotherapy drugs and radiation attempt to selectively kill cancer cells as they divide, taking advantage of their relatively rapid rate of division. These treatments almost always kill other rapidly dividing, but normal, cells, potentially causing severe side effects and even death. In some patients, this can be minimized by highly targeted approaches to radiation treatment and researchers are working on more targeted approaches to delivery chemotherapy. Mechanistic drugs, on the other hand, are designed to specifically attack particular genomic or metabolic pathways in cancer cells, significantly reducing their side effects but also potentially the response rates of patients.

In summary, cancer is a disease of the genome and related cellular mechanisms and is commonly treated by broadly or more selectively attacking the genetic or metabolic mechanisms in cancer cells. It is therefore logical that the likely success of a particular selective (mechanistic) cancer drug in a specific patient will depend on the complex interplay between the drug and genomics of that patient and those of their cancer. Yet, for decades, the drug choice was often based on the type of cancer and its appearance under a microscope or, at best, this histologic information along with one or a few genetic factors in the cancer and/or the patient. Given the complexity of the patient and the cancer's genome, physicians are therefore almost certainly grouping patients who will react differently to a therapy but are treating them the same. Indeed, this has been the clinical result, and on average, only about 28 percent of patients respond to a specific mechanistic drug (Lehrach 2013).

Physicians might get better results and harm patients less if they individually selected each patient's therapy based on the genomic factors in that specific patient and those of their specific cancer. Since physicians cannot experiment with each patient by trying all possible therapies, a personalized therapy approach may well be the likely future of cancer care. Using this approach in clinical practice could be greatly facilitated by a model that can consider all the factors that have been discussed (and others that have not been discussed) along with the known literature on all available cancer treatments.

Developing such a model is the goal of Alacris Pharmaceuticals, a company derived from research done at Germany's Max Planck Institute for Molecular Genetics. The company's Virtual Patient System™ is based on a detailed model of tumors within patients. The overall model (figure 10.4a) is driven by specific data obtained from clinical samples from patients and their cancers. This data set defines a "state" based on the specifics of the DNA and RNA and targeted information from the samples' protein and regulatory network content. This information drives a patented biological network modeling system developed by one of the company's scientific founders, professor Hans Lehrach. The complex model is based on all available research that describes the interactions among genes, the elements of the gene expression control network, and proteins and other molecules (the "components" of cells) (figure 10.4b).

In a specific example, data from 800 of a patient's genes (that code for both proteins and elements of the gene expression control network) yielded over 5,000 components (Lehrach 2013). Similar data is obtained by sequencing the predominant tumor cell type (and also, if possible, from tumor stem cells).

The result is a patient and cancer specific model that the company believes is able to predict the results of proposed treatment with mechanistic drugs. Dr. Lehrach cited an early test patient who was treated with success using a drug the model predicted would work, but the patient eventually developed a new metastasis that did not respond clinically

Figure 10.4a   A diagrammatic representation of the cellular biochemical pathways that drive the Virtual Patient System™ illustrates that the complexity involved is beyond consideration or analysis by human care providers. A detailed view of the outlined area follows in figure 10.4b.

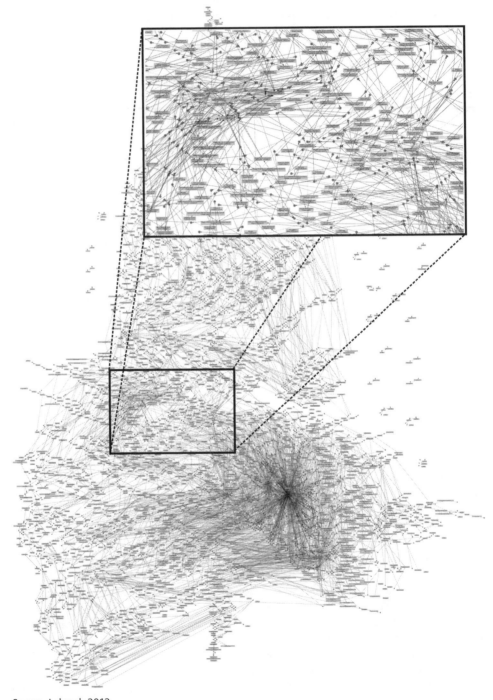

Source: Lehrach 2013

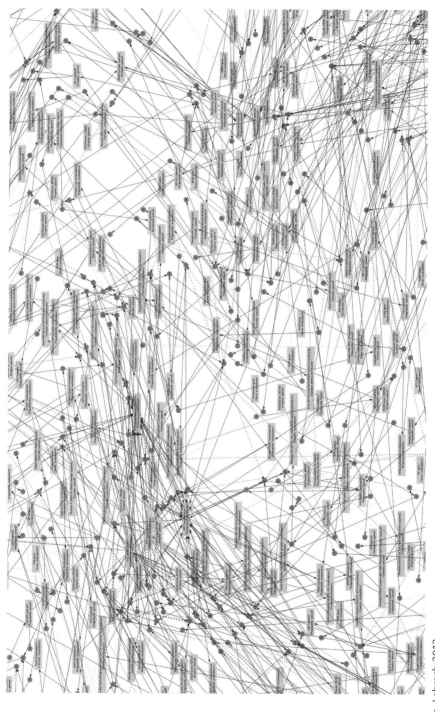

Figure 10.4b A close-up diagrammatic representation of an outlined part of the cellular biochemical pathways that drive the Virtual Patient System™. The boxes are components and the circles represent their reactions.

Source: Lehrach 2013

to the treatment (Lehrach 2013). Reanalysis using data from the metastasis predicted that the drug would fail showing that the model can make distinctions that are difficult or even impossible to make using traditional clinical approaches.

Other interesting potential applications of the model are in selecting drugs for clinical trials and the best patients for those trials. Today patients that meet certain criteria are entered into a double-blind clinical trial to see if a proposed new drug is clinically effective. There is a description of this type of trial earlier in this chapter. Clinical trials are expensive and time consuming, which can lead to slow progress. As a result, pharmaceutical companies often have to make decisions about whether or not to further test a drug based on economic factors. If a "virtual clinical trial" could be performed using the model, the risk factors could potentially be better understood before an expensive human trial is begun. It is also possible that, once patients are enrolled in a trial, many of them or their tumors have characteristics that the model would use to say the drug will not work. If all prospective patients for the trial were screened using the model, it might turn out that a drug was far more clinically effective in a specific subgroup of patients than would otherwise be known. Such a drug might be approved for use based on a more selective clinical trial, which could cut the time, costs, and risk for the development of new drugs, and help many more drugs to reach the market, even if they work on a smaller subset of cancer patients.

While this fascinating use of modeling is not yet routine, it appears to show promise. It certainly suggests the role that modeling will play in personalizing cancer and other treatments and possibly even in smarter, more efficient, effective, and less costly clinical trials.

Case Study: Evidence-based Design

Healthcare is delivered to actual patients within real physical spaces, such as exam and hospital rooms and surgical suites. These, in turn, exist within the larger space of a clinic or hospital. Can analytic techniques help improve the design of these spaces to promote safer, more efficient, and more patient-friendly care? This is the focus of Georgia Tech's SimTigrate Lab, which adds a novel dimension to the application of big data to healthcare. The SimTigrate team gathers data about care environments and processes and uses it to build models that can inform better decisions about the design of care spaces, the placement of furniture and fixtures, and even the optimal mobile computing devices to be used within those spaces.

A recent example of the SimTigrate approach was a hospital contemplating the expansion of its surgical floor. The key questions were:

- How many supporting spaces (other than the rooms where surgery is performed) of three types (preoperative holding area (POHA), postanesthesia care unit (PACU), and Level 2 recovery) were needed, and in what combination, to support current and anticipated future volume and case mix (the types of patients being cared for)?

- What factors might affect the amount of space needed to support anticipated future volume?

- What design solutions would work best for these supporting spaces?

Three design solutions were considered:

- One bed type: a universal bed that could serve to provide all three functions
- Two bed types: one for PACU and the other for either POHA or Level 2 care
- Three bed types: one each for the three supporting space types

To inform this decision, data were collected on approximately 1,000 surgical procedures, representing one month of cases. These data were used to create a model of the current state of the surgical area using medBPM (Ramudhin et al. 2006) a healthcare specific modeling tool.

Similar models were created for each of the proposed design solutions, taking advantage of the temporal data on the operative processes and their use of space. These were used to simulate a typical day for the three care areas, to determine the peak demand for beds in each area, which of course, ultimately drives the capacity that must be built to. The model was then run using the three proposed bed type solutions, and the results are summarized in figure 10.5, which shows that the universal bed solution substantially reduces the space requirements, while still meeting the current and anticipated future capacity needs of the hospital.

The ability to more cost effectively make substantial design decisions that are both difficult and costly to change once they have been implemented in physical buildings has the potential to help reduce healthcare costs. Other projects undertaken by the SimTigrate team suggest that design can also impact both the quality and efficiency of care and the quality of the patient experience.

Case Study: IBM's Watson

In February 2011, IBM's software program, Watson, defeated two expert human opponents in the TV game show *Jeopardy* (Markoff 2011). The *New York Times* said that this was "proof that the company has taken a big step toward a world in which intelligent machines will understand and respond to humans, and perhaps inevitably, replace some of them" (Markoff 2011). It is rapidly becoming clear that, with the help of systems like Watson, physicians can make better decisions that are very specifically tailored to each patient.

Almost as impressive, if not more impressive than Watson winning against expert human opponents, was the nature of the game because, again quoting the *New York Times*, "I.B.M. researchers were tackling a game that requires not only encyclopedic recall, but

Figure 10.5 Aggregation of the data from a model of a proposed surgical suite shows that the universal bed minimizes the bed requirement.

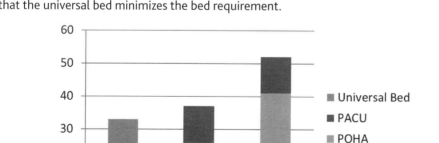

Source: Courtesy of Professor Craig Zimring

also the ability to untangle convoluted and often opaque statements, a modicum of luck, and quick, strategic button pressing" (Markoff 2011). If Watson could do that, could it make sense of the unstructured text that can constitute up to 80 percent of the typical electronic medical record (Nazarko 2013)? Again, the answer appears to be yes. In fact, Watson is being used by oncologists at Memorial Sloan-Kettering, one of the leading cancer treatment centers in the United States, to help make the best treatment decisions for patients with non-small cell adenocarcinoma, the most common form of lung cancer. Work is ongoing to train Watson to help with breast, colon, and prostate cancers, which together with lung cancer, are the most commons forms of the family of diseases collectively called cancer.

Memorial Sloan-Kettering (MSK) uses the EPIC hospital information system, commonly found in large health systems across the country. When a physician wishes to "consult" with Watson, the record of their patient is exported from EPIC, using that company's standard and application program interface (API) tools—typically as text documents that may even include PDFs. Generally, except for the Continuity of Care Document (CCD) mandated by Meaningful Use, commercial systems do not provide export of entire records in a more structured (and easier to use) form, such as an Extensible Markup Language (XML) document. The record can then be de-identified using either the hospital's software or tools provided by IBM and submitted to Watson via a web service. The Watson servers for this application are actually housed and operated by MSK, but at present, four other cancer treatment centers are using the tool via a web service (Nazarko 2013).

Watson's clinical opinion is typically returned in a few minutes in the form of the patient's record with annotations and a clinical summary with hyperlinks that, when clicked, show the information in the original record that led Watson to conclude that the patient has whatever the text in the link describes. In a substantial majority of cases, Watson then provides treatment recommendations ranked in the order that Watson feels they should be considered. These documents are formatted in XML to facilitate parsing of the information for storage in the EHR or visualization in formats most usable by the referring physicians.

However, Watson is not yet omniscient. It can consider only medical treatments for cancer (typically antineoplastic medications) but not surgical treatments, which are a key part of cancer care. Moreover, unlike the research project at Cornerstone described earlier in this chapter, Watson considers only clinical outcomes and not cost. This is an increasingly important topic in cancer, where medications costing hundreds of thousands of dollars may only prolong life by a few weeks or months. The reason for these "gaps" in Watson's knowledge base are that they require more specificity in the relationship between the data found in the EHR and therapeutic decisions than is currently available for surgical decisions and the cost benefit of care.

Case Study: Process Mining of Stroke Care

How do physicians actually care for their patients? Does that care fall within generally accepted practice guidelines? How do individual physicians vary in caring for similar patients and are those variations clinically justified? Which of those variations actually produces the most cost-effective results? These are a few of the questions that are driving the increasing interest in healthcare processes and have fostered an interest in finding ways to more precisely describe clinical processes. Developing formalisms to describe processes (such as those discussed in chapter 5) is one aspect of the problem, but could the actual determination of the processes be automated by analyzing digital data from EHRs and other sources?

Sifting through large data sets and using statistical techniques to find patterns and make inferences about the data is called data mining, a field that may revolutionize business and industry practices over the next several decades. Process mining (or care flow mining) is a subset of this field that could be used to describe, examine, and analyze business and clinical processes in healthcare now that sufficient storehouses of digital clinical data are becoming available (Van der Aalst 2011).

In process mining, XML-formatted event or activity logs are used to reconstruct sequential activity-based models for various business practices. This approach has been applied to analyze clinical decisions using EMR data. Clinical events are converted to activity log formats, which can then be passed to process mining software that summarizes and visualizes the clinical data in useful ways.

There are many potential applications of process mining in healthcare. Different models can be constructed for individual physicians to facilitate standardization and eliminate inefficiencies. Costs of various decisions can also be modeled, and then used in comparative effectiveness research. Process mining would make it easier to measure the adherence of physicians to evidence-based guidelines by automating the analysis. In addition to cost-effectiveness, process models may eventually be enhanced to consider the influence of medical test results on clinical decision making. Process mining could then be used to refine or even generate clinical guidelines that could be more objective and accurate then existing guidelines.

The potential is illustrated by a study from the Netherlands in which stroke care clinical processes are mined and compared using two data sets representing events pre- and post-hospitalization for 368 consecutive patients with a confirmed diagnosis of first-ever ischemic stroke (blockage of an artery to the brain) (Mans et al. 2008). The prehospital behavior data was collected through direct interviews with 234 patients and includes events that occurred from stroke onset until the patient's arrival in the hospital. The data set contains temporal information about the actions taken by patients, their relatives, and the referring physician. Post-hospitalization data for the diagnostic and treatment procedures, complications, and other factors are labeled according to the time elapsed from the onset of symptoms. It is important to note that the needed temporal (time and date) information may not be routinely or accurately recorded in current EHR systems even if they provide for it.

Figure 10.6 shows only the main flow (relationships between events) of the process for frequently occurring events. Events are depicted by activity boxes. The numbers in the boxes indicate the occurrence frequency of the activity. For example, hospital 1, on the left, had 15 admissions while hospital 2 had 31 admissions. Boxes are connected by arcs. The top number associated with each arc indicates the reliability (strength) of the relationship between the activities. For example, for hospital 1 the reliability of admission followed by neuroprotection (treatment to halt or at least slow the loss of neurons due to the oxygen deprivation caused by the blocked artery) is 0.917. The lower number on the arcs represents the number of times this activity pattern occurred in the log.

The process differences between these two hospitals are striking. For example, hospital 2 performs hypertension therapy earlier and much more than hospital 1 (and the other hospitals in the study). While antihypertensive treatment is a common practice, it is not clearly justified by scientific evidence. According to the researchers, hospital 1 seems to practice more on the basis of medical evidence as shown by its use of therapeutic protocols such as neuroprotection. Hospital 1 is also more compliant with the more recent guidelines that recommend early physical therapy.

There are many potential benefits of evidence-based practice guidelines. However, actually developing and implementing them within the complex adaptive system of healthcare is challenging, as illustrated by this quote from *Guidelines for Clinical Practice*:

Figure 10.6   The main process flow in two hospitals for frequently occurring events (depicted by boxes) involved in the treatment of ischemic stroke. The numbers in the boxes are the frequency of the event. The arcs show event relationships (activity), the top number indicates the relationship reliability, the lower number is the occurrences of this activity.

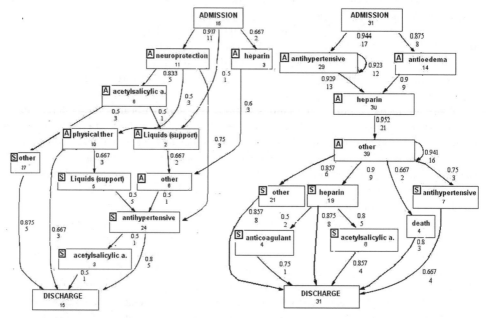

Source: Courtesy Mans et al. 2008

Guidelines for the provision of clinical care have been linked in recent years to almost every major problem and proposed solution on the American health policy agenda. Practice guidelines have been tied in some way, by some individual or organization, to costs, quality, access, patient empowerment, professional autonomy, medical liability, rationing, competition, benefit design, utilization variation, bureaucratic micromanagement of health care, and more. The concept has acted as a magnet for the hopes and frustrations of practitioners, patients, payers, researchers, and policy makers.

The broadest hopes of all parties are that practice guidelines will raise the quality of care and improve both the real and the perceived value obtained for health care spending. Beyond such widely held aspirations, individual groups differ in the emphasis they place on other narrower objectives. For example, administrators, regulators, and purchasers tend to stress cost control and reduced variation in practice patterns much more than physicians do. Practitioner groups tend to emphasize professionally developed guidelines as a means to maintain autonomy and to free professional decision making from external micromanagement. Consumer and patient advocates focus on guidelines to inform patients' decisions, clarify patient preferences, and strengthen patient autonomy.

Each group that has positive objectives for practice guidelines also fears their misuse. Their fears are essentially the obverse of their hopes—less sensitivity to patient needs, poorer outcomes, increased costs, lower quality, reduced autonomy or "cookbook" medicine, more bureaucracy, and greater inequity in resource use. In particular, many physicians, especially those longer in practice, see guidelines as a challenge to clinical judgment and resist them as a threat to the most fundamental element of professional autonomy. (IOM 1992)

Process mining and the other analytic tools discussed in this chapter offer the hope of developing more extensive, objective, and effective clinical guidelines that can be used to inform clinical decision support at the point-of-care. These tools also offer the potential to provide insights and guidance for a redesigned and reengineered care delivery system, along with the facilities and information technology needed to support it. That would be a signature accomplishment for the second, and potentially the most impactful, informatics powered revolution in healthcare.

Challenges

Three challenges can stand in the way of realizing the potential of digital health data:

- No strong incentives or champions for its use within clinician groups or hospitals
- Privacy concerns
- EHR platforms that are fragmented and have limited interoperability (Murdoch et al. 2013)

The changes in financial incentives that are needed have been discussed in detail and are underway which would potentially overcome the first challenge. Privacy concerns were covered in chapter 4. Chapters 3 and 5 focus on information exchange and standards, key issues to overcoming part of the third issue.

A fourth aspect of this difficult problem is access to data. Health systems and even providers often view their data as proprietary and are reluctant to share it. Yet, in most domains, to be potentially transformative, data must meet Dr. Hidalgo's metrics of size, resolution, and scope that have been discussed early in this chapter (Hidalgo 2012). This almost always implies sharing and combining data from many sources. Doing this requires not only a willingness to share but overcoming the interoperability and data standards issues. The critical importance of this issue was highlighted by the newly appointed national coordinator for health information technology, Dr. Karen DeSalvo when she said that interoperability will be the "top priority for 2014," at the Fourth Annual Health Care Innovation Day in Washington, DC, hosted by ONC and the West Health Institute. (Manos 2014)

The technologies of distributed query have been discussed, but before concluding, it is useful to look at Linked Life Data (LLD), an interesting and illustrative example from the life sciences field. LLD introduces the concept of a data-as-a-service platform that provides access to 25 public biomedical databases through a single access point (Linked Life Data 2013). The service allows writing of complex data analytical queries that can answer complex bioinformatics questions, such as "give me all human genes located in Y-chromosome with the known molecular interactions." LLD allows its users to simply navigate through the information, or export subsets like "all approved drugs and their brand names." One can only imagine the benefits that might be obtained if all the major health systems around the country (or the world) contributed properly de-identified data to a similar resource.

The premier example of this is the Clinical Practice Research Datalink (CPRD) maintained by the National Health Service (NHS) in the United Kingdom. CPRD, known as the General Practice Research Database (GPRD) until March 2012, contains de-identified primary care data for over eight million patients over more than 50 million person years (CPRD 2013). The discussion of health maintenance organizations (HMOs) pointed out that primary care physicians in them typically serve as gatekeepers and care coordinators. This is the model throughout the NHS, so data from these practices can provide an extensive overview of the care of their patients. Obtaining access to this data requires a research agreement and is not free. Another example, the Centers for Medicare and Medicaid Services' (CMS) public chronic conditions data warehouse provides publically available health data obtained from Medicare and Medicaid claims since 1999 and pharmacy claims since 2006 (CMS 2013).

Conclusion

Informatics, like everything in US healthcare, operates within an extraordinarily complex industry, which until now has proven exceptionally resistant to change. The industry may be finally open to transforming itself under the pressure of new policies, incentives, and the increasing awareness that the current US healthcare system is unsustainable. This chapter is intended to demonstrate the potential of health informatics to use the digital data created as providers adopt electronic records to assist and guide those providers, as well as decision and policy makers, to make wise decisions. The end result both in terms of the adoption of these recommendations and their ultimate impact on care quality and efficiency remains to be seen but should become clearer over the coming years.

REFERENCES

Bennett, C.C. and K. Hauser. 2013. Artificial intelligence framework for simulating clinical decision-making: A Markov decision process approach. *Artificial Intelligence in Medicine* 57(1):9–19. http://www.sciencedirect.com/science/article/pii/S0933365712001510

Centers for Medicare and Medicaid Services. 2013. Chronic Conditions Data Warehouse. https://www.ccwdata.org/

Clinical Practice Research Datalink. 2013. http://www.cprd.com

Ginsburg, G.S. and J.J. McCarthy. 2001. Personalized medicine: revolutionizing drug discovery and patient care. *TRENDS in Biotechnology* 19(12).

Hidalgo, C. 2012. What is Value? What is Money? http://edge.org/conversation/what-is-value

Institute of Medicine, Committee on Clinical Practice Guidelines. 1992. *Guidelines for Clinical Practice: From Development to Use*. Edited by M.J. Field and K.N. Lohr. National Academy Press.

Kumar, R.K. 2011. Technology and healthcare costs. *Annals of Pediatric Cardiology*. 4(1): 84–86.

Lehrach, H. 2013 (August). Personal communication with author.

Linked Life Data. 2013. http://linkedlifedata.com/

Manos, D. 2014. DeSalvo: Interoperability 'top priority'. *Health IT News*. http://www.healthcareitnews.com/news/desalvo-interoperability-top-priority

Mans, R., H. Schonenberg, G. Leonardi, S. Panzarasa, A. Cavallini, S. Quaglini, and W. van der Aalsta. 2008. Process Mining Techniques: An Application to Stroke Care. *eHealth beyond the Horizon—Get IT There*, Edited by S.K. Andersen, et al. IOS Press. http://

person.hst.aau.dk/ska/MIE2008/ParalleSessions/PapersForDownloads/07.LM&S/SHTI136-0573.pdf

Markoff, J. 2011 (February 17). Computer wins on 'Jeopardy!': Trivial, it's not. *New York Times*. http://www.nytimes.com/2011/02/17/science/17jeopardy-watson.html?pagewanted=all&_r=0

Miller, S.D. B.L. Duncan, J. Brown, J.A. Sparks, and D.A. Claud. 2003. The outcome rating scale: A preliminary study of the reliability, validity, and feasibility of a brief visual analog measure. *Journal of Brief Therapy* 2:2:91–100. http://macmhb.org/StateWide%20Trauma%20Seminar/60%20Outcome%20Rating%20Scale%20p.88%20-%20already%20on%20p.82.pdf

Murdoch, T.B., and A.S. Detsky. 2013. The inevitable application of big data to health care. *JAMA* 309(13):1351–1352.

Nazarko, E. 2013 (April). Personal communication with author.

Park, H., T. Clear, W.B. Rouse, R.C. Basole, M.L. Braunstein, K.L. Brigham, and L. Cunningham. 2012. Multilevel simulations of health delivery systems: A prospective tool for policy, strategy, planning, and management. *Service Science* 4:253–268. http://pubsonline.informs.org/doi/pdf/10.1287/serv.1120.0022

Ramudhin, A., E. Chan, and A. Mokadem. 2006. A framework for the modeling, analysis and optimization of pathways in healthcare. *2006 International Conference on Service Systems and Service Management* (ICSSSM 2006) 698–702.

Sanger Institute. 2012. Human Genome Far More Active than Thought. http://www.sanger.ac.uk/about/press/2012/120905.html

Singer, E. 2013. Tracking the evolution of cancer, cell by cell. *Quanta Magazine*. https://www.simonsfoundation.org/quanta/20131113-tracking-the-evolution-of-cancer-cell-by-cell

Stahl, J.E. 2008. Modelling methods for pharmacoeconomics and health technology assessment: An overview and guide, *Pharmacoeconomics* 26(2):131–48.

Sun, J., J. Hu, D. Luo, M. Markatou, F. Wang, and S. Edabollahi. 2012 (November 3). Combining Knowledge and Data Driven Insights for Identifying Risk Factors using Electronic Health Records. AMIA Annu Symp Proc. 2012; 2012: 901–910. http://www.ncbi.nlm.nih.gov/pmc/articles/PMC3540578/

van der Aalst, W.M.P. 2011. *Process Mining: Discovery, Conformance and Enhancement of Business Processes*. Springer Verlag.

Wilson, P.W.F., R.B. D'Agostino, D. Levy, A.M. Belanger, H. Silbershatz, and W.B. Kannel. 1998. Prediction of coronary heart disease using risk factor categories. Circulation 97:1837–1847.

RECOMMENDED READING AND RESOURCES

The Outcome Rating Scale is available here but requires registration: http://scottdmiller.com/performance-metrics/.

A website devoted to healthcare process mining can be found here: http://www.healthcare-analytics-process-mining.org/.

Linked Life Data (LLD): http://linkedlifedata.com/. Use of this site requires expertise in SPARQL, a specific RDF database query language. The Resource Description Framework (RDF) is a method for modeling web information and relationships (somewhat like SNOMED).

The Clinical Practice Research Datalink, the largest available data warehouse, is derived from primary care medicine in the United Kingdom: http://www.cprd.com/.

The CMS public chronic conditions data warehouse can be found here: https://www.ccwdata.org/web/guest/home.

An up-to-date review of the informatics tools and strategies developed over a number of research efforts to improve the data infrastructure to facilitate research on clinical effectiveness, improved outcomes for patients and quality improvement: http://repository.academyhealth.org/edm_briefs/11.

Lenz, R., S. Miksch, M. Peleg, M. Reichert, D. Riaño, and A. ten Teije. 2012. Process Support and Knowledge Representation in Health Care. *Lecture Notes in Computer Science*, Vol. 7739 2013. http://link.springer.com/book/10.1007/978-3-642-36438-9/page/1.

Glossary of Health and Health Information Technology Terms

Accountable Care Organization (ACO): MEDICARE's outcomes-based contracting approach

American Recovery and Reconstruction Act (ARRA): the Obama administration's 2009 economic stimulus bill

Arden Syntax: an approach to specifying medical knowledge and clinical decision support rules in a form that is independent of any electronic health record (EHR) and thus sharable across hospitals

Blue Button: an ASCII text-based standard for heath information sharing first introduced by the Veteran's Administration to facilitate access to records stored in VistA by their patients. The newer Blue Button + format provides both human and machine readable formats

Bluetooth: a short range wireless technology increasingly used to communicate with medical devices in the home

Biosense: the CDC's electronic surveillance network for disease outbreaks and bioterrorism

Care Coordinator: a professional who engages with and monitors patients between visits to what is often a patient centered medical home model practice

Centers for Disease Control and Prevention (CDC): the federal agency focused on disease in the community

Centers for Medicare and Medicaid Services (CMS): the component of the Department of Health and Human Services that administers the Medicare and Medicaid programs

Certificate Authority (CA): an entity that digitally signs certificate requests and issues X.509 digital certificates that link a public key to attributes of its owner

Client-Server Computing: a computing paradigm in which the hardware and software required to automate a business entity is dedicated and located onsite (or at a remote hosting center but still dedicated to one entity)

Clinical Context Object Workshop (CCOW): an HL7 standard for synchronizing and coordinating applications to automatically follow the patient; user (and other) contexts allow the clinical user's experience to resemble interacting with a single system when the user is using multiple, independent applications from many different systems

Clinical Data Repository: a database specifically designed to support ad hoc query and usually populated with data from EHRs and other clinical support systems in a hospital or health system

Clinical Decision Support: the provision of evidence-based medical advice to providers, ideally within the context of decision making using their EHR

Clinical Document Architecture (CDA): an XML-based markup standard intended to specify the encoding, structure, and semantics of clinical documents

Clinical Information Modeling Initiative (CIMI): an independent collaboration of major health providers to improve the interoperability of healthcare information systems through shared and implementable clinical information models

Cloud Computing: the concept of providing unlimited, on-demand computing resources as a service

CommonWell Alliance: a group of major HIT companies that is working to achieve interoperability among their respective software products and services

Complete EHR: an EHR software product that, by itself, is capable of meeting the requirements of certification and Meaningful Use

Computer-based Physician Order Entry (CPOE): the direct entry of patient orders by physicians. CPOE often provides an opportunity to offer timely clinical decision support

CONNECT: ONC supported open source software for managing the centralized model of HIE

Consolidated Clinical Document Architecture (CCDA): the second revision of HL7's CDA that attempts to introduce more standardized templates to facilitate information sharing (a mandate of Meaningful Use 2)

Continuity of Care Document (CCD): an XML-based patient summary based on the CDA architecture

Continuity of Care Record (CCR): an XML-based patient summary format that preceded CDA

Cross-Enterprise Document Sharing (XDS): the use of federated document repositories and a document registry to create a longitudinal record of information about a patient

Current Procedural Terminology (CPT): the American Medical Association's standard for coding medical procedures

Deidentified Patient Health Information: PHI from which all data elements that could allow the data to be traced back to the individual patient have been removed

Digital Imaging and Communications in Medicine (DICOM): a widely used standard for creation and exchange of medical images

Direct: a set of ONC-supported standards for secure exchange of health information using e-mail

Domain Name System (DNS): the naming system for computers, services, or any resource connected to the Internet (or a private network). Among other things, it translates domain names (for example, eBay.com) to the numerical IP addresses needed to locate Internet connected resources.

EDI/X12: a format for electronic messaging that utilizes cryptic but compact notation primarily to support computer-to-computer commercial information exchange

eHealth Exchange: a set of standards, services, and policies that enable secure nationwide, Internet-based HIE using CONNECT or one of the commercial HIE products that support eHealth Exchange

Electronic Health Record (EHR): a stakeholder-wide electronic record of a patient's complete health situation

Electronic Health Record Certification: a set of technical requirements developed by ONC that, if met, qualify an EHR to be used by an eligible professional to achieve Meaningful Use

Electronic Medical Record (EMR): an electronic record used by a licensed professional care provider

Eligible Professionals (Medicaid): health providers who are eligible for Medicaid Meaningful Use payments: doctors of medicine, osteopathy, dental surgery, dental medicine, nurse practitioners, nurse certified nurse-midwives, and physician assistants who work in a federally qualified health center or rural health clinic that is led by a physician assistant

Eligible Professionals (Medicare): health providers who are eligible for Medicare Meaningful Use payments: doctors of medicine, osteopathy, dental surgery, dental medicine, podiatry, optometry, and chiropractic

EMPI: an enterprise master patient index that establishes patient identity across all the parts of an integrated healthcare delivery system

Electronic Healthcare Network Accreditation Commission (EHNAC): an independent, federally recognized, standards development organization focused on improving the quality of healthcare transactions, operational efficiency and data security

e-Prescribing: the electronic ordering of prescription medications, ideally through an EHR, and the transmission of that order to a connected pharmacy of the patient's choosing

Extensible Markup Language (XML): a widely used standard for machine- and human-readable electronic documents and the language used to define CDA templates

External Data Representation (XDR): an operating system and transport method agnostic mechanism for exchanging data that is encoded/decoded into/from the XDR format

Fast Health Interoperable Resources (FHIR®): an HL7 initiative that seeks to use modern web standards and technologies to simplify and expedite real world interoperability solutions

Gatekeeper: a provider (usually a primary care physician in an HMO) with overall responsibility for a patient's care and who controls access to specialist physicians

GELLO: a programming language intended for use as a standard query and expression language for clinical decision support. Now compatible with the HL7 Version 3.0 Reference Information Model (RIM)

Health eDecisions: an ONC workgroup to identify, define, and harmonize standards for shareable clinical decision support interventions including standards to structure medical knowledge in a shareable and executable format and that define how a system can interact with and utilize an electronic interface that provides helpful, actionable clinical guidance

Health System: a network of providers that are affiliated for the more integrated delivery of care

Health Information Exchange (HIE): the sharing of digital health information by the various stakeholders involved, including the patient

Health Information Service Provider (HISP): a component of Direct that provides a provider directory, secure e-mail addresses, and public-key infrastructure (PKI)

Health Information Technology (HIT): the set of tools needed to facilitate electronic documentation and management of healthcare delivery

Health Insurance Portability and Accountability Act of 1996 (HIPAA): legislation intended to secure health insurance for employees changing jobs and simplify administration with electronic transactions. It also defines the rules concerning patient privacy and security for PHI.

Health Level 7 (HL7): a not-for-profit global organization to establish standards for interoperability

Health Maintenance Organization (HMO): an organization that provides managed healthcare on a prepaid basis. Employers with 25 or more employees must offer federally certified HMO options if they offer traditional healthcare options.

Healthcare Information Technology Standards Panel (HITSP): a public and private partnership to promote interoperability through standards

Healtheway: an ONC-supported public-private partnership to promote nationwide HIE via the eHealth Exchange

HIMSS: describes itself as a "a global, cause-based, not-for-profit organization focused on better health through information technology (IT)"[1]

HITECH Act: a law that authorizes expenditures of approximately $20 billion over five years to promote the adoption and use of electronic health record technologies that would be connected through a national health information network

HL7 Development Framework (HDF): the framework used by HL7 to produce specifications for data, messaging process, and other standards

hQuery: an ONC-funded, open source effort to develop a generalized set of distributed queries across diverse EHRs for such purposes as clinical research. It is now part of the more comprehensive Query Health Project initiated by ONC

---

[1]HIMSS. 2014. Healthcare Information and Management Systems Society (HIMSS). http://www.himss.org/AboutHIMSS/

Hypertext Transfer Protocol (HTTP): a query-response protocol used to transfer information between web browsers and connected servers. HTTPS is the secure version

i2b2 (Informatics for Integrating Biology and the Bedside): a scalable query framework for exploration of clinical and genomic data for research to design targeted therapies for individual patients with diseases having genetic origins

IHE Cross-Enterprise Document Media Interchange (XDM): a standard mechanism for including both documents and meta-data in zip format using agreed upon conventions for directory structure and location of files

International Classification of Diseases (ICD): the World Health Organization's almost universally used standard codes for diagnoses. The current version is ICD-10, but ICD-9 is used in most US institutions. The conversion date is October 1, 2014

International Health Terminology Standard Development Organisation (IHTSDO): the multinational organization that maintains SNOMED

Interoperability: the ability of diverse information systems to seamlessly share data and coordinate on tasks involving multiple systems

IP Address: a 32-bit (the standard is changing to 128-bit to accommodate Internet growth) number assigned to each device in an Internet Protocol network that indicates where it is in that network

Lightweight Directory Access Protocol (LDAP): a protocol for accessing (including searching) and maintaining distributed directory information services (such as an e-mail directory) over an IP network

Logical Observation Identifiers Names and Codes (LOINC): the Regenstrief Institute's standard for laboratory and clinical observations

Massachusetts General Utility Multi-Programming System (MUMPS): an integrated programming language and file management system designed in the late 1960s for medical data processing that is the basis for some of the most widely installed enterprise health information systems

Master Patient Index (MPI): software to provide correct matching of patients across multiple software systems, typically within a health enterprise

Meaningful Use: a set of usage requirements defined in three stages by ONC under which eligible professionals are paid for adopting a certified EHR. The three stages are often referred to as MU1, MU2, and MU3

MEDCIN: a proprietary vocabulary of point-of-care terminology, intended for use in electronic health record systems (as a potential alternative to SNOMED-CT) maintained by Medicomp Systems.

Medicaid: the joint federal and state program to provide healthcare services to poor and some disabled US citizens

Medical Dictionary for Regulatory Activities (MedDRA): the International Conference on Harmonisation's classification of adverse event information associated with the use of biopharmaceuticals and other medical products

Medical Logic Module (MLM): the basic unit in the Arden Syntax that contains sufficient medical knowledge and rules to make one clinical decision

Medicare: the federally operated program to provide healthcare services to US citizens over the age of 65

mHealth: the use of mobile communication devices, such as mobile phones, by patients and providers for health services and information

Multipurpose Internet Mail Extensions (MIME): the Internet standard for the format of e-mail attachments used in Direct. S/MIME is the secure version.

Modular EHR: a software component that delivers at least one of the key services required of a Certified EHR

National Drug Codes (NDC): the Food and Drug Administration's numbering system for all medications commercially available in the United States

Nurse Practitioner (NP): a highly trained licensed nursing professional who may be able to practice independently of a physician, depending on state laws. Some NPs can prescribe medications and even diagnose diseases

Office of the National Coordinator for Health Information Technology (ONC): the agency created in 2004 within the Department of Health and Human Services to promote the deployment of HIT in the United States

Outcomes-Based Contract: an approach to pay for healthcare that rewards physician performance against certain defined quality metrics when combined with a lower-than-predicted cost of care

Patient-Centered Medical Home (PCMH): a team-based healthcare delivery model often particularly focused on the management of chronic disease

Pay for Performance (P4P): an approach to pay for healthcare that rewards physician performance against certain defined quality metrics

Patient Portal: a secure website that gives patients access to personal health information. Data typically include: recent provider visits, hospital discharge summaries, and clinical information such as medications and lab results. More advanced portals provide functions like e-mail to the provider, appointment scheduling, and prescription renewal requests

Personal Health Record (PHR): typically a web page where health data and information related to their care is maintained by the patient

Physician's Assistant (PA): a trained and licensed professional who typically engages in patient care with supervision as part of a medical office

Primary Care Physician (PCP): the generalist in a patient's care team who assumes overall responsibility for all their health issues and often the gatekeeper who must generate referrals to specialists

Private Key: the protected (known only to its owner) part of the special pair of numbers used to encrypt documents using PKI

Protected Health Information (PHI): any health or health-related information that can be related back to a specific patient. PHI is subject to HIPAA regulations

Provider: health professionals, including physicians, nurse practitioners, physicians' assistants, that are engaged in direct patient care

Public Key: the public part of the special pair of numbers used to encrypt documents using PKI

Public Key Infrastructure (PKI): a widely used system for protection of documents, messages, and other data that rests on a pair of public and private keys to allow for a variety of use cases

Query Health Project: ONC's workgroup to identify the standards and services for distributed population health queries to certified EHRs and other patient data sources, such as HIEs

Read Codes: a hierarchical clinical terminology system used in general practice in the United Kingdom

Reference Information Model (RIM): a pictorial representation of the HL7 clinical data (domains) that illustrates the life cycle of an HL7 message or groups of related messages

Registration Authority (RA): an entity that collects information for the purpose of verifying the identity of an individual or organization and produces a certificate request

Resource Description Framework (RDF): a method for describing or modeling information on the web using subject-predicate-object expressions (triples) in the form of subject-predicate-object expressions that could be used to represent health ontologies (SNOMED, ICD-10)

Representational State Transfer (REST): web interoperability principles, proposed by Roy Fielding, as a simple, consistent implementation of HTTPS basic commands (GET, PUT, POST, or

DELETE) for transfer of media (which can be data, images, or other forms of digital information) between a server and a client. The ease and speed of REST development and led to its growing use for web interoperability. REST is FHIR's preferred transport protocol implementation for exchanging FHIR Resources

Semantic Web: the proposed next generation of web in which technologies like RDF would create a "web of data" in which browsers (and other tools) could "understand" the content of webpages

Simplified Mail Transport Protocol (SMTP): the Internet standard for e-mail used by Direct. The secure version is S/SMTP

Standards and Interoperability Framework: an ONC-supported initiative that uses volunteer participants to collaborate on interoperability challenges critical to meeting Meaningful Use objectives

Specialist Physician: a physician who delivers care that is usually focused on diseases of one organ system or body component

Systemized Nomenclature of Medicine (SNOMED): a comprehensive, hierarchical healthcare terminology system

Systemized Nomenclature of Medicine Clinical Terms (SNOMED CT): SNOMED subset for the EHR

Synthetic Health Data: facsimile clinical data created by a software system to realistically resemble actual patient data

Telemedicine: the use of telecommunications-based technologies to deliver remote medical care, monitor patients, or provide other healthcare services

Templates: the reusable basic XML-based building blocks of a CCDA document that can represent the entire document, its sections, or the data entries within a section

Transition of Care Initiative (ToC): the effort to develop a standard electronic clinical summary for transitions of care from one venue to another

Treatment, Payment, or Operations (TPO): HIPAA exception for providers, insurance companies, and other healthcare entities to exchange information necessary for treatment, payment, or operations of healthcare businesses

Unified Medical Language System (UMLS): a set of resources maintained by the National Library of Medicine that "brings together many health and biomedical vocabularies and standards to enable interoperability between computer systems"[2]

Veterans Health Information Systems and Technology Architecture (VistA): the Veteran's Administration's system-wide, MUMPS-based health information infrastructure

View, Download, Transmit (VDT): a requirement of Meaningful Use Stage 2 that patients view, download, or transmit their health information

X.509 Digital Certificate: the technical name for an electronic document issued by a CA that uses a digital signature to bind a public key with an identity based on information from an RA

XMPI: a cross-organizational master patient index capable of dealing with many unaffiliated hospitals and health systems

[2]NLM. 2014. UMLS Quick Start Guide. http://www.nlm.nih.gov/research/umls/quickstart.html

Index